Stereotactic Neurosurgery

VOLUME 2: CONCEPTS IN NEUROSURGERY

EDITOR

M. PETER HEILBRUN, M.D.

Professor and Head
Division of Neurological Surgery
University of Utah Health Sciences Center
Salt Lake City, Utah

SERIES EDITORS

Fremont P. Wirth, M.D.
Robert A. Ratcheson, M.D.

SERIES ASSOCIATE EDITORS

Robert L. Grubb, Jr., M.D.
Julian T. Hoff, M.D.
Martin H. Weiss, M.D.

Sponsored by the
Congress of Neurological Surgeons

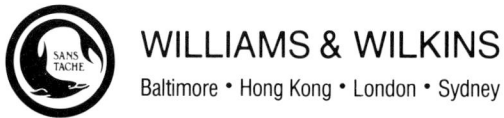

WILLIAMS & WILKINS
Baltimore • Hong Kong • London • Sydney

Copyright © 1988

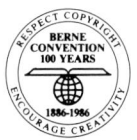

THE CONGRESS OF NEUROLOGICAL SURGEONS

Library of Congress cataloged this serial as follows:

Stereotactic neurosurgery.

  (Concepts in neurosurgery; v. 2)
  Includes bibliographies and index.
  1. Nervous system—Surgery. 3. Stereoencephalotomy.
I. Heilbrun, M. Peter. II. Congress of Neurological
Surgeons. III. Series. [DNLM: 1. Neurosurgery—
methods. 2. Stereotaxic Technics. W1 CO459RK v.2/
WL 368 S838]
RD593.S75 1988   617'.48   87-21685
ISBN 0-683-03954-7

All rights reserved. This book is protected by copyright. No part of this book may be reproduced in any form or by any means, including photocopying, or utilized by any information storage and retrieval system without written permission from the copyright owner.

Accurate indications, adverse reactions, and dosage schedules for drugs are provided in this book, but it is possible that they may change. The reader is urged to review the package information data of the manufacturers of the medications mentioned.

Printed in the United States of America

Stereotactic Neurosurgery

VOLUME 2: CONCEPTS IN NEUROSURGERY

A good surgeon is trained in his craft during his apprenticeship and later in the practical school of operative experience. He soon learns that technique is a thing that he must alter progressively as greater understanding comes to him. The writer who believes that he can describe the finally perfected surgical technique has entered the "fixed period" of his life which is, or should be, the signal for his retirement!

                      Wilder Penfield, M.D.
                      From Penfield W: Surgical therapy. In Penfield W, Jasper H (eds): *Epilepsy and the Functional Anatomy of the Human Brain.* Boston: Little, Brown & Co, 1954.

To my wife, Robyn,
and my secretary, Janet Goldstein,
for their editorial expertise.

To Bob Ratcheson, Phil Wirth, and the officers of the Congress of Neurological Surgeons for initiating the Concept series and for convincing me to edit this volume.

Series Foreword

The Congress of Neurological Surgeons was founded in 1951 with the prime purposes being to maintain high standards of neurosurgery and to promote continuing education. While the emphasis has been on the needs of the resident in training and the younger neurosurgeon, the programs of the Congress have benefited not only neurosurgery but also the neuroscience fields in general.

To help provide for the continuing education needs of its members, the Congress began publication in 1953 of an annual volume entitled, *Clinical Neurosurgery*, which presents in detail the invited presentations made at the annual meeting of the organization. This volume has become an important reference source for neurosurgeons. Then in 1977, after several years of planning, the Congress began publication of a monthly journal entitled, *Neurosurgery*, which proved to be an outstanding addition to the medical literature.

Now, under the direction of Doctors Fremont P. Wirth and Robert A. Ratcheson, the Congress is embarking on another publication series entitled, *Concepts in Neurosurgery*. The goals of this publication, as proposed by Dr. Ratcheson during his term as President of the Congress, are to provide a monograph that will cover a specific area in depth with basic scientific knowledge and theory applied to practical neurosurgical issues. For the resident in training this publication can supplement the educational program or provide knowledge in an area that might not be covered in depth in a training program. For the trained neurosurgeon, each monograph will provide the opportunity to review recent knowledge about a practical subject and supply up-to-date information in an important area of neurosurgery.

The Congress has selected Doctors Wirth and Ratcheson as editors, two individuals who have been members of the Executive Committee for several years and have recently been officers, who have also had considerable experience with educational programs. They will be aided by associate editors, Doctors Robert L. Grubb, Julian T. Hoff, and Martin Weiss, who also have had broad experience with publications and continuing education endeavors.

The Congress is again providing a leadership role in an important area that will benefit all of neurosurgery.

Robert G. Ojemann, M.D.

Foreword

This book, the second in the series *Concepts in Neurosurgery,* which is sponsored by the Congress of Neurological Surgeons, represents the continued commitment of the Congress to neurosurgical education. This work, under the editorship of Dr. M. Peter Heilbrun, describes the theory and practice of modern stereotactic surgery. A well-chosen group of experts has effectively conveyed the technical advances of this field and renewed the promise and excitement which stereotactic surgery held in the 1960s.

This monograph well fulfills the intent of *Concepts in Neurosurgery.* It will provide neurosurgeons and neurosurgical trainees with modern concepts and serve as an exceptional resource for basic and practical information in this field. The publication of this important book by the Congress will benefit all of Neurosurgery and our patients.

Robert A. Ratcheson, M.D.
Fremont P. Wirth, M.D.

Preface

STEREOTACTIC NEUROSURGERY—A PERSONAL REFLECTION

The ability to conceptualize a position in three-dimensional space is an essential skill of neurosurgeons. Yet, no matter how skilled the neurosurgeon may be, free-hand approaches to intraaxial brain lesions cannot achieve the repeatable precision and accuracy of current stereotactic methods.

In 1970, when I completed my neurosurgical residency, I recognized the inherent accuracy of stereotactic guidance systems, but my neuroanatomic and neurophysiologic knowledge of positional variability of basal ganglia structures made me skeptical of a fixed schema of localization based on formulae derived from variable distances of the AC/PC line. Also, by that time, L-dopa had become the treatment of choice for parkinsonian tremor, bringing a precipitous drop in the number of stereotactic cases for tremor. As these unilateral tremor cases were decreasing, referrals for stereotactic treatment of more complex movement disorders, such as dystonia muscularum deformans, were increasing. However, the results of destructive lesions in these types of cases were not always satisfactory, and complications were common. Finally, the available instrumentation required conceptually complicated conversions from two-dimensional AP and lateral radiographs to mathematical calculations in order to transform points on x-rays to projected three-dimensional coordinates in space and unseen positions within the brain. Thus, at that point in my career, I determined to leave considerations of stereotactic surgery to others, especially since the greatest practical and technical neurosurgical challenges seemed related to subarachnoid hemorrhage and carotid occlusive disease.

Before the decade was over, my reservations were outdated. The CT scanner inspired new considerations for the stereotactic method, and innovative neurosurgeons quickly recognized that the classic stereotactic conversion for accessing a projected target within the brain could now be accomplished by CT guidance to discretely measurable and verifiable points.

The intention of this volume is to reintroduce neurosurgeons of all generations to stereotactic localization and its innumerable applications. The chapters contain individual perspectives on stereotactic technique from classical management of movement disorders to the more recent management of intraaxial tumors. I would like to thank each contributor for the work involved in compiling these chapters.

The book is divided into two sections. The first section presents an overview of stereotactic surgery, descriptions of instrumentation, and reviews of the primary applications, including intraaxial tumors, functional disorders, pain, and epilepsy. The second section contains eight chapters that describe more specialized applications of the stereotactic method. These chapters describe diverse procedures from the treatment of trigeminal neuralgia and somatic pain to stereotactically directed radiation for vascular malformations and computer-assisted laser resection of tumors, as well as interstitial brachytherapy.

By the time this book is published, some of the methods and instrumentation will, inevitably, be supplanted as neurosurgeons continue to search for even better techniques and solutions.

M. Peter Heilbrun, M.D.

Contributors

SERIES EDITORS

Fremont P. Wirth, M.D.
Neurological Institute of Savannah
Director, Neurosurgical and Neurological
Intensive Care Unit
St. Joseph's Hospital
Savannah, Georgia

Robert A. Ratcheson, M.D.
Professor and Chief, Division of Neurological
  Surgery
Case Western Reserve University
University Hospitals of Cleveland
Cleveland, Ohio

SERIES ASSOCIATE EDITORS

Robert L. Grubb, Jr., M.D.
Professor of Neurological Surgery
Washington University School of Medicine
St. Louis, Missouri

Julian T. Hoff, M.D.
Professor of Surgery
Head, Section of Neurosurgery
University of Michigan Hospital
Ann Arbor, Michigan

Martin H. Weiss, M.D.
Professor and Chairman
Department of Neurosurgery
LAC/USC Medical Center
Los Angeles, California

VOLUME EDITOR

M. Peter Heilbrun, M.D.
Professor and Head
Division of Neurological Surgery
University of Utah Health Sciences Center
Salt Lake City, Utah

CONTRIBUTORS

Michael L. J. Apuzzo, M.D.
Professor of Neurosurgery
University of Southern California School of
  Medicine
Director of Neurosurgery
Kenneth R. Norris Cancer Hospital and
  Research Institute
Los Angeles, California

Nicholas M. Barbaro, M.D.
Assistant Professor
Department of Neurological Surgery
School of Medicine
University of California
San Francisco, California

J. L. Barcia-Salorio, M.D.
Department of Neurosurgery
University of Valencia
Valencia, Spain

Robert E. Breeze, M.D.
Clinical Instructor
Department of Neurosurgery
University of Southern California School of
  Medicine
Los Angeles, California

Parakrama T. Chandrasoma, M.D.
Associate Professor of Pathology
Department of Neuropathology
University of Southern California School of Medicine
Surgical Pathologist
Kenneth R. Norris Cancer Hospital and Research Institute
Los Angeles, California

Robert J. Coffey, M.D.
Assistant Professor
Department of Neurological Surgery
University of Pittsburgh
Pittsburgh, Pennsylvania

Deirdre M. Cohen, M.D.
Assistant Clinical Professor
Department of Radiation Oncology
Kenneth R. Norris Cancer Hospital and Research Institute
Los Angeles, California

William A. Friedman, M.D.
Associate Professor
Department of Neurological Surgery
University of Florida
Gainesville, Florida

Edward Ganz, M.D.
Assistant Professor of Neurosurgery and Radiology
Case Western Reserve University
School of Medicine
Cleveland, Ohio

Philip L. Gildenberg, M.D., Ph.D.
Clinical Professor of Neurosurgery
University of Texas Medical School at Houston
Houston, Texas

S. J. Goerss, B.S.
Department of Neurosurgery
Mayo Clinic and Mayo Foundation
Rochester, Minnesota

Philip H. Gutin, M.D.
Associate Professor
Departments of Neurological Surgery and Radiation Oncology and the Brain Tumor Research Center of the Department of Neurological Surgery
School of Medicine
University of California
San Francisco, California

Edward R. Hitchcock, Ch.M.F.R.C.S., F.R.C.S.Ed.
Head, Department of Neurosurgery
The University of Birmingham
Birmingham, England

B. A. Kall, M.S.
Department of Information Processing and Systems
Mayo Clinic and Mayo Foundation
Rochester, Minnesota

Patrick J. Kelly, M.D.
Professor of Neurological Surgery
Department of Neurosurgery
Mayo Medical School
Rochester, Minnesota

Yik San Kwoh, Ph.D.
Director of Research
Memorial Medical Center
Long Beach, California

Lauri Laitinen, M.D.
Associate Professor
Department of Neurosurgery
University Hospital
Umea, Sweden

Steven A. Leibel, M.D.
Associate Professor
Department of Radiation Oncology
School of Medicine
University of California
San Francisco, California

Dan G. Leksell, M.D.
Department of Head and Neck Surgery
Huddinge University Hospital
Karolinska Institute
Stockholm, Sweden

Gary Luxton, Ph.D.
Radiation Physicist
Kenneth R. Norris Cancer Hospital and Research Institute
Los Angeles, California

Amitabha Mazumder, M.D.
Associate Professor of Medicine
University of Southern California School of Medicine
Medical Oncology
Kenneth R. Norris Cancer Hospital and Research Institute
Los Angeles, California

Michael Sapozink, M.D., Ph.D.
Kenneth R. Norris Cancer Hospital and
  Research Institute
Los Angeles, California

Dennis D. Spencer, M.D.
Professor and Chief
Section of Neurological Surgery
Yale University School of Medicine
New Haven, Connecticut

Ronald F. Young, M.D.
Professor and Chief
Division of Neurological Surgery
University of California
Irvine, California

Contents

Series Foreword vii
Robert G. Ojemann, M.D.
Foreword ix
Robert A. Ratcheson, M.D. and Fremont P. Wirth, M.D.
Preface xi
Contributors xiii

CHAPTER 1
Stereotactic Surgery: Present and Past 1
Philip L. Gildenberg, M.D., Ph.D.

CHAPTER 2
Stereotactic Applications: General Overview 17
Robert J. Coffey, M.D., and William A. Friedman, M.D.

CHAPTER 3
Stereotactic Surgical Instrumentation 55
William A. Friedman, M.D., and Robert J. Coffey, M.D.

CHAPTER 4
Applications of Image-Directed Stereotactic Surgery in the Management of Intracranial Neoplasms 73
Michael L. J. Apuzzo, M.D., Parakrama T. Chandrasoma, M.D.,
Robert E. Breeze, M.D., Deirdre M. Cohen, M.D., Gary Luxton, Ph.D., and
Amitabha Mazumder, M.D.

CHAPTER 5
Contemporary Stereotactic Ventralis Lateral Thalamotomy in the Treatment of Parkinsonian Tremor and Other Movement Disorders 133
Patrick J. Kelly, M.D.

CHAPTER 6
Stereotactic Methods in the Management of Pain 149
Ronald F. Young, M.D.

CHAPTER 7
Stereotactic Methods in the Management of Epilepsy 161
Dennis D. Spencer, M.D.

CHAPTER 8
Special Stereotactic Techniques: Trigeminus Stereoguide for Trigeminal and Glossopharyngeal Neuralgia ... 179
Lauri Laitinen, M.D.

CHAPTER 9
Special Stereotactic Techniques: Stereotactic Lesions of the Spinal Cord and Pons for Pain ... 185
Edward R. Hitchcock, M.D.

CHAPTER 10
Special Stereotactic Techniques: Stereotactic Radiosurgery ... 195
Dan G. Leksell, M.D.

CHAPTER 11
Special Stereotactic Techniques: Single-Beam Photon Radiosurgery ... 211
J. L. Barcia-Salorio, M.D.

CHAPTER 12
Special Stereotactic Techniques: Robotic Methods Applied to Stereotactic Surgery ... 219
Yik San Kwoh, Ph.D.

CHAPTER 13
Special Stereotactic Techniques: Hyperthermia Techniques ... 227
Michael Sapozink, M.D., Ph.D.

CHAPTER 14
Special Stereotactic Techniques: Stereotactic Laser Resection of Deep-Seated Tumors ... 233
Patrick J. Kelly, M.D., B. A. Kall, M.S., and S. J. Goerss, B.S.

CHAPTER 15
Special Stereotactic Techniques: Stereotactic Interstitial Brachytherapy ... 241
Philip H. Gutin, M.D., Nicholas M. Barbaro, M.D., and Steven A. Leibel, M.D.

CHAPTER 16
Future Developments in Stereotactic Neurosurgery ... 247
Edward Ganz, M.D.

Index ... 257

Chapter 1

Stereotactic Surgery: Present and Past

PHILIP L. GILDENBERG, M.D., Ph.D.

In the last 80 years, stereotactic surgery has progressed from an innovation in the laboratory study of neuroscience to an ever-increasing part of the practice of neurosurgery. The now burgeoning field of human stereotactic surgery began only 40 years ago, and its rapid rate of progress has often been dictated by developments in other clinical and nonclinical fields, particularly contributions from radiology, neurophysiology, electronics, metallurgy; more recently, neuropathology, computer science, computerized tomographic (CT) scanning, and magnetic resonance imaging; and soon neuropharmacology and embryology.

The first recorded use of guided probes in the neurophysiology laboratory was in 1873, when Dittmar in Ludwig's laboratory applied a uniquely designed guiding device to the medulla oblongata, but it did not constitute a universally usable stereotactic system (23).

Stereotactic surgery, as we know it, began with a monumental contribution by Horsley and Clarke in 1908 in a landmark paper detailing the design of their new apparatus to study cerebellar function in the monkey (Fig. 1.1) (45). Not only did they provide complete plans for their stereotactic apparatus, but included instructions for developing a stereotactic atlas and a study (which has to this day not been surpassed) of the effects of electrolytic lesions on nervous tissue.

Their technique was based on the reproducibility of the relationships between landmarks on the skull (external auditory canals, inferior orbital rims, midline) and anatomical structures within the brain of the experimental animal. However, extension of their technique for use in patients was fraught with great difficulty, due to the great variability between skull landmarks and cerebral structures in the human. Variability in animals can be compensated for by sacrificing the animals after the experiment, studying the brains histologically, and discarding results from any animal in which the electrode was imperfectly placed. Such a luxury is not available in patients, where every electrode insertion must be accurate. Interestingly, an adaptation of the Horsley-Clarke stereotactic apparatus based on those principles was developed by Mussen in 1918 for use in humans, but it was probably never used (88).

It was not until 1946 that Spiegel and Wycis devised a practical human stereotactic apparatus. Their original stereoencephalotome is now in the Smithsonian Institute. Their design was centered on a plaster cap that was fitted to each individual patient. A head ring was suspended from the plaster cap, and an electrode carrier, which was very similar to the Horsley-Clarke design and could be moved laterally, vertically, and horizontally, was mounted to the head ring (Fig. 1.2) (110). Their unique contribution was the idea of relating anatomical targets to landmarks within the brain itself—hence the name "stereoencephalotomy." The landmarks that were the basis for Spiegel and Wycis' original human stereotactic atlas were the pineal gland and the foramen of Monro, visualized by preoperative or intraoperative pneumoencephalograms (104). With the later advent of positive contrast agents for ventriculography, the anterior and posterior commissures and the connecting intercommissural line

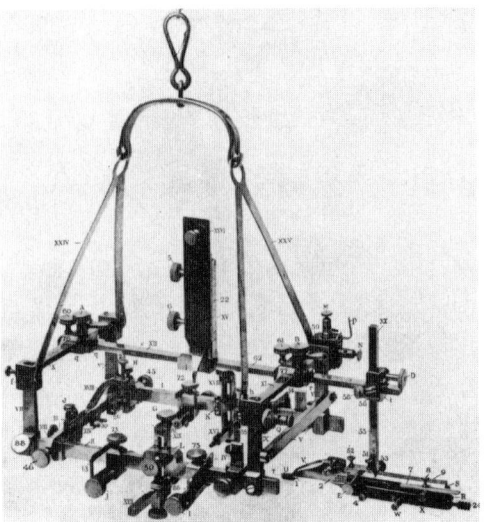

Figure 1.1. Horsley and Clarke's original animal stereotactic apparatus. (From Horsley, V., and Clarke, R. H. The structure and functions of the cerebellum examined by a new method. Brain *31:* 45-124, 1908.)

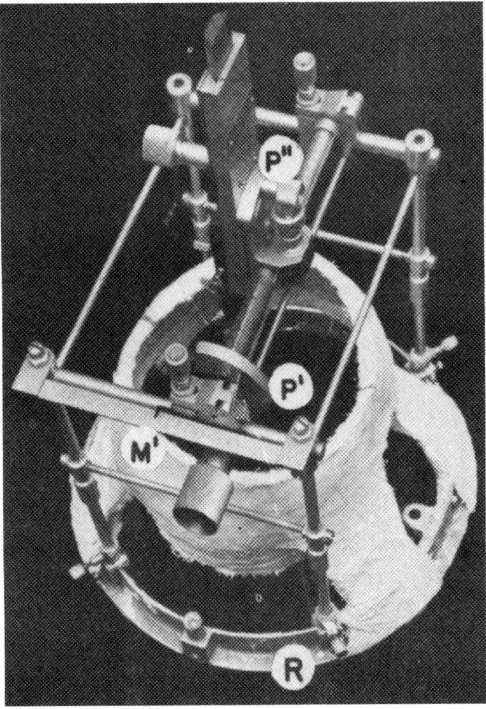

Figure 1.2. Spiegel and Wycis' original human stereotactic apparatus. Note the resemblance to the Horsley-Clarke apparatus. (From Spiegel, E. A., Wycis, H. T., Marks, M., and Lee, A. St. J. Stereotaxic apparatus for operations on the human brain. Science *106:* 349-350, 1947.)

became the most commonly used internal cerebral landmarks.

TYPES OF STEREOTACTIC APPARATUS

Within the next few years a number of other stereotactic apparatus were described, a few of which were probably under development even before Spiegel and Wycis' first publication. The question of who developed the second human apparatus has never been resolved. The Leksell apparatus was first described in 1949 (57) and the Narabayashi system in 1951 (78, 26). The Riechert apparatus was introduced in 1951 (97), and a modification by Mundinger appeared in 1955 (95). Obrador's apparatus was described in 1957 (85).

Originally these apparatus fell into three distinct categories, depending on how the electrode carrier was mounted (Fig. 1.3). In the Spiegel-Wycis apparatus, like the Horsley-Clarke device, the electrode carrier was held vertical and moved by a translational system in two dimensions, with a microdrive to advance the electrode in the third. Later models (six Spiegel-Wycis models were eventually developed) incorporated precision lockable hinges to adjust angles in the anteroposterior and lateral planes as well.

The Talairach system is closely related, but includes a grid system to introduce a large number of electrodes from the lateral position. The system was designed particularly for the introduction of multiple electrodes to study seizure foci in the temporal lobes (114, 115).

The Leksell system is an example of the second category, an arc or polar coordinate system employing an electrode carrier fitted to an arc in such a way that it always points to the center of the arc (57, 58). Thus, by aligning the target point with the center of the arc by adjusting the attachment of the arc, the electrode advances to the target, regardless of the angle of insertion. The Todd-Wells apparatus also is an arc system, but it is designed reciprocally so that the arc system is fixed and the patient's head is moved in a controlled fashion to align it with the target point (124).

The Riechert system (97), and its later

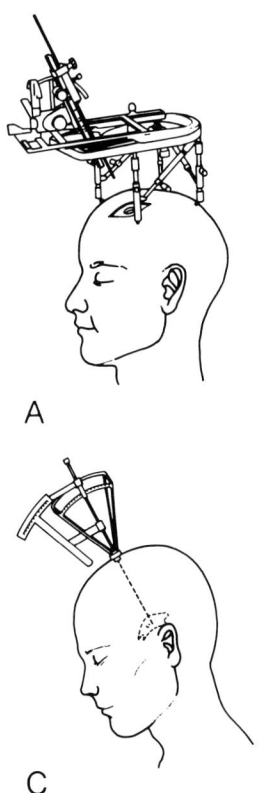
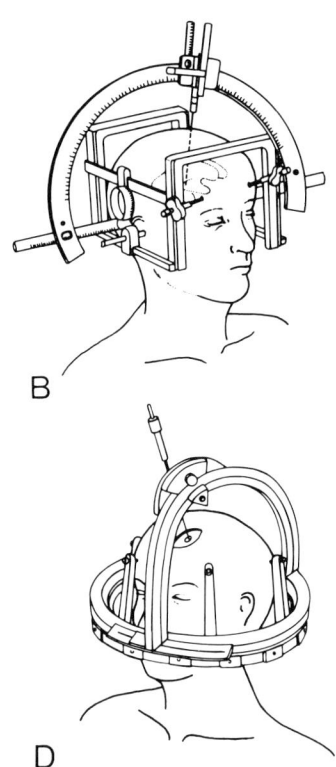
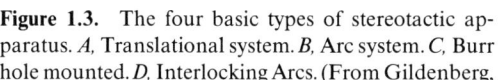

Figure 1.3. The four basic types of stereotactic apparatus. *A,* Translational system. *B,* Arc system. *C,* Burr hole mounted. *D,* Interlocking Arcs. (From Gildenberg, P.L. Whatever happened to stereotactic surgery? Neurosurgery *20:* 983-987, 1987.)

modifications with Mundinger (95), is likewise an arc system, but, instead of the target being at the center of the arc, the electrode carrier is offset, and it is desirable to use a phantom (or later a computer) to adjust the apparatus. The phantom mechanically simulates the placement of the arc system on the head and the coordinates of the target.

Burr hole-mounted systems consist of a fulcrum attached to the burr hole to which is fixed an electrode carrier with angular adjustments to point to the target and a microdrive to advance the electrode (4). Such systems were inherently less accurate, but were popular during the time when many neurosurgeons with little stereotactic background were doing a large number of thalamotomies for Parkinson's disease. A recent modification of this system mounts the fulcrum more securely to a base plate attached to the skull, and a phantom is used to aim the device, but it is used primarily for CT-stereotactic surgery (see below) (12).

Recently, a fourth type of stereotactic system was introduced (to digress out of chronological order). The Brown-Roberts-Wells apparatus was designed primarily for CT-stereotactic surgery and consists of interlocking arcs (44). Because of the complexity of adjusting the individual arcs to define a specific trajectory, it is necessary to use a computer to define the coordinates of the target point and the adjustment necessary to reach the target.

STEREOTACTIC ATLASES

In order to use a stereotactic apparatus, however, it is necessary to know the relationship between the landmarks and any given anatomical target and to have information about how much these measure-

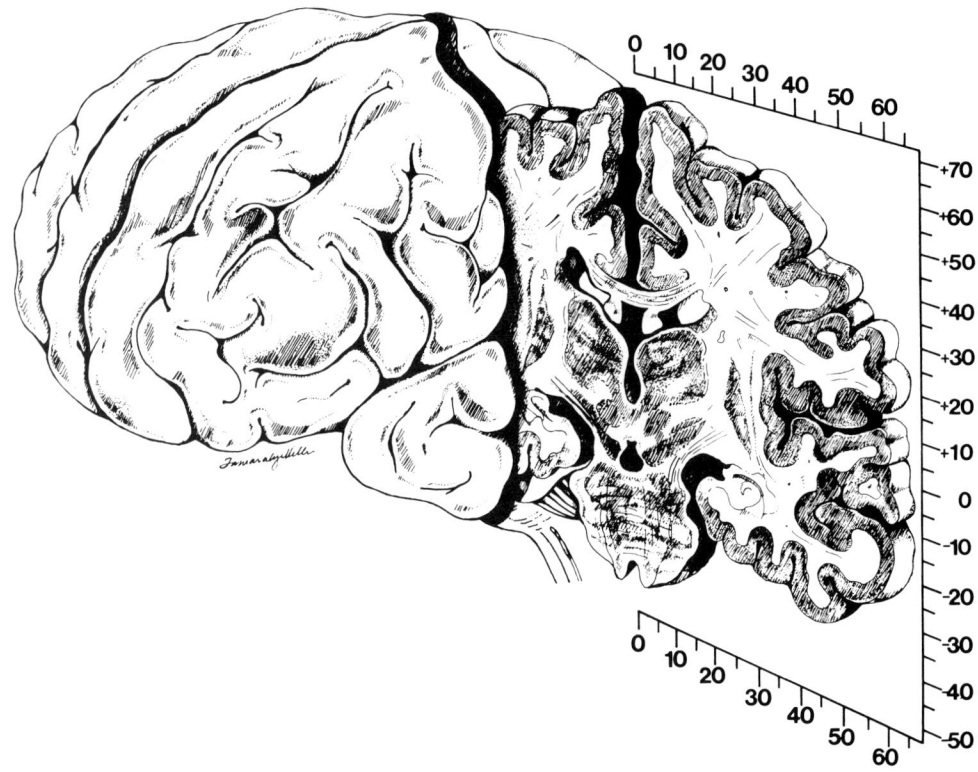

Figure 1.4. Each page in a stereotactic atlas represents a brain slice taken at a measured position within the brain. (From Gildenberg, P. L., Surgery for seizures. In *Modern Stereotactic Surgery,* edited by L. D. Lunsford, Martinus Nighoff; Hingham, MA, 1987.)

ments vary in a patient population. Horsley and Clarke included information about a monkey atlas in their historical publication (45). Likewise, Spiegel and Wycis developed a human stereotactic atlas, which they published in 1952 (104), based on the same principle, that is, a series of precise brain sections at measured intervals containing a grid system to relate the coordinates of any point to the intracerebral landmarks (Fig. 1.4). This was followed soon after by a number of human stereotactic atlases. Schaltenbrand and Bailey's atlas contained transparent pages on which the anatomical nuclei were drawn, overlying stained sections of the brain, with particular emphasis on the area around the thalamus (101). The Talairach atlas (114) contains information about the location of blood vessels and was designed with an accent on epilepsy surgery. Later atlases by Andrew and Watkins (3) and Van Buren and Borke (127) contained greatly enlarged drawings defining the relationships of subnuclei, particularly those of the thalamus. Afshar's atlas concerns the brainstem and cerebellar nuclei (1), and Tasker's atlas (120) contains much physiological as well as anatomical information for localization.

The use of computers in the past 10 yr has greatly affected the development of stereotactic atlases. Computer-based stereotactic atlases presently consist of graphic illustrations derived from published atlases. The computer atlas representation may be purposefully distorted to fit the measurements of the individual patient's landmarks or nuclei, as demonstrated on x-ray or CT scan (51), or magnified and manipulated in the operating room to provide information and views helpful to the surgeon (40). It may provide a repository for information obtained in the operating room by physiological testing or stimulation, or may be correlated with results (43, 77, 118, 120).

LESION PRODUCTION

During the early days of stereotactic surgery, there was considerable controversy about the best way to make a lesion. The earliest work was done with the same electrolytic technique that had been described by Horsley and Clarke 50 yr earlier (45). However, the passage of a direct current through the patient was not without risk if the current varied suddenly. Also, the lesions were very small and discrete (both an advantage and a disadvantage), and it was necessary to replace electrodes regularly as the tips became pitted and electrolyzed.

Mechanical methods of producing lesions with leukotomes or wire loops have been employed since the earliest days of stereotactic surgery (85, 86) and are still employed. However, there is a danger of interruption of blood vessels with such devices, although techniques restricting the arc through which the wire loop is rotated theoretically minimize this danger.

One early technique to produce lesions involved the injection of alcohol, which was used by Spiegel and Wycis (103) only briefly, but championed by Cooper (15, 17) for several years. However, the distribution of the alcohol varies greatly when injected, since it tends to follow tracts or diffuse back up the needle tract (26). An attempt was made to produce a cavity with temporary inflation of a balloon, but that did not improve the lesion and, in fact, the blunt tip of the balloon-cannula itself produced damage (25). The idea of using a thicker substance prompted the development of Etopalin, which was a mixture of ethylcellulose and alcohol (15), but that did not significantly improve the configuration of the lesion (25). A procaine-oil-wax mixture introduced by Narabayashi et al. appeared more desirable and is still used by a few surgeons.

The production of extremely low temperatures to produce subcortical lesions was suggested by both Mark et al. (67) and Cooper and Lee (21) in 1961. Although Mark's group discontinued the use of this technique several years later because of the complication of hemorrhage (68), the latter investigators continued to use it. Cooper commissioned Arnold Lee, a bioengineer, to develop an apparatus to control the flow of liquid nitrogen through a "cryoprobe" to regulate the tip temperature accurately (21). Lee is one of the lesser known important figures in the development of stereotactic neurosurgery. He is the same individual who worked with Spiegel and Wycis on the development of their original apparatus, coauthored the historical paper in *Science* (110), and worked with Austin on his burr hole-mounted apparatus (14).

There was some interest in the use of focused ultrasound for the production of subcortical lesions (73). However, because the technique involves very expensive and elaborate equipment, requires the use of a large dural exposure, and prohibits prelesion stimulation or recording, it never gained popularity.

Although high-frequency sine wave generators for the production of subcortical lesions were introduced as early as 1945 by Wyss (130) in a device further refined in 1953 (49), control of current and adequacy of insulation (26, 28) were problems in these early radiofrequency systems. It was not until Mundinger *et al.* (75) used an electrode with an incorporated thermocouple to control current and improved insulation was developed that the use of radiofrequency current became the most commonly used technique to produce subcortical lesions (22, 27, 28).

A variation of radiofrequency heating involves the introduction of metallic pellets that become hot when the head is placed in a high-frequency inductive coil, so-called inductive heating (11, 93, 128). Although this provides the theoretical advantage of being able to supplement the size of the lesion as the effect on symptoms is monitored, it has not been used generally. More recent work involving the use of microwave hyperthermia in treatment of brain tumors may revive some interest in this technique (98, 99).

Interest in the use of irradiation for the production of discrete subcortical lesions began early in stereotactic history with techniques described by Leksell and coworkers (58, 60), using roentgen rays, and Tobias et al. (123), using deuterons, both in 1955. Later, Leksell et al. (61) and Kjellberg et al. (55) described the use of proton beams to make subcortical lesions for functional neurosurgery, but the lesions were not as stable or controllable as hoped. Kjellberg's group still employs this technique for the management of tumors, vascular malformations, and other mass lesions. Leksell, meanwhile, developed a device that uses directed gamma rays from several hundred cobalt sources, all focused on a small volume, which has been used to produce functional neurosurgical lesions as well as to treat mass lesions (59).

STEREOTACTIC TARGETS AND INDICATIONS

Even prior to the use of human stereotactic surgery, neurophysiological information had been available to theorize how interruption of pathways within the brain might serve to alter abnormal function (71, 72). The procedure most widely used, of course, was the interruption of thalamofrontal projections by undercutting the frontal lobes, the classical leukotomy of psychosurgery, which was important in the days before tranquilizers were available (24). Indeed, it was because of the frequently severe intellectual changes that often accompanied this procedure that Spiegel pursued stereoencephalotomy, in hopes of refining psychosurgery and putting it on a scientific basis and achieving the desired therapeutic result without the intolerable side effects. However, this indication soon became overshadowed by many others of more lasting clinical significance.

The first movement disorder treated stereotactically was Huntington's chorea (103), and choreoathetosis was treated soon after (108).

The use of stereotactic surgery for Parkinson's disease was at first considered inadvisable. It was recognized experimentally that lesions in the globus pallidus or the pallidofugal fibers caused a hypertonus in certain experimental animals. Since parkinsonian patients already had hypertonus, there was concern that they would be made worse by interrupting the extrapyramidal pathways. It was recognized, however, that cutting into the cerebral peduncle might alleviate some parkinsonian symptoms, but with a great risk of paralysis (71, 72). While undertaking this operation in a patient in 1951, Cooper inadvertently interrupted the anterior choroidal artery and aborted the attempt to incise the peduncle. When the patient awoke with no paralysis and also without his tremor, Cooper used this observation as the basis for the recommendation, in 1953, for ligation of the anterior choroidal artery to treat the symptoms of Parkinson's disease (13, 14). Since the distribution of the artery is variable (89), however, the results and side effects were inconsistent. He deduced that the effect was because of the infarction of the globus pallidus and advocated injecting alcohol into that structure in parkinsonism, thereby reducing the mortality rate, but still with inconsistent effectiveness (16-18). At about the same time, a number of other neurosurgeons had begun to make selective lesions stereotactically, such as Narabayashi and Okuma in the globus pallidus (80) and Spiegel and Wycis in the emerging fibers of the ansa lenticularis (106), with good results. When, at autopsy in approximately 1958, the lesions in several of Cooper's patients with excellent results proved to be in the ventral lateral nucleus of the thalamus (Cooper was not using stereotactic techniques to guide his lesion), Cooper moved his intended lesion to that structure (20). In the meantime, however, other neurosurgeons were already advocating the interruption of this same pathway at various places for the treatment of the symptoms of Parkinson's disease (63).

Thus, although the recommended lesion for the treatment of Parkinson's disease (as well as other movement disorders) changed through these early years, it always involved the interruption of the same pallidothalamic pathway at various points—the globus pallidum (pallidotomy) (15, 80, 108), the ventral lateral nucleus of the thalamus (thalamotomy) (17, 117), or the intervening connecting pathway in the ansa lenticularis (ansotomy) (106, 107). Spiegel, Wycis, et al. (111, 112) later recommended making the lesion in the pathway at a different point closer to the thalamus where the fibers of the ansa lenticularis and the lenticular fasciculus funneled together in Forel's field H (campus Foreli, hence the name campotomy) where a very small lesion interrupted the maximum amount of this pathway (111). Attention has more recently been directed back to the thalamus, where the subnucleus Ventrointermedius is generally considered to be the ideal target for tremor (thalamotomy) (87, 119, 121). However, the coordinates by which various neurosurgeons expect to find that structure to alleviate parkinsonian tremor vary considerably (56). Also, despite the guise of a scientific approach, it must be conceded that the lesion for most movement disorders treated by ablative subcortical lesions involves essentially the same targets, with only minor variations (for summary, see 30).

Perhaps the next most active field became the treatment of epilepsy. Not only was it possible to record from the awake human brain during surgery, and thereby help identify deep epileptogenic foci, but it became possible to interrupt those pathways thought important in the propagation of the epileptic activity to prevent the activity from becoming generalized (50, 109), or to ablate the focus itself stereotactically (79).

It is difficult to determine just who performed the first stereotactic operation for each clinical indication. Series were slow to accumulate, so publication had to await a large enough group of patients; even then, series for most disorders were quite small. Procedures were done with poor results, whereas later minor modification in target point or technique provided good relief of symptoms. The literature is overcrowded with reports indicating the intended anatomical target, with no documentation of the location of the lesion and no coordinates so other investigators could verify or replicate results. Many significant reports were presented in obscure journals, sometimes regional publications in a variety of countries. It is impossible in a brief review such as this to have a complete overview of the field as a whole, or to recognize all who made significant contributions.

An amazingly large amount of clinical experimentation for an incredible number of indications was done on a remarkably small number of patients during the first decade of the stereotactic era, much by Spiegel and Wycis (102, 107). Indeed, it is rare to read a report for a "new" ablative procedure without discovering the precedent for it in their early writings.

In addition to ablative procedures to alleviate symptoms of various neurological disorders, a surprising variety of nonfunctional procedures were done in the early years of stereotactic surgery—implantation of radioisotopes (92) or lesion production for pituitary tumors (96, 113), hypophysectomy (96, 113, 131), removal of foreign bodies (92), coagulation of the lumen of aneurysms (2), and relief of hydrocephalus (91). Instillation of isotopes into craniopharyngioma cysts began as early as 1948 (62) and was soon followed by other reports involving interstitial radiation of brain tumors (76, 129).

The use of stereotactic surgery for intractable pain paralleled other techniques used for pain. In the early days of the field, it seemed only logical that interruption of pathways concerned with pain perception would alleviate that complaint. It was found, however, that if patients with chronic pain of benign origin lived long enough, the pain almost always recurred, sometimes with disabling side effects as well (102). Interruption of pain pathways can be an excellent supplement to the management of cancer pain, however, and some of the earlier techniques are still employed.

The first such technique that proved to be extremely successful was the interruption of the spinothalamic tract at the level of the mesencephalon (mesencephalotomy) (82, 105). This can provide analgesia over the contralateral body, face, and head, and is especially useful if the pain involves shoulder, head, or neck. Incorporation of the extralemniscal pathways within the thalamus in the intralaminar area (basal or intralaminar thalamotomy) may also provide relief from the suffering or aching neuropathic pain that accompanies cancer pain, especially if neural structures are involved (summarized in 30). Pain of thalamic syndrome or anesthesia dolorosa may be helped by lesions in the posterior part of the internal medullary lamina (100), although deep brain stimulation may be more helpful (see below) (48).

One cannot review stereotactic management of pain without digressing to another aspect of functional neurosurgery, the use of implanted stimulators to inhibit pain perception. When it was discovered in the late 1960s that stimulation of large somatosensory fibers might inhibit transmission of pain via the small axons (70), stimulation, with a surgically implanted stimulating device, of the large fibers where they are uniquely gathered in the dorsal columns of the spinal cord became a recognized procedure (dorsal column stimulation or spinal cord stimulation) (65). These implantable devices were consequently available when it was discovered, in 1973, that there are sites within the brain that inhibit pain perception when stimulated, so-called stimulation-produced analgesia (64, 69). The natural progression has been the development of implanted devices to stimulate the periventricular or periaqueductal pain-inhibitory areas (deep brain stimulation) (46, 90). It has subsequently been appreciated that similar stimulation of the somatosensory areas of the thalamus or internal capsule might afford relief from denervation pain (46, 47, 125). Currently ablative procedures are being recommended for cancer pain, whereas stimulation procedures might be considered for chronic pain of benign origin, but only within part of a comprehensive pain program (36, 37).

THE "STEREOTACTIC SOCIETY"

The increasing activity in the field required a forum to disseminate information about new procedures, techniques, and results to a growing number of scientist-neurosurgeons whose interests were often out of the mainstream of neurosurgery or even neurology. Coincidentally, Spiegel had been founder and editor of a journal dedicated to these borderlands of neurology, *Confinia Neurologica,* which became the major source of information in the field of stereotactic surgery. The journal began publication in 1938, and up to that time had published the proceedings of the Harvey Cushing Society (now the American Association of Neurological Surgeons) and the Philadelphia Neurological Society. In 1975, the title was changed to *Applied Neurophysiology* when Gildenberg became editor, and it is now in its fiftieth volume. In 1985, the subtitle, *Journal of Stereotactic and Functional Neurosurgery,* was added.

In addition, *Acta Neurochirurgica* has become the major European publication concerned with stereotaxis. In it are published the proceedings of the meetings of the European Society for Stereotactic and Functional Neurosurgery. In the US, many articles have also appeared in the *Journal of Neurosurgery* and in *Neurosurgery.*

The increasing interest in this field led to the formation of a new society, which was done in conjunction with the First International Symposium on Stereoencephalotomy held in Philadelphia in October, 1961. The International Society for Research in Stereoencephalotomy held its Second International Symposium partly in Copenhagen and partly in Vienna in 1965. The Third International Symposium was held in Madrid in 1967, the Fourth in New York in 1969, and the Fifth in Freiburg in 1970.

The Sixth International Symposium held in Tokyo in 1973 marked a turning point. There was considerable discussion as to whether the acceptable spelling should be "stereotactic" or "stereotaxic." "Stereo-" is from the Greek root meaning "three-dimensional," and it was agreed to be appropriate. By majority vote, "stereotactic," combining the Latin root "to touch," rather than "stereotaxic," from the Greek root for an "arrangement," was accepted as the official spelling, since surgery involves introducing a probe to the target, rather than merely defining the relationships.

At the same meeting, it was also agreed to change the name from International Society for Research in Stereoencephalotomy to the World Society for Stereotactic and Functional Neurosurgery, indicating that the members were interested in all aspects of functional neurosurgery, i.e., surgery designed to change the function of the nervous system, in addition to just stereotactic techniques, thereby including epilepsy surgery and the new field of chronic stimulation of the spinal cord. Shortly thereafter, the various branches were renamed as the American, European, and Japanese Societies for Stereotactic and Functional Neurosurgery.

The Seventh Meeting was held in Sao Paulo in 1977, the Eighth in 1981 in Zurich, and the Ninth in 1985 in Toronto. The Tenth Meeting, representing 40 years of progress, is planned for Tokyo in 1989. In addition, the American and European Societies meet in alternate years in which there is no World Society meeting, and the Japanese Society meets annually.

The proceedings of all these meetings, with the exception of the independent European Society meetings, are published in *Confinia Neurologica* or *Applied Neurophysiology*.

A perusal of the programs of the meetings offers some insight into the progress of the field of stereotactic and functional neurosurgery. The first meeting in 1961 was mainly devoted to a display of each participant's personal apparatus (about three dozen different apparatus had been produced by then) and discussion of basic techniques, such as lesion production, electrode design, or x-ray visualization. It was noted at that time that more than 5,000 operations had already been reported in the world literature. In 1965 there was a review of the indications for stereotactic surgery, each participant contributing the histories of a few patients with this or that problem. The 1965 meeting was held at the height of the use of stereotactic surgery for the treatment of Parkinson's disease, each speaker emphasizing the size of his series, and it was estimated that almost 26,000 stereotactic operations had been performed.

The general tenor of the 1967 meeting in Madrid was one of reflection, with many basic science papers searching for more scientific approaches to future developments, as well as an emphasis on lesions in the cerebellum.

By 1969, an additional 11,000 procedures had been performed, bringing the total to roughly 37,000, but the imminent decline of surgical treatment of Parkinson's disease was already apparent. There were many papers on clinical experimentation, as participants used the opportunity of stereotactic surgery to investigate the pathophysiology of the conditions under treatment. L-dopa, which had come into use the previous year, was a major topic, several reports even involving injection of L-dopa directly into the basal ganglia. The decline of activity in the field was apparent in the topics at the meeting the following year, as scientists reported the use of stereotactic techniques in a multitude of new conditions with varying, and sometimes very limited, success.

Nineteen seventy-three brought the first few papers about CT-stereotactic surgery, as well as reports of expansion of the use of computers in the operating room, especially to enhance physiological observations.

The 1980 Meeting of the American Society was devoted to discussion of individual techniques for CT-stereotactic surgery, with many custom-designed apparatus. Nineteen eighty-one brought a discussion of new indications for CT-stereotactic surgery (as well as many presentations about stimulation of various parts of the nervous system, both stereotactic and nonstereotactic). In 1985 were presented series of CT-stereotactic operations, each larger than the others, a pattern that appeared to repeat that of the first three stereotactic meetings. That most recent meeting was also marked by reports of many technical, computer, and electronic advances, as well as a return to the use of thalamotomy for movement disorders.

THE PRESENT

Present indications for functional stereotactic procedures have not changed significantly in the last decade and are summarized below.

The most commonly treated movement disorder is still Parkinson's disease. There was a significant decrease in the number of parkinsonian patients presenting for surgery when L-dopa became available in the late 1960s (32, 35, 53, 102). Interestingly, L-dopa has been superior for the management of bradykinesia and rigidity, which are most often the disabling symptoms of this disease, whereas stereotactic surgery is still the most effective treatment for tremor. Which therapy is indicated, or whether a combination of both is preferred, depends on the individual patient's symptoms (32, 53, 74).

Nonparkinsonian tremor, such as essential tremor or that occurring after a stroke or trauma, may respond quite well to stereotactic thalamotomy (94) and is one of the most common indications at the present time.

Hemiballismus usually resolves spontaneously, when it occurs after a stroke, but, if not, thalamotomy is still the procedure of choice (94). The occasional patient with athetosis may likewise respond, as may the patient with dystonia musculorum deformans, but the results are inconsistent and large lesions may be required (19, 107).

The history of psychosurgery, which is now most often stereotactic in nature, has been markedly and adversely influenced by political and social controversy. Although the need for such surgery is significantly less than in the pretranquilizer days and the techniques are more precise with far fewer adverse side effects, there was an instigated movement against psychosurgery in the 1970s. It was alleged that psychosurgery was used to control violence in socially deprived patients, that it had no benefit, that it had objectionable side effects, and that it was used against minorities (10). A government commission was formed to study these allegations, each of which was found to be false (83). Indeed, an objective assessment of patients who had undergone psychosurgery found that they were performing much better socially and intellectually after their operation (122). Unfortunately, this field has never recuperated from the injuries sustained at that time, and activity remains relatively quiescent. Nevertheless, psychosurgery can be endorsed for intractable depression and obsessive-compulsive behavior (6). Although the original target point was the dorsomedial nucleus or the frontal fibers projecting from it (102), the most commonly used target now is the cingulate gyrus (cingulotomy or cingulumotomy) (6, 122).

Stereotactic surgery is still used in the management of epilepsy, but not generally to produce lesions to interrupt propagation of seizure activity. It is more often used in conjunction with more classical protocols to identify temporal lobe foci for craniotomy and temporal lobectomy, which sometimes requires the use of implanted depth-recording electrodes (34).

CT-STEREOTACTIC SURGERY

Undoubtedly the most important recent development in the field of stereotactic surgery has been its marriage to CT scanning to form the entirely new field of CT-stereotactic surgery (29, 31).

The science of CT scanning is based on the same type of cartesian coordinate system as the stereotactic system, i.e., each point in space is defined in three dimensions. Consequently, it is inherent that any point identifiable on a CT scan can be related to stereotactic coordinates, as long as the relationship between the scan and the stereotactic apparatus is known.

The identification of the anteroposterior (AP) and lateral coordinates is not difficult, because they can be identified on the individual CT slice and relate well to the usual stereotactic AP and lateral coordinate system. The problem arises in the identification of the position of that CT slice in relationship to the stereotactic apparatus. Several techniques have been employed to establish that relationship.

The earliest such attempt involved securing the Leksell apparatus to the scanner table and using the translational measurements of the table to identify the vertical coordinate (8). Other stereotactic apparatus have been adapted or designed to be incorporated onto the scanner table (66) in a similar manner.

Other early techniques involved the use of x-ray opaque lines of varying lengths attached to the patient's head or to the stereotactic apparatus (7). The number of lines intersected by the CT slice could be seen on that slice and used to calculate the position of the slice relative to the patient's head or to the apparatus.

Another technique employed the Scout-View or translational CT-scan image. The image looks like a lateral skull x-ray on the CT console, and the location of each slice can be indicated. By identifying the landmarks through which a slice passes at the base of the skull and by knowing the distance between that slice and the slice bearing the target, it becomes possible to indicate the position of both slices on a lateral x-ray taken in the operating room, thus establishing the vertical coordinate. By using this technique, any stereotactic apparatus can be used for CT-stereotactic surgery (39).

The most significant advance was the use of an N-shaped localizer system (44), which is described in detail elsewhere in this volume. The localizer frame is attached to the stereotactic device during the scan, so that the three limbs of the N are intersected, and the ratio between the distances separating the limbs can be used to calculate the height of the scan above the base of the apparatus. This system is now employed in a number of CT-stereotactic systems, including the modified Todd-Wells, the Brown-Roberts-Wells, and the modified Riechert apparatus, the most commonly used devices (38).

Numerous indications for CT-stereotactic neurosurgery have been presented in the decade since its inception. The most commonly used technique is the biopsy of intracranial mass lesions (38), a technique of growing importance with the increasing number of AIDS patients. As interstitial irradiation becomes more widespread (9, 41, 42), the combination of biopsy followed by irradiation will become more common. As more lesions are seen on CT scan in such conditions as epilepsy, biopsies of previously nonidentifiable lesions becomes practical (29, 31). Intracerebral hematomas have been successfully evacuated (5, 116), and combining that technique with instillation of urokinase (84) opens new indications for surgical management of intracranial bleeding. CT-stereotactic surgery can be a valuable adjunct to open surgical procedures, by allowing insertion of tubing or other marking devices that allow more efficient identification and visualization of resectable lesions. The adaptation of laser to the stereotactic frame allows not only controlled resection of mass lesions, but computerized correlation of the resection with the volume of the lesion seen on CT or magnetic resonance scans (52, 54). As com-

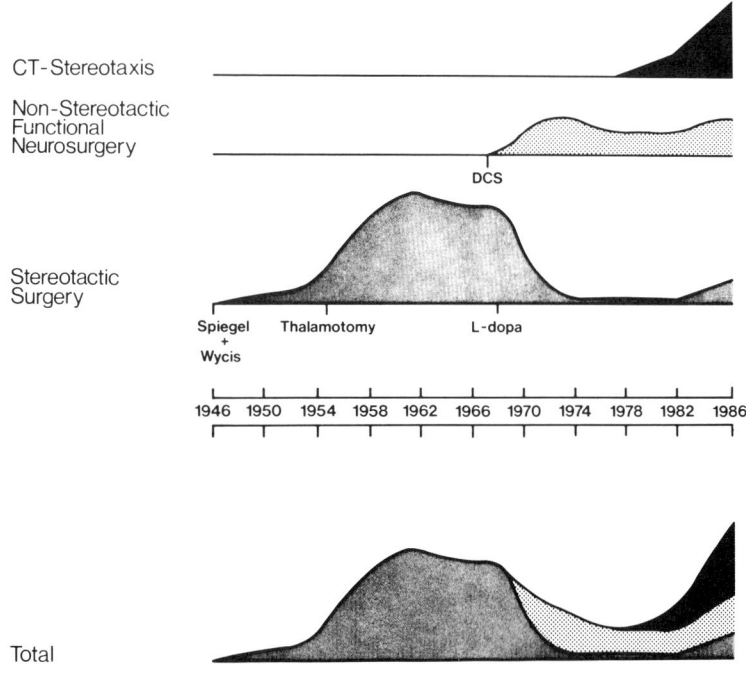

Figure 1.5. Variation in the level of stereotactic and functional neurosurgery throughout its history. (From Gildenberg, P. L. Whatever happened to stereotactic surgery? Neurosurgery 20: 983–987, 1987.)

puter techniques become more sophisticated, they will provide more and more opportunity for the development of new stereotactic techniques. (54).

SUMMARY

If one reviews the history of human stereotactic surgery, variations in the level of activity related to developments can be seen (Fig. 1.5). The field began with the introduction of Spiegel and Wycis' apparatus in 1947. The next 5 years were a period of slow development, when other pioneers introduced various types of apparatus and basic techniques were established. The early part of the 1950s saw a gradually increasing use of these techniques in several centers throughout the world. The decade and a half before the introduction of L-dopa saw a rapid expansion of the field, which overflowed into the realm of general neurosurgery, as thousands of patients with Parkinson's disease were treated stereotactically. Implantable stimulating devices brought nonstereotactic functional neurosurgery into the arena, coincident with a great decrease in the use of stereotactic surgery in the last few years of the 1960s. However, the mid-1970s brought about the inception of CT-guided stereotactic surgery, which has been growing at an ever increasing rate and becoming a more and more important part of neurosurgery as a whole. There is more activity in the field of stereotactic surgery now than ever, and it promises to be even more active in the future.

REFERENCES

1. Afshar F, Watkins ES, Yap JC: *Stereotaxic Atlas of the Human Brainstem and Cerebellar Nuclei.* New York, Raven Press, 1978.
2. Alksne JF, Fingerhut AG, Rand RW: Magnetic probe for the stereotactic thrombosis of intracranial aneurysm. *J Neurol Neurosurg Psychiatr* 30: 159-162, 1967.
3. Andrew J, Watkins ES: *Stereotactic Surgery. A Stereotaxic Atlas of the Human Thalamus,* Baltimore, Williams & Wilkins, 1969.
4. Austin B, Lee AA: plastic ball and socket type of stereotaxic detector. *J Neurosurg* 15: 264-268, 1958.
5. Backlund E, von Holst H: Controlled subtotal evacuation of intracerebral hematomas by stereotactic technique. *Surg Neurol* 9: 99-101, 1978.
6. Ballentine HT Jr, Giriunas IE: Advances in psychiatric surgery. In Rasmussen T, Marino R, (eds): *Functional Neurosurgery.* New York, Raven Press, 1979, pp 155-164.
7. Barcia-Salorio JL, Broseta J, Hernandez G, Roldan P, Bordes V: A new approach for directed CT localization in stereotaxis. *Appl Neurophysiol* 45: 383-386, 1982.
8. Bergstrom M, Greitz J: Stereotaxic computed tomography. *AJR* 127: 167-170, 1976.
9. Bernstein M, Gutin PH: Interstitial irradiation of brain tumors: a review. *Neurosurgery* 9: 741-750, 1981.
10. Breggin PR: The return of lobotomy and psychosurgery. *Congressional Record* 118(26): Feb. 24, 1972.
11. Burton CV, Mozley JM, Walker AE, Braitmann HE: Inductive heating. *IEEE Trans Biomed Engin* 13: 114, 1966.
12. Carol MA: true "advanced imaging assisted" skull-mounted stereotactic system. *Appl Neurophysiol* 48: 69-72, 1985.
13. Cooper IS: Ligation of the anterior choroidal artery for involuntary movements of parkinsonism. *Psychiatr Q* 27: 317-319, 1953.
14. Cooper IS: Surgical alleviation of parkinsonism; effects of occlusion of the anterior choroidal artery. *J Am Geriatr Soc* 11: 691-717, 1954.
15. Cooper IS: *Chemopallidectomy Science* 121: 217, 1955.
16. Cooper IS: Clinical results and follow-up studies in a personal series of 300 operations for parkinsonism. *J Am Geriatr Soc* 4: 1171-1181, 1956.
17. Cooper IS: Chemopallidectomy and chemothalamectomy for parkinsonism and dystonia. *Proc R Soc Med* 52: 47-60, 1959.
18. Cooper IS: Results of 1000 consecutive basal ganglia operations for parkinsonism. *Ann Intern Med* 52: 483-499, 1960.
19. Cooper IS: *Involuntary Movement Disorders.* New York, Hoeber, 1969.
20. Cooper IS, Bravo G, Riklan M, Davidson N, Gorek E: Chemopallidectomy and chemothalamectomy for parkinsonism. *Geriatrics* 13: 127-147, 1958.
21. Cooper IS, Lee A: StJ Cryostatic congelation. *J Nerv Ment Dis* 33: 259-263, 1961.
22. Cosman ER, Nashold BS Jr, Bedenbaugh P: Stereotactic radiofrequency lesion making. *Appl Neurophysiol* 46: 160-166, 1983.
23. Dittmar C: Ueber die Lage des sogenannten Gefaesszentrums in der Medulla oblongata. *Ber saechs Ges Wiss Leipzig (Math phys)* 25: 449-469, 1873.
24. Freeman W, Watts JW: *Psychosurgery.* Springfield, IL, Charles C Thomas, 1942.
25. Gildenberg PL: Variability of subcortical lesions produced by a heating electrode and Cooper's balloon cannula. *Conf Neurol* 20: 53-65, 1960.
26. Gildenberg PL: Clinical and Physiological Applications. In Speigel EA, Wycis HT (eds):

Stereoencephalotomy. Part II. New York, Grune & Stratton, 1962, pp 41-49.
27. Gildenberg PL: Survey of stereotactic and functional neurosurgery in the United States and Canada. *Appl Neurophysiol* 38: 31-37, 1975.
28. Gildenberg PL: Radiofrequency lesion making procedures. *Symp Appl Neurophysiol* 39: 69-132, 1976.
29. Gildenberg PL: Computerized tomography and stereotactic surgery. In Spiegel EA (ed): *Guided Brain Operations,* Basel, Karger, 1982, pp 24-34.
30. Gildenberg PL: Functional neurosurgery. In Schmidek HH, Sweet WH (eds): *Operative Neurosurgical Techniques,* New York, Grune & Stratton, 1982, Vol II, pp 993-1043.
31. Gildenberg PL: Stereotactic neurosurgery and computerized tomographic scanning. *Appl Neurophysiol* 46: 170-179, 1983.
32. Gildenberg PL: The present role of stereotactic surgery in the management of Parkinson's disease. *Adv Neurol* 40: 447-452, 1984.
33. Gildenberg PL: General concepts of stereotactic surgery. In Lunsford LD (ed): *Modern Stereotactic Surgery,* Hingham, MA, Martinus Nijhokff, 1987.
34. Gildenberg, P. L. Surgery for seizures. In Frost EAM (ed): *Anesthesia in Neurosurgery???.* New York, Butterworth, 1987, pp. 293-316.
35. Gildenberg PL: Whatever happened to stereotactic surgery? *Neurosurgery* 20: 543-553, 1987.
36. Gildenberg PL, DeVaul RA: Management of chronic pain refractory to specify therapy. In: Youmans JR (ed): *Neurological Surgery,* Philadelphia, WB Saunders, 1981, pp 3749-3768.
37 Gildenberg PL, DeVaul RA: *The Chronic Pain Patient. Evaluation and Management.* Basel, Karger, 1985.
38. Gildenberg PL, Franklin PO: Survey of CT-guided stereotactic surgery. *Appl Neurophysiol* 48: 477-480, 1985.
39. Gildenberg PL, Kaufman HH, Murthy KSK: Calculation of stereotactic coordinates from the computed tomographic scan. *Neurosurgery* 10: 580-586, 1982.
40. Giorgi C, Cerchiari U, Broggi G, Birk P, Struppler A: Digital image processing to handle neuroanatomical information and neurophysiological data. *Appl Neurophysiol* 48: 30-33, 1985.
41. Gutin PH, Hosobuchi Y, Phillips TL, Stupar TA: Stereotactic interstitial irradiation for the treatment of brain tumors. *Cancer Treat Rep* 652: 103-106, 1981.
42. Gutin PH, Leibel SA: Stereotaxic interstitial irradiation of malignant brain tumors. *Neurol Clin* 3: 883-893, 1985.
43. Hardy TL, Koch J, Lassiter A: Computer graphics with computerized tomography for functional neurosurgery. *Appl Neurophysiol* 46: 217-266, 1983.
44. Heilbrun MP: Computed tomography-guided stereotactic systems. *Clin Neurosurg* 31: 564-581, 1984.
45. Horsley V, Clarke RH: The structure and functions of the cerebellum examined by a new method. *Brain* 31: 45-124, 1908.
46. Hosobuchi Y: Combined electrical stimulation of the periaqueductal gray matter and sensory thalamus. *Appl Neurophysiol* 46: 112-115, 1983.
47. Hosobuchi Y: Subcortical electrical stimulation for control of intractable pain in humans. Report of 122 cases (1970-1984). *J Neurosurg* 64: 543-553, 1986.
48. Hosobuchi Y, Adams JE, Rutkins B: Chronic thalamic stimulation for the control of facial anesthesia dolorosas. *Arch Neurol* 29: 158-161, 1973.
49. Hunsperger RW, Wyss OAM: Ausschaltung von Nervengewebe durch Hochfrequenz-Koagulation. *Helv Physiol Pharmacol Acta* 11: 283-304, 1953.
50. Jinnai D, Nishimoto A: Stereotaxic destruction of Forel H for treatment of epilepsy. *Neurochirurgia* (Stuttgart) 6: 164-176, 1963.
51. Kall BA, Kelly PJ, Goerss BS, Frieder G: Methodology and clinical experience with computed tomography and a computer resident stereotactic atlas. *Neurosurgery* 17: 400-407, 1985.
52. Kelly PJ, Alker GJ Jr: A method for stereotactic laser microsurgery in the treatment of deep seated CNS neoplasms. *Appl Neurophysiol* 43: 210-215, 1960.
53. Kelly PJ, Gillingham FJ: The long-term results of stereotaxic surgery and L-dopa therapy in patients with Parkinson's disease. A 10-year follow-up study. *J Neurosurg* 53: 332-337, 1980.
54. Kelly PJ, Kall BA, Goerss S, Earnest F: Present and future developments of stereotactic technology. *Appl Neurophysiol* 48: 1-6, 1985.
55. Kjellberg RN, Koehler AM, Preston WM, Sweet WH: Stereotaxic instrument for use with the Bragg peak of a proton beam. *Conf Neurol* 22: 183-189, 1962.
56. Laitinen LV: Brain targets in surgery for Parkinson's disease. Results of a survey of neurosurgeons. *J Neurosurg* 62: 349-351, 1985.
57. Leksell LA: stereotaxic apparatus for intracerebral surgery. *Acta chir scand* 99: 229-233, 1949.
58. Leksell L: *Stereotaxis and Radiosurgery. An Operating System.* Springfield, IL, Charles C Thomas, 1971.
59. Leksell L: Stereotactic radiosurgery. *J Neurol Neurosurg Psychiatry* 46: 797-803, 1983.
60. Leksell L, Herner T, Liden K: Stereotaxic radiosurgery of the brain. *K fysiogr Saellsk Lund Foerh* 25: 1-10, 1955.
61. Leksell L, Larsson B, Andersson P, Rexed B, Sourander P, Mair W: Lesions in the depth of the brain produced by a beam of high energy protons. *Acta Radiol* 54: 251-264, 1960.
62. Leksell L, Liden K: A therapeutic trial with radioactive isotopes in cystic brain tumour. *Radioisotope Tech.* 1: 1-4, 1951.
63. Levy A: Stereotaxic brain operations in Parkinson's syndrome and related motor disorders. Comparison of lesions in the pallidum and thalamus with those in the internal capsule. *Conf Neurol* (Suppl.) 29: 1-70, 1967.

64. Liebeskind JC, Gilubaum G, Besson JM, Oliveras JL: Analgesia from electrical stimulation of the periaqueductal grey in the cat. Behavior observations and inhibitory effects on spinal cord interneurons. *Brain Res* 50: 441-446, 1973.
65. Long DM, Erickson DE: Stimulation of the posterior columns of the spinal cord for relief of intractable pain. *Surg Neurol* 41: 134-141, 1975.
66. Lunsford LD: A dedicated CT system for the stereotactic operating room. *Appl Neurophysiol* 45: 374-378, 1982.
67. Mark VH, Chato JC, Eastman FG, Aronow S, Ervin FR: Localized cooling in the brain. *Science* 134: 1520-1521, 1961.
68. Mark VH, Chiba T, Ervin FR, Hamlin H: The comparison of heat and cold for the production of localized lesions in the central nervous system. *Conf Neurol* 26: 178-184, 1965.
69. Mayer DJ, Liebeskind JC: Pain reduction by focal electrical stimulation of the brain. An anatomical and behavioral analysis. *Brain Res* 68: 73-93, 1974.
70. Melzack R, Wall PD: Pain mechanisms: A new theory. *Science* 150: 971-979, 1965.
71. Meyers R: The modification of alternating tremors, rigidity and festination by surgery of the basal ganglia. *Res Publ Ass Res Nerv Ment Dis* 21: 602-665, 1942.
72. Meyers R: Historical background and personal experiences in the surgical relief of hyperkinesia and hypertonus. In Fields W, (ed): *Pathogenesis and Treatment of Parkinsonism.* Springfield, IL, Charles C Thomas, 1958.
73. Meyers R, Fry WJ, Fry FJ, Dreyer LL, Schultz DF, Noyes RF: Early experiences with ultrasonic irradiation of the pallidofugal and nigral complexes in hyperkinetic and hypertonic disorders. *J Neurosurg* 16: 32-54, 1959.
74. Miyamoto T, Bekku H, Moriyama E, Tsuchida S: Present role of stereotactic thalamotomy for parkinsonism. Retrospective analysis of operative results and thalamic lesions in computed tomograms. *Appl Neurophysiol* 48: 294-304, 1985.
75. Mundinger F, Riechert T, Gabriel, E: Untersuchungen zu den physikalischen und technischen Voraussetzungen einer dosierten Hochfrequenz-Koagulation bei stereotaktischen Hirnoperationen. *Zentralbl Chir* 85: 1051-1063, 1960.
76. Murtagh F, Wycis HT, Robbins R, Spiegel-Adolph M, Spiegel EA: Visualization and treatment of cystic brain tumors by stereoencephalotomy. *Acta Radiol* 46: 407-414, 1956.
77. Nagaseki Y, Horikoshi T, Fukamachi A: A three-dimensional display of stereotactic V.im thalamotomy reproduced with a personal computer. *Appl Neurophysiol* 49: (in press).
78. Narabayashi H: Stereotaxic instrument for operation on the human basal ganglia. *Psychiatr Neurol Jpn* 54: 669-671, 1952.
79. Narabayashi H, Mizutani T: Epileptic seizures and the stereotaxic amygdalotomy. *Conf Neurol* 32: 289-297, 1970.
80. Narabayashi H, Okuma T: Procaine oil blocking of the globus pallidus for the treatment of rigidity and tremor of parkinsonism. *Proc Jpn Acad* 29: 310-318, 1953.
81. Narabayashi H, Shimazu H, Fujita Y, Shikiba S, Nagao T, Nagahata M: Procaine-oil-wax pallidotomy for double athetosis and spastic states in infantile cerebral palsy. *Neurology* 10: 61-69, 1960.
82. Nashold BS Jr: Brainstem stereotaxic procedures. In: Schaltenbrand G, Walker AE (eds): *Stereotaxy of the Human Brain.* Stuttgart, Georg Thieme Verlag, 1982, pp 475-483.
83. National Commission for the Protection of Human Subjects of Biomedical and Behavioral Research: Report and Recommendations, Psychosurgery. DHEW Publication No. (05) 77-0001, Washington, DC, US Government Printing Office, Feb 24, 1977.
84. Niizuma H, Otsuki T, Jonkura H, Nakazato N, Suzuki J: CT-guided stereotactic aspiration of intracerebral hematoma. Results of a hematoma lysis method using urokinase. *Appl Neurophysiol* 48: 427-430, 1985.
85. Obrador S: A simplified neurosurgical technique for approaching and damaging the region of the globus pallidus in Parkinson's disease. *J Neurol Neurosurg Psychiatry* 20: 47-49, 1957.
86. Obrador S, Dierssen G:. Cirugia de la region palidal. *Revta Clin Esp Ano* XVII 61: 229-237, 1956.
87. Ohye C, Hirai T, Miyazaki M, Shibazaki T, Nakajima H: V.im thalamotomy for the treatment of various kinds of tremor. *Appl Neurophysiol* 45: 275-280, 1982.
88. Olivier A, Bertrand G, Picard C: Discovery of the first human stereotactic instrument. *Appl Neurophysiol* 46: 84-91, 1983.
89. Rand RW, Brown WJ, Stern WE: Surgical occlusion of anterior choroidal arteries in parkinsonism. Clinical and neuropathologic findings. *Neurology* 6: 390-401, 1956.
90. Richardson DE, Akil H: Pain reduction by electrical brain stimulation in man. II. Chronic self-administration in the periventricular grey matter. *J Neurosurg* 47: 184-194, 1977.
91. Riechert T: Die Entfernung von Hirnstecksplittern mit Hilfe des stereotaktischen Operationsverfahrens. *Zentralbl. Neurochir* 15: 159-164, 1955.
92. Riechert T: Die stereotaktischen Hirnoperationen in ihrer Anwendung bei den Hyperkinesen (mit Ausnahme des Parkinsonismus), bei Schmerzzuständen und einigen weiteren Indikationen (Einfüren von radioaktiven Isotopen usw.). *Acta Med Belg* 121-160, 1957.
93. Riechert T: Moderne Chirurgie des Zentralnervensystems (inductive heating). *Therapiewoche* 9: 430-435, 1959.
94. Riechert T: *Stereotactic Brain Operations. Methods, Clinical Aspects, Indications.* Bern, Stuttgart, Vienna, Hans Huber, 1980.
95. Riechert T, Mundinger F: Beschreibung uind Anwendung eines Zielgeraetes fuer stereotaktische Hirnoperationen (II. Modell). *Acta Neurochir. Wien* (Suppl.) 3: 308-337, 1955.
96. Riechert T, Mundinger F: Indications, technique

and results of the stereotactic operations upon the hypophysis using radio-isotopes. *J Nerv Ment Dis* 13: 1-9, 1960.
97. Riechert T, Wolff M: Ueber ein neues Zielgeraet zur intrakraniellen elektrischen Abteilung und Ausschaltung. *Arch Psychiatr Z Neurol* 186: 225-230, 1951.
98. Salcman M: Feasibility of microwave hyperthermia for brain tumor therapy. *Prog Exp Tumor Res* 28: 220-231, 1984.
99. Salcman M, Samaras GM: Interstitial microwave hyperthermia for brain tumors. Results of a phase-1 clinical trial. *J Neurooncol* 1: 225-236, 1983.
100. Sano K, Yoshioka M, Ogashiwa M, Ishijima B, Ohye C: Thalamolaminotomy. A new operation for relief of intractable pain. *Conf Neurol* 27: 63-66, 1966.
101. Schaltenbrand G, Bailey P: *Introduction to Stereotaxis with an Atlas of the Human Brain.* Stuttgart, Thieme, 1959.
102. Spiegel EA: *Guided Brain Operations.* Basel, Karger, 1982.
103. Spiegel EA, Wycis HT: Pallidothalamotomy in chorea. *Arch Neurol Psychiatr* Chicago 64: 495-496, 1950.
104. Spiegel EA, Wycis HT: *Stereoencephalotomy, Part I.* New York, Grune & Stratton, 1952.
105. Spiegel EA, Wycis HT: Mesencephalotomy in the treatment of "intractable" facial pain. *Arch Neurol* 69: 1-13, 1953.
106. Spiegel EA, Wycis HT: Ansotomy in paralysis agitans. *Arch Neurol Psychiatry* 71: 598-614, 1954.
107. Spiegel EA, Wycis HT: *Stereoencephalotomy. Part II. Clinical and Physiological Applications.* New York, Grune & Stratton, 1962.
108. Spiegel EA, Wycis HT, Baird HW: Effect of thalamic and pallidal lesions upon involuntary movements in choreoathetosis. *Trans Am Neurol Assoc* 75: 234, 1950.
109. Spiegel EA, Wycis HT, Baird HW: Pallidotomy and pallidoamygdalotomy in certain types of convulsive disorders. *Arch Neurol Psychiatr* Chicago, 80: 714-728, 1958.
110. Spiegel EA, Wycis HT, Marks M, Lee A: StJ Stereotaxic apparatus for operations on the human brain. *Science* 106: 349-350, 1947.
111. Spiegel EA, Wycis HT, Szekely EG, Adams J, Flanagan M, Baird H W: Campotomy in various extrapyramidal disorders. *J Neurosurg* 20: 871-881, 1963.
112. Spiegel EA, Wycis HT, Szekely EG, Soloff L, Adams J, Gildenberg PL, Zanes C: Stimulation of Forel's field during stereotaxic operations in the human brain. *EEG Clin. Neurophysiol.* 16: 537-548, 1964.
113. Talairach J, Aboulker J, Tournoux P, David M: Technique stereotaxique de la chirurgie hypophysaire par voie nasale. *Neurochirurgie* 2: 3-23, 1956.
114. Talairach J, David M, Tournoux P, Corredor H, Krasina T: *Atlas d'Anatomie Stereotaxique.* Paris, Masson, 1957.
115. Talairach J, Hecaen M, David M, Monnier M, Ajuriaguerra J: Recherches sur la coagulation therapeutique des structures sous-corticales chez l'homme. *Rev Neurol* 81: 4-24, 1949.
116. Tanikawa T, Amano K, Kawamura H, Kawaratake H, Notani M, Iseki H, Shiwaku T, Nagao T, Iwata Y, Tairo T, Umezawa Y, Shimizu T, Kitamura K: CT-guided stereotactic surgery for evacuation of hypertensive intracerebral hematoma. *Appl Neurophysiol* 48: 431-439, 1985.
117. Tasker R R: Thalamic stereotaxic procedures. In Schaltenbrand G, Walker AE (eds): *Stereotaxy of the Human Brain.* Stuttgart, New York, Georg Thieme Verlag, 1982, pp 484-497.
118. Tasker RR, Hawrylshyn P, Rowe IH, Organ LW: Computerized graphic display of results of subcortical stimulation during stereotactic surgery. *Acta Neurochir* (Suppl.) 24: 85-98, 1977.
119. Tasker RR, Organ LW, Hawrylshyn P: Investigation of the surgical target for alleviation of involuntary movement disorders. *Appl Neurophysiol* 45: 261-274, 1982.
120. Tasker RR, Organ LW, Hawrylshyn PA: *The Thalamus and Midbrain of Man. A Physiological Atlas Using Electrical Stimulation.* Springfield, IL, Charles C Thomas, 1982.
121. Tasker RR, Siqueira J, Hawrylshyn P, Organ LW: What happened to V.im thalamotomy for Parkinson's disease? *Appl Neurophysiol* 46: 68-83, 1983.
122. Teuber HL, Corkin S, Twitchell TE: *A study of Cingulotomy in Man.* DHEW Publications No. (05) 77-0002. Washington, DC, US Government Printing Office, Feb 24, 1977.
123. Tobias CA, Roberts JE, Lawrence JH, Lew-Beer BVA, Anger HO, Born JL, McCombs R, Huggins C: Peaceful uses of atomic energy. *Proc Int Conf,* Geneva 10: 95, 1955.
124. Todd EM: Stereotaxic surgery of the basal ganglia. In: *Todd-Wells Manual of Stereotaxic Procedures.* Randolph, MA, Codman and Shurtleff, 1967.
125. Tsubokawa T, Maejima S, Yamamoto T, Katayama Y: Pain control with deep brain stimulation. Differences in clinical effects between thalamic relay nucleus stimulation and periaqueductal gray stimulation. *Appl Neurophysiol* 49: 296-297, 1986.
126. Uchimura Y, Narabayashi H Stereoencephalotom. *Psychiatr Neurol Jpn* 52: 265, 1951.
127. Van Buren JM, Borke RC: *Variations and Connections of the Human Thalamus. 2. Variations of the Human Diencephalon.* New York, Springer, 1972.
128. Walker AE, Burton CV: Radiofrequency telethermocoagulation. *JAMA* 197: 108-112, 1966.
129. Wycis HT, Robbins R, Spiegel-Adolph M, Meszaros J, Spiegel E A: Studies in stereoencephalotomy III. Treatment of a cystic craniopharyngioma by injection of radioactive P-32. *Conf Neurol* 14: 193-202, 1954.
130. Wyss OAM: Hochfrequenz Koagulationsgeraet zur reizlosen Ausschaltung. *Helv Physiol Pharmacol Acta* 3: 437-443, 1945.
131. Zervas NT: Technique of radio-frequency hypophysectomy. *Conf Neurol* 26: 157-160, 1965.

Chapter 2

Stereotactic Applications: General Overview

ROBERT J. COFFEY, M.D. AND WILLIAM A. FRIEDMAN, M.D.

TRADITIONAL STEREOTACTIC APPLICATIONS

Introduction

The application of stereotactic techniques to neurological disorders is best discussed under two broad headings: functional and anatomical (77). In functional stereotactic surgery, an intracerebral site is selected for destruction (59, 166), stimulation, or physiological monitoring. The disorder under investigation or treatment may be the result of a localizable lesion (stroke, injury), a widespread neurotransmitter defect (parkinsonism), or some process with an unclear anatomical or physiological basis (psychoses, certain painful states). The actual target in the majority of functional stereotactic operations is normal brain tissue according to usual radiographical or histological criteria. Its location must be indirectly calculated by recourse to a standard brain atlas, followed by plotting the target's location according to a standard set of intracranial references, usually the intercommissural line and the midsagittal plane.

Radiographical confirmation of final probe position is essential in traditional stereotactic surgery for both anatomical and functional disorders. Variations in the dimensions of the third ventricle and deep nuclei are, additionally, significant enough that correct radiographical probe placement can still result in an improperly placed lesion if physiological control of some sort is not used (90, 137). Phenomena observed during electrical stimulation, macro- or microelectrode recording, impedance monitoring, local cooling, and local anesthetic injection have been used to help confirm that the probe tip is actually at its intended physiological target (27–29, 34, 43, 79, 107, 126, 145, 146, 169, 170, 192–195).

Stereotactic surgery for anatomical disorders involves the application of precision-guidance instrumentation to the categories of neurological illness that more commonly confront neurosurgeons. Among these entities to which traditional stereotactic surgery has been applied are mass lesions, vascular malformations or aneurysms, hydrocephalus, and foreign bodies. In contrast to functional stereotactic surgery, the target tissue in anatomical stereotactic surgery is almost always radiographically and histologically abnormal. A target for traditional anatomical stereotactic surgery, unless it is radiodense and visible on plain films, is inferred from stereotactic ventriculograms or angiograms. The target coordinates referable to the instrument being used can then be calculated without a brain atlas.

In anatomical operations, physiological control is optional. Histological control in the form of immediate frozen section or cytological examination is helpful in biopsy cases by ensuring that the tissue obtained is indeed pathological.

FUNCTIONAL STEREOTACTIC SURGERY

Involuntary Movement Disorders

Parkinson's Disease

Stereotactic ablations of various targets within the extrapyramidal system for involuntary movement disorders (IMDs) comprised the largest category of operations performed during the first two decades of traditional functional stereotactic surgery. In 1940, Meyers (122) was the first to demonstrate that involuntary tremors could be eliminated by operations at the level of the basal ganglia and pallidothalamic connections without producing motor weakness. His open transventricular operations had a considerable complication rate (mortality 15%). During 1950 to 1952, Spiegel, Wycis, et al. (183), Cooper, during 1954 to 1958 (54, 56–58), and Hassler and Riechert, 1955 (89), developed stereotactic interventions upon the basal ganglia and/or thalamus for the relief of movement disorders.

Targets within the rostral part of the lateral thalamic nuclear mass (VL thalamotomy), variably including ventrooralis anterior (VOa), ventrooralis posterior (VOp), and ventrointermedius (VIm), were favored by most surgeons (111), sometimes in combination with other extrapyramidal targets (198). Often, a lesion was incrementally enlarged until the patient's tremor was abolished or side effects appeared. Other targets have been used; one of Cooper's early targets was the medial globus pallidus. Stereotactic pallidotomy with ansotomy (section of the ansa lenticularis), reportedly relieved parkinsonian rigidity early, but had a delayed favorable effect on tremors that took up to 3 months to appear.

The target favored by Spiegel, Wycis et al. (183), was located more ventral and medial than the usual thalamic site. Their "campotomy" operation severed pallidothalamic fibers in Forel's field H and could include some dentatothalamic fibers as well, if enlarged posteriorly. Ojemann (111) also favored a target below the intercommissural line, but located more posteriorly, below the VL nucleus and situated within the region of the zona incerta and thalamic fasciculus. In practice, lesions located either within VL or more ventrally at the level of its afferents have equivalent therapeutic effects. Tremor is more favorably affected by a posteriorly placed lesion that interrupts dentatothalamic inputs, while rigidity is reduced by more anterior lesions within the pallidothalamic circuits.

The results of unilateral thalamotomy for parkinsonism were encouraging (119, 174, 175). Cooper obtained relief of tremor and rigidity in over 90% of his "good risk" patients both initially and at follow-up (57). Walker, in a smaller series, had a similar success rate (204). Mundinger, Reinker et al. reported more modest early results, with relief of tremor in 78% of patients and relief of rigidity in 67% (204). Their more recent results were improved (130). In 1983, Tasker (196) reported 82% elimination of tremor by VIm thalamotomy, with an additional 7% of patients having "almost no tremor" on the operated side.

In a recent review, Gildenberg stated that 85 to 93% of patients should obtain relief of tremor on the operated side, with greater than 50% obtaining long-lasting relief of rigidity (82). He suggested that thalamotomy be considered early in the management of patients whose most disabling symptom is tremor, since this manifestation of parkinsonism is the least likely to respond satisfactorily to medication. In patients disabled by bradykinesia, thalamotomy should be considered if maximal medical management is complicated by L-dopa intolerance or the on-off effect. Operation often resulted in better tolerance of therapeutic doses of L-dopa while preventing the appearance of drug-induced dyskinesias.

A discussion of side effects and complications of thalamotomy for parkinsonism applies to stereotactic surgery for other conditions as well. In 1965, Bravo et al. (40), in a review of 650 selected cases, found 88 neurological side effects for an incidence of 13%. Hemiballismus was seen in 26 cases and was always transient. Others have also described postoperative hyperkinetic phenomena (125). Pathological examination has disclosed no accidental lesion in the subthalamic nucleus. Dystonia occurred in 17 patients. In contrast to the transient nature of most hyperkinetic side effects, postoperative dystonic limb symptoms, usually an equinovarus foot deformity, tended to be permanent. Sensory deficits occurred in 15 patients, of which seven were permanent, while a thalamic pain syndrome occurred in three patients. Hemiparesis was seen in 12 cases and was permanent in five (<1%). Bravo (40) suggested that, despite adequate radiographical and physiological controls, postoperative neurological deficits were due to improper placement of the lesioning instrument.

In other series, language disturbance after dominant or bilateral thalamotomy was the most frequently seen side effect of surgery. This occurred in 13.1 to 42% of patients undergoing thalamotomy for parkinsonism. The duration and severity of language disturbances varied in all series. The incidence of this complication increased with age in the parkinsonian population. The incidence in the cerebral palsy group, with involuntary movements treated by thalamotomy, has been extremely high (41, 42).

Bilateral lesions encroaching on the genu of the internal capsule can lead to severe dysarthria and dysphagia. The desire to avoid these complications accounts for the relatively low proportion of bilaterally operated patients in many series (25–33%). In cases where both sides are equally involved, a number of authors recommend thalamotomy on the dominant side first, in order to give the patient maximal benefit from a single operation (82, 121). A period of at least 2 to 3 months should elapse before performing a contralateral operation. Management strategies include making a smaller lesion on the second side or, alternatively, avoiding the thalamus altogether and selecting a target in the globus pallidus.

The occurrence of clinically significant intracerebral hematomas after thalamotomy has probably been underestimated in the large series operated before the advent of CT scanning. In 1974, Crevier reviewed, by questionnaire, 20,000 stereotactic operations (60). He found an 0.8% incidence of hematomas, diagnosed either surgically or at autopsy. Fifty-six percent of these hematomas were fatal, while 32% of the survivors were hemiplegic. The incidence of post-stereotactic motor deficits of undetermined etiology in this review was 1.4%, and certainly included hematomas not large enough to warrant operation or cause death. Close control of the patients' blood pressure to a level of <150 mm Hg systolic intraoperatively and in the first postoperative days lessened the likelihood of hematoma formation (204).

Infectious complications of stereotactic surgery are rare. Many large series do not mention even a single case of postoperative infection. In 1981, Hood and Yap (99) reported three infections in a personal series of 365 operations performed with the Bennett frame. This system requires the long-term implantation of a perforated plate in the subgaleal space, and would be expected to yield a higher than usual infection rate. Their incidence was still <1%.

In 1977, Bernoulli, Siegfried et al. (25) reported the transmission of Jakob-Creutzfeld (J-C) disease to two patients by a depth electrode that had been used on a prior patient with undiagnosed J-C disease. At the time of these mishaps, the now standard procedures for sterilization of instruments exposed to the slow virus were unknown.

A generalized encephalopathy of variable severity and duration, including somnolence, confusion, and memory disturbance, follows thalamotomy in 5 to 10% of cases overall. Males are affected with this psychoorganic syndrome more than twice as often as females, with the risk increasing to 15% with age >55 years and the presence of underlying systemic illness (162). A number of authors have noted that air or positive-contrast ventriculography, rather than thalamotomy, precipitates this encephalopathy. For this reason, the actual operation has often been performed by reapplication of the stereotactic frame at a second stage 5 to 10 days following ventriculography. The development of CT- and MRI-guided systems, capable of the accuracy needed for functional stereotactic surgery, may eliminate the need for ventriculography and, hence, these complications.

Pneumonia, pulmonary embolism, cardiac, and other medical complications occur after stereotactic operations, especially in the elderly population. Pathological respiratory patterns seen in a high proportion of patients with advanced parkinsonism predispose such patients to bronchopneumonia, especially if a postoperative encephalopathic state keeps them bedridden for a prolonged period.

Tremor

Some forms of tremor other than the parkinsonian variety are also relieved by stereotactic thalamotomy (79, 122–124, 148, 180). The results can be excellent, provided accurate diagnosis and careful case selection are employed. Intraoperative abolition of familial or "essential" tremors can be accomplished in >90% of patients with a long-term cure rate of >80% (57, 58, 201). Most surgeons favor an intrathalamic target within the VL-VIm complex, at or above the intercommissural line, similar to the target in parkinsonism.

Cerebellar intention tremor is most often seen as a manifestation of multiple sclerosis, but can be familial, posttraumatic, poststroke, or idiopathic. Some of the best results of thalamotomy are seen in the posttraumatic and idiopathic groups. Recent series of VL thalamotomy for posttraumatic tremor and other involuntary movements show improvement to some degree in all patients followed long term (5, 6, 47). Transient increased paresis and dysarthria (especially after dominant-side lesioning) were seen in a significant number of patients.

While VL thalamotomy can dramatically reduce or abolish the severe intention tremor of multiple sclerosis (MS) intraoperatively in 75 to 100% of patients, lasting relief is achieved only 73% of the time (57, 80). Despite these moderately favorable figures, most patients with MS do not improve in overall disability rating or functional status after surgery. The presence of multifocal deficits, which progress with time, and the tendency of ventriculography and surgery to provoke an acute exacerbation of demyelination (163) contribute to a general pessimism regarding the benefits of surgery in patients with MS. Postoperative pneumonia, dysarthria, and micturition disturbances also occur with relative frequency in this group.

Cerebral Palsy

The involuntary movements associated with cerebral palsy (CP) include tremor, athetosis, dystonia, and spasticity in all combinations. Patients with CP classically present with a static neurological picture, often manifesting widespread damage in the pyramidal as well as extrapyramidal systems. The situation is in some ways similar to that of MS, in that stereotactic surgery can reduce or eliminate some target symptoms, but the actual benefits to the patient in terms of increased functional abilities are usually modest at best. As standard VL thalamotomy alone is often ineffective in these cases, various staged approaches have evolved. Most involve bilateral surgery, and many include pulvinotomy or dentatotomy as part of the multitarget strategy (84, 85, 118).

The results of VL/VIm thalamotomy, often done bilaterally in stages or as a single procedure, have been best in those cases where tremor was a prominent symptom (41, 42, 147). The "considerable improvement" seen in 72.7% of Broggi's cases (41) represents the best result in any recent series. In 1975, Ramamurthi and Davidson (154) reported centromedian thalamotomy as an element of multitarget thalamic surgery in 62 cases of CP. The long-term results of this protocol showed that less than 50% sustained improvement despite a much higher early success rate.

In 1969, Nashold and Slaughter (140), studied the effects of stimulation and ablation of the deep cerebellar nuclei in six patients with involuntary movement disorders (IMDs), two of whom suffered from CP. Both of these patients benefited from surgery. The authors also reported their anatomical studies, giving stereotactic radiographical coordinates for the dentate nucleus via a suboccipital transcerebellar trajectory. Since physiological confirmation of probe position has been unreliable in most surgeons' experience, radiographical landmarks alone have been used. Subsequent workers have revised Nashold and Slaughter's original coordinates as more experience with this operation has accumulated.

Siegfried (176–178) reported his results with dentatotomy in 50 patients, 42 with spastic CP. Thalamotomy and pulvinotomy were performed in some patients. "Good results" seen initially in 60% of patients diminished to 32% in the long term. Nursing care was made easier by surgery in 50% of patients. Hitchcock (96) also performed dentatotomy for ipsilateral or bilateral spasticity in CP, using VL thalamotomy as well, if athetosis was present. In neither of these series, nor in others, were cures or dramatic improvements noted (138). One important caveat with respect to bilateral dentatotomy, especially if large lesions are inflicted at a single sitting under general anesthesia, is that profound hypotonia may result, leaving the patient unable to stand or support himself.

In 1977, Zervas (211) stated that CP is not helped by dentatotomy, and that its further use in that condition was not warranted. Although the place for dentatotomy in the treatment of movement disorders remains controversial, a number of prominent surgeons employ the technique for the relief of spasticity of supraspinal origin. Expectations regarding overall functional improvement after surgery for CP should be kept modest. A realistic objective of surgery is to provide the patient with a more favorable motor foundation upon which to base intensive physiotherapy.

Dystonia

Dystonia refers to a state of local or generalized increased muscle tone of central origin. Simultaneous agonist-antagonist muscle contractions often result in bizarre limb or trunk postures. The dystonic postures may be undulating in the early stages of disease, and are usually made worse by attempts at voluntary movement. Dystonia musculorum deformans (DMD, hereditary or torsion dystonia), is a variably progressive syndrome classically appearing in Ashkenazic Jews with a positive family history. Dystonic limb and trunk postures are also seen as a component of other movement disorders.

As the effects of the disease are usually bilateral, most authors on the subject favor a treatment strategy beginning with dominant VL thalamotomy. A contralateral thalamotomy is performed 3 months later if contralateral or axial symptoms persist (55, 78, 156, 178, 211). Late recurrence of symptoms may warrant repeat thalamotomy, with close physiological monitoring and incremental lesion-making techniques. The need to destroy additional targets within the thalamus (pulvinotomy), or deep cerebellar nuclei (dentatotomy), is controversial.

Cooper (57) reported the largest series (226 cases) undergoing thalamotomy for dystonia. Most patients required multiple bilateral operations. The mean follow-up was 7.9 yr. Of the entire group, 24.5% were markedly improved, and 45.2% were moderately improved, for a 69.7% overall success rate. Twelve percent were worse at the end of the follow-up period, while 18.3% were unchanged. The best results were obtained in the classic hereditary DMD group, with 85% either markedly or moderately improved. In the sporadic, non-Jewish group, 56% of patients were improved.

In 1975, Fraioli and Guidetti (78) reported marked or moderate improvement in all 16 patients subjected to dentatotomy for dystonic syndromes other than classic hereditary DMD. Their two patients with classic DMD were unchanged postoperatively. Siegfried (176–178) also had unfavorable results with dentatotomy in classic DMD. Zervas, who reviewed the use of dentatotomy with skepticism for CP, performed the operation on four patients with DMD who had undergone thalamotomy previously and were still symptomatic. Two of the three patients available for long-term follow-up obtained significant lasting benefit from dentatotomy.

These figures should be interpreted in the context of the natural history of the hereditary generalized dystonias, in which a significant proportion of those affected deteriorate to a state of total disability over time. As in other progressive diseases (parkinsonism, for example), patients who sustain modest improvement or even no change on long-term follow-up have, to some degree, beaten the odds with respect to the natural history of their disorder.

Spasmodic Torticollis

Spasmodic torticollis, as an isolated movement disorder unassociated with progressive dystonia, has been one of the more controversial indications for stereotactic surgery. Some experienced stereotacticians feel that thalamotomy does not work in torticollis and instead recommend peripheral denervation procedures. In contrast, others report good results after unilateral thalamotomy. The thalamus ipsilateral to the hypertrophied sternocleidomastoid muscle is lesioned (that is, the thalamus contralateral to the direction the face turns in the horizontal component of the torticollis).

Hassler recommends the thalamic fasciculus (H1 of Forel) as the target for turning movements and medial basal portion of ventrooralis internus (VOi) for tilting movements. Additional vestibulothalamic connections in VIm are lesioned only in resistant cases as "motor neglect" of the contralateral extremities, seen in 16.1% of patients in his series, is a potential complication. Hassler and Dieckmann (88) reported good or excellent relief in 66.7% of 92 patients followed from 1 to 14 yr. Twenty-three percent had fair results, and 10.3% were unchanged. None were made worse. In 24% of these patients, peripheral denervation of a persistently hypertrophied sternocleidomastoid muscle was necessary before a satisfactory result was obtained.

von Essen et al. reported 75% or greater improvement in 11 of 17 patients (64.7%) operated by unilateral thalamotomy (202). The torticollis was cured in four patients. Maximal improvement was sometimes delayed for 3 months to 3 yr with the horizontal component responding best. One patient suffered transient hemiparesis and aphasia.

Bilateral, multitarget stereotactic operations have been advocated by some for this condition. Andrew et al. lesioned as many as nine targets in a single patient with torticollis (5). Five of his six cases included bilateral VIm thalamotomy. All patients experienced early improvement, which was long lasting in 50%. Cooper (57) cautiously recommended staged bilateral VL and CM thalamotomies for torticollis, reporting a 70% long-term success rate. Dysarthria occured in 20% of his patients and was severe and permanent in 5%.

Pain

The sensation of acute pain as a warning or result of tissue injury has adaptive value in an organism's struggle to survive. In humans, chronic pain of known etiology rarely, if ever, has such adaptive value. When overlaid with the affective component of suffering, chronic pain becomes a disabling disease severely compromising the patient's lifestyle. A variety of stereotactic operations has been employed, with varying success, for this problem. A brief enumeration of current indications for stereotactic surgery for relief of chronic pain follows (80, 187, 190).

Paramount in obtaining the expected result from surgery is correct diagnosis, especially with respect to the category of pain from which the patient suffers. Somatic or nociceptive pain can often be alleviated by interruption of the classic neospinothalamic pathways at any level of the neuraxis. The operation must produce analgesia in the painful zone to be effective. Dysesthetic, deafferentation, or central pain can result from injury to the nervous system at any level. A loss of sensation is often found in the spontaneously painful zone (anesthesia dolorosa). Examples include the pain of zoster ophthalmicus, anesthesia dolorosa after surgery for trigeminal neuralgia, and the pain sometimes seen after brainstem or thalamic stroke, spinal cord injury, or limb amputation. Special categories of pain include the failed-back syndrome and the pain of multiple bone metastases in hormonally sensitive adenocarcinomas.

Destructive Operations
Thalamus

For both somatic and dysesthetic pain syndromes, targets have been lesioned in the conducting, nonspecific, and limbic thalamic nuclei. Good results were achieved in 46 to 82% of over 800 patients in pooled series reviewed by Tasker (190). The variable success rate correlated with target selection. The most common thalamic target in this review (696 patients) was the intralaminar nuclear complex. Although one series reported 70% good results, others were less encouraging (46–66% success). Richardson (159), encouraged by the earlier favorable reports of Leksell and Myerson, explored the centromedian (CM), parafascicularis (PF), and medial pulvinar (110) nuclei with stimulating electrodes before inflicting lesions for pain relief. His findings were similar to Tasker's, in that no reliable responses were found at conventional stimulus intensities. Lesions reportedly produced relief of chronic pain in the contralateral hemibody without loss of epicritic or protopathic sensation. Both Richardson and Tasker found that most patients obtained initial relief, but that pain returned in many.

Lesions in the somatosensory relay nuclei (VPL, VPM) cause an initial polymodal sensory loss over the contralateral hemibody, which shrinks over days to include only the area corresponding to the site within the thalamic homunculus in which the lesion was inflicted. As in other operations interrupting the neospinothalamic tract, the analgesia must cover the painful region completely to be effective. More than 80% of patients obtain relief of somatic pain from a VP lesion. The results of a solitary lesion in this area are superior to a multitarget approach. Others have achieved equivalent results from medial pulvinotomy (110), the physiological basis of which remains unexplained. Unfortunately, the incidence of neurological side effects is relatively high with the VP target. Nearly one-third of patients suffer either a postoperative sensory ataxia or late dysesthetic pain. The incidence of these side effects is lower with lesions in the intralaminar-CM/PF complex (10–20%), but so is the success rate.

The thalamic targets for dysesthetic pain include not only the somatosensory and intralaminar nuclei used in somatic pain, but also a greater proportion of limbic system targets (dorsomedial nucleus, DM). The proportion of multitarget operations performed in this category of afflictions is relatively high.

In 1977, Mundinger and Becker (131, 132), reviewed 64 patients available for follow-up out of a series of 138 patients treated by thalamotomy for a variety of dysesthetic pain syndromes. A multitarget approach was used, including the somatosensory, intralaminar-CM/PF nuclei and pulvinar. In 22 patients with phantom pain or "stump causalgia," all were improved, with 60% pain-free at 4 to 6 yr. In trigeminal neuralgia (anesthesia dolorosa?) and zoster ophthalmicus, 70% of 18 patients were improved, with 50% totally pain-free postoperatively.

At 1 to 2 yr follow-up, 60% remained improved. Similar results were obtained in 17 patients with thalamic syndrome, a pain entity notoriously difficult to treat surgically.

The aforementioned results are among the best reported in any series for treatment of dysesthetic pain. Pooled data reviewed by Tasker (191) showed good results in only 29 to 36% of patients submitted to multitarget surgery for the same group of conditions. The inclusion of the dorsomedial nucleus in multitarget surgery did not appear to increase the chances of successful pain relief. The significantly higher success rates with the various thalamic targets for somatic pain compared with dysesthetic pain may be in part artifactual. Many of the patients with somatic pain have terminal cancer and, therefore, may not outlive the beneficial effects of thalamotomy.

Midbrain

Wycis and Spiegel (208) performed stereotactic mesencephalotomy for both somatic and dysesthetic pain syndromes beginning in 1947. Their targets were the spinothalamic and quintothalamic tracts in the midbrain tegmentum, 1 to 5 mm below the posterior commissure and 7.5 mm lateral to the midline. They took into account the spinoreticular connections at this level medially, and tailored the lesions to include these fibers. In 1962, they reported the long-term results of mesencephalotomy in 54 patients. A number also underwent dorsomedial thalamotomy for "emotional overlay," and a few had undergone prefrontal lobotomy before referral.

The majority of patients suffered from dysesthetic pain of various etiologies: facial anesthesia dolorosa after unsuccessful denervation for atypical facial pain, zoster ophthalmicus, tabetic crisis, spinal cord injury, stump or phantom pain, and post-stroke thalamic pain. Three-fourths of these patients obtained significant early pain relief from surgery, but lasting relief was seen in only one-third of patients. This figure is remarkably similar to those in the multitarget thalamotomy series reviewed above (191) and to Tasker's mesencephalotomy (± intralaminar thalamotomy) patients with dysesthetic pain.

Nashold (139, 141, 142) reported the physiological findings and clinical results of stimulation and lesioning of the medial (quintothalamic tract and periaqueductal gray), or lateral (spinothalamic tract) midbrain tegmentum. They were able to achieve long-term relief of dysesthetic pain in 50% of their patients. Stimulation at the medial target (5 mm lateral to the aqueduct), which included the lateral margin of the periaqueductal gray, induced affective and autonomic effects not seen at the lateral target (10 mm lateral to the aqueduct). Lesioning at the medial target relieved suffering as well as pain.

Schvarcz (171) reported stereotactic paraqueductal mesencephalotomy in five cases of facial central pain after brainstem stroke, with an 80% favorable postoperative result. He placed the lesion 2 mm lateral to the aqueduct at the midcollicular level. Stimulation at the target site yielded autonomic and emotional responses similar to those reported by Nashold *et al.* (142). The high success rate in this small series is exceptionally good for any destructive operation treating dysesthetic pain.

The early series of Wycis and Spiegel contained 12 patients with cancer and other somatic pain syndromes (208). Postoperatively, 75% obtained early pain relief. Four patients were not helped by surgery. In contrast to the dysesthetic pain group, almost all of the patients with an early good result had some lasting relief until death, from days to years postoperatively. Similar results were seen by Voris and Whisler (203) in a series of 90 chronic pain patients, 32 of whom suffered from malignancies. Of this cancer group, 25 patients underwent mesencephalotomy either unilaterally (21 patients), bilaterally (2 patients), or with cingulotomy (2 patients). Only one patient was not helped by surgery. Twenty-one of the remaining 24 patients had pain relief until death for an 84% success rate. This is on a par with the best results of thalamotomy in the somatic pain category. As in other series, the majority of this group of patients died of malignancy within 1 yr of operation. In the same series, the results of mesencephalotomy in patients without cancer were as disappointing as other series. Only 5 of 13 patients (38%) were relieved of pain for greater than 1 yr, dropping to 3 of 13 patients (23%) pain-free at 3 yr.

The specific complications and side effects of stereotactic mesencephalotomy result from the compact anatomy of the region (52). In Wycis and Spiegel's series (208), mortality was 7.4% (4 of 54 patients). Two deaths resulted from apparent hemorrhage in patients with poorly controlled hypertension. Two other early deaths occurred in cachectic cancer patients. In later series, the mortality rate has been reduced to 5% or less. As the operative mortality rate for open lateral mesencephalic tractotomy was 24%, the stereotactic series represented an improvement.

Contralateral deafness due to interruption of the brachium of the inferior colliculus was seen in 50% of Wycis and Spiegel's (208) earliest operations, with a target at the pineal level. Moving the target to the level of the posterior commissure reduced the incidence of this complication to 16.6%. Extraocular motion disorders occured in nearly all patients after mesencephalic tractotomy. The most common permanent deficit was loss of upgaze, which was not bothersome in the majority of cases. Transient diplopia, as well as a temporary complete Parinaud's syndrome, also occurred. Permanent symptomatic diplopia was much less common (on the order of 5% of cases).

Hemiparesis, resulting either from injury to pyramidal fibers within the cerebral peduncle ventral to the target or from damage by the probe at a more proximal point along its trajectory, occurred in 9% of Wycis and Spiegel's patients, (208) but was permanent in only 4%. Selection of an entry point away from the motor cortex reduced the incidence of postoperative paralysis. Postoperative dysesthesiae appeared in 15% of patients, but were bothersome in only 3.7%. The fear of causing a late postoperative dysesthetic pain syndrome should, therefore, not dissuade the surgeon from offering mesencephalotomy to a patient with intractable head and neck pain due to an ultimately fatal malignancy.

Recently, Amano *et al.* (4) reported the long-term results of rostral mesencephalic reticulotomy (RMR) in 34 patients operated on since 1973. The target was 5 mm lateral to the aqueduct and 5 mm below the posterior commissure, placing it at the border of the periaqueductal gray and medial reticular formation. A lesion was inflicted on the side contralateral to the patient's worst pain. Of 28 patients who suffered from "denervation pain," 64% obtained good relief. This figure is nearly as good as the outstanding results in Mundinger's thalamotomy (131, 132) series. Pain relief occurred in 83% of patients (5 of 6) with somatic pain. The operative mortality was zero. Parinaud's sign appeared in 26% of patients postoperatively and was the only morbidity reported in the series.

Pons, Medulla, and High Cervical Cord

Destructive stereotactic operations at brainstem levels below the mesencephalon have been reported infrequently. The older atlases did not include useful coordinates for nuclei and tracts at the pontine or medullary levels. The situation has improved recently, but early workers employing cerebellar targets for movement disorders or lower brainstem targets for pain had to chart their own courses.

A theoretical advantage of pontine tractotomy over high cervical cordotomy is the spatial separation of sensory and autonomic (respiratory, micturition, etc.) fibers in the brainstem. An advantage over the more established mesencephalic tractotomy is that many of the paleospinothalamic fibers mediating slow pain linked to suffering have not yet separated from the neospinothalamic tract at the pontine level. Both systems are accessible to stimulation and lesioning at approximately the same target. This anatomical feature was also felt to reduce the potential for postoperative dysesthesiae.

In 1973, Hitchcock (97) reported the first cases of stereotactic pontine spinothalamic tractotomy for the treatment of pain. He began by establishing coordinates for the spinothalamic tract relative to the floor of the fourth ventricle and the perpendicular line dropped from the fastigium of the fourth ventricle. Using his own frame, Hitchcock's preferred trajectory was trans-cerebellar, via a suboccipital burr hole. An additional frontal burr hole was required for positive-contrast ventriculography in order to establish frame alignment and to calculate target coordinates. One patient who could not flex his neck for the suboccipital approach because of a tracheostomy was operated via a parietal burr hole and transtentorial approach. Intraoperative stimulation was always carried out, with sensory phenomena in the painful zone as the physiological parameter for confirming correct probe position.

Of the six patients with malignancy, the site of pain was the thorax and/or upper extremity in four patients, and the hip or sacrum in two patients. The pattern of postoperative sensory loss varied from a contralateral upper extremity monoanalgesia to complete hemibody analgesia. All patients had good early pain relief, lasting until death in four patients (9 days to 8 months postoperatively). Two patients developed recurrent pain accompanying shrinkage of the region of sensory loss over weeks to months after surgery. A single patient, with lower extremity dysesthetic pain after a lumbar wound infection, arachnoiditis, and unsuccessful rhizotomies and cordotomy, had a good therapeutic result from surgery. She was the only long-term survivor in the series.

Neurological complications included motor deficits in three patients (50%), consisting of hemiparesis, ataxia, hypotonia, or tremor. Cranial nerve deficits appeared in four patients (66%), including dysphagia, V, VI, or VII nerve palsies, and ptosis. Hitchcock (97) cautiously recommended the procedure for selected patients in whom cordotomy or other more conventional operations were contraindicated.

Barbera *et al.* (23) reported their results in five further cases performed according to Hitchcock's method. Their target was 6 mm ventral to the fourth ventricular floor and 7.5 mm lateral to the midline on a plane where the fastigial line intersects the fourth ventricular floor at right angles. All five patients suffered from somatic pain associated with metastatic malignancy involving the upper body. One patient with bilateral upper and lower extremity pain underwent bilateral operation at a single stage. All patients experienced good pain relief in the upper body for the duration of their survival. The single patient with total body pain experienced an early recurrence of severe lower back and hip pain that was not helped by any subsequent procedures. A late postoperative dysesthetic pain syndrome, much less distressing than the patient's original pain, occurred in the single long-term survivor. This was the only morbidity reported in the series. Barbera et al. (23) were able to accomplish Hitchcock's earlier prediction (97) that further experience and smaller electrodes would improve the results and lower the complication rate.

Stereotactic explorations and ablations at the spinomedullary junction have been reported by only a few individuals (81), and relate to two specific operations: trigeminal tractotomy and extralemniscal myelotomy. Schvarcz (172), building on earlier work by Hitchcock (97a), performed stereotactic trigeminal tractotomy via posterior puncture at the occipitoatlantal junction. He recorded, stimulated, and coagulated through the same electrode wire in order to minimize technical and neurological complications. The initial series contained eight patients suffering from intractable somatic pain in cranial nerve sensory territories as a consequence of skull base or orofacial neoplasms. The results were excellent, with all patients relieved of pain until death or long-term follow-up at 12 to 16 months.

In another 17 patients with a variety of dysesthetic facial pain syndromes, largely following prior denervation operations, results were remarkably good. All but one patient with longstanding trigeminal anesthesia dolorosa obtained excellent pain relief. Side effects were few and transient, including ipsilateral ataxia in two patients and contralateral hypalgesia in an unspecified number. The analgesia was selective in all cases, leaving touch and corneal reflexes intact. The somesthetic afferents of the vagus and glossopharyngeal nerves enter the subnucleus caudalis of Cranial Nerve V at the level of surgery and were thus accessible to lesioning in cases of oropharyngeal cancer pain without risk of causing swallowing or phonation problems.

Extralemniscal myelotomy, reported separately by Hitchcock (97b), Schvarcz (170a) and Eiras et al. (72a), involves the placement of a small lesion in the high cervical spinal cord just ventral to the dorsal columns. The target is usually 5 mm deep to the dorsal surface of the cord as defined by pantopaque cisternography. The Riechert-Mundinger and Hitchcock frames or the Rosomoff cordotomy guide have all been used with x-ray or fluoroscopic guidance. The unique feature of a small lesion in this region is the production of deep bilateral analgesia without an accompanying cutaneous sensory loss in most cases.

Eiras et al. (72a) reported a series of 12 patients with advanced cancer suffering from bilateral or midline pain. Good initial relief was obtained in all patients, and was complete in seven patients. Narcotics were required by three patients for pain control 6 to 12 months postoperatively. Transient ataxia and dysmetria, lasting as long as 2 weeks, occurred in all patients after surgery. Nondermatomal sensory loss or paresthesiae were seen in seven patients. No other morbidity or operative mortality was reported.

Trigeminal tractotomy and extralemniscal myelotomy are operations with a growing body of physiological and empirical evidence supporting their efficacy. These procedures have, however, been performed almost exclusively by a few surgeons with considerable experience in stereotactic interventions at the spinomedullary junction.

The introduction of implantable neurostimulation and drug delivery systems has reduced the number of destructive stereotactic operations done for the relief of chronic pain. A number of the operations at the brainstem level still offer patients suffering from ultimately lethal malignancies of the head, neck, upper extremities, and torso an excellent chance of relief with an acceptably low complication rate. Lesion-making operations have the additional benefit of not requiring a patient with a short life expectancy to purchase expensive implantable devices for use over a relatively brief period of time.

Deep Brain Stimulation

Acute and chronic focal stimulation at various limbic system and basal ganglia sites had been known to relieve pain for periods outlasting the actual stimulation (65, 66). Reynold's report, in 1969, of analgesia produced by stimulation in the rat periaqueductal gray (PAG), was the first to demonstrate selective pain inhibition without emotional side effects (158). Subsequent studies determined that the caudal perithird ventricular gray (PVG) was also an effective area for stimulation-produced analgesia.

The anatomical substrate of this effect appears to be pathways connecting the PAG to the nucleus raphe magnus in the medulla. The raphe is the origin of a descending serotonergic inhibitory pathway that modulates pain transmission at the level of the spinal cord dorsal horn. The role of endorphins in stimulation-produced analgesia is not as clear as was once believed. CSF levels of β-endorphins have not correlated with the onset of stimulation or its effectiveness in recent studies.

Most recent patients have been implanted with multicontact electrodes and the leads externalized for a period of trial stimulation lasting days to weeks. Different stimulus parameters can be tried in the ambulatory patient to optimize relief before final internalization of the implantable receiver unit. A number of targets for deep brain stimulation (DBS) have been employed since the early 1960s. Selection of the implantation site has been based on pain category, pharmacological testing, or personal experience. Although opinions are far from unanimous, it has been the experience of many that stimulation of PAG-PVG targets relieves somatic pain, while stimulation of the somatosensory system within the thalamus or posterior limb of the internal capsule (IC) favorably affects dysesthetic or deafferentation pain. The rationale is that PAG-PVG stimulation requires intact neural pathways down to the level of the dorsal horn. Somatosensory stimulation sufficient to produce paresthesias may relieve pain by some not yet understood modulation of sensory transmission analogous to the gate theory. One must be cautious in presenting any apparently cohesive scheme for pain patient selection and evaluation, as other algorithms have not proven to have a sound scientific basis.

Thalamic Targets

Since the early 1960s, Mazars has accumulated a large series of patients treated with temporary (until 1972) and permanent implantation of thalamic electrodes in the VPL/VPM nuclei (189). He soon found that patients with somatic pain associated with malignancy did not benefit from stimulation at those targets. In a series of 101 patients with various forms of dysesthetic-deafferentation pain, reported in 1976, he achieved an overall long-term success rate of 84%. Six patients with thalamic syndrome were not helped by thalamic DBS. Mazars' success rate for facial anesthesia dolorosa treated by VPM stimulation was only 45%.

The results of Roldan et al. (165) and Plotkin (152) were similar to Mazars'. Most forms of deafferentation pain were relieved, with the exception of thalamic syndrome, which was never helped. Dieckmann et al. (68) and Mundinger and Neumuller (136), in separate series, shared Mazars' lack of success with post-herpes zoster ophthalmicus (HZO) neuralgia. Others have had remarkably better results from VPM stimulation in this entity. Rodman and Siegfried, reviewed by Dieckmann (68), reported 100% and 80% success respectively. Within a larger recent series, including a number of other target sites, Young et al. implanted thalamic electrodes alone in six patients selected on the basis of a negative response to opiate infusion tests (210). Only two of these patients experienced relief.

Dieckmann (68), in reviewing his own experience, expressed skepticism regarding the utility of thalamic stimulation for deafferentation pain. In his 29 patients, 16 (55%) were helped by surgery. Like Mundinger, he had poor results in facial anesthesia dolorosa and thalamic syndrome. His success rate, exclusive of those conditions, was 75%, more on a par with other workers in the field.

In summary, thalamic DBS of VPL/VPM is effective in a variety of dysesthetic pain syndromes (in 75 to 100% of selected patients). Although thalamic stimulation does not appear to be effective in pain of thalamic syndrome, Hosobuchi (100) reported that 8 of 10 patients responded well to IC stimulation in that disorder. Results vary widely in facial anesthesia dolorosa, with investigators reporting from 0 to 100% success.

PAG/PVG and Combined PAG/PVG-Thalamic/IC Targets

The PAG/PVG has been used alone and in combination with the thalamus or IC as a target for DBS in patients with chronic pain. Richardson and Akil (160, 161) reported a 75% excellent or good long-term response to chronic PAG/PVG stimulation in an early series of eight patients. At that time, an additional 15 patients with short follow-up had experienced similar results.

More recently, other investigators have reported the results of single- or dual-target electrode implantations in larger numbers of patients. Hosobuchi (101) reported 11 patients with chronic noncancer pain. Nine patients suffered from the failed-back syndrome, and two had dysesthetic-deafferentation pain syndromes. Two electrodes were implanted in each patient: one in the left PAG, and the other in the thalamic sensory nucleus contralateral to the side of the patient's worst pain. All patients had a favorable response to stimulation at 1 to 3 years postoperatively. All took L-tryptophan supplementation.

Young et al. (209, 210) implanted PAG/PVG electrodes in 26 patients, combined PAG/PVG-thalamic electrodes in 14 patients, and PAG/PVG-IC electrodes in two patients. Pharmacological selection criteria were used in lieu of selection on the basis of pain category. On the basis of a major or partial response to opiate infusion, patients were implanted in the PAG/PVG region alone or in combination with another target, respectively. Patients implanted in the thalamus alone were discussed above. As in Hosobuchi's series, a relatively large number of patients suffered from the failed-back syndrome (16). The results of Young et al. (209, 210) were good overall, with 72% of patients experiencing complete or partial relief. Of the 16 patients with dual electrodes, 75% were helped, but only one patient was considered an excellent result. Analysis by etiology revealed an 87.5% favorable response in the failed-back category, with >50% in this group experiencing an excellent result.

The operative mortality and number of patients made worse by DBS operations is zero in most series. Complications requiring reoperation are most often hardware related, including lead breakage, disconnection, or pain at receiver or connector implantation sites. Deep infections requiring removal of the system are infrequent, occurring in one of 48 patients in the series of Young et al. (209, 210).

Reoperations for unwanted neurological side effects are rarely mentioned. The common use of multicontact electrodes allows a limited degree of flexibility in stimulation site selection during the trial period. Some patients initially implanted in the PAG experience troublesome eye movement disturbances or fearful affective reactions at stimulation parameters producing analgesia. Replacement of the lead into a PVG target was helpful in three such cases reported by Young et al. (209, 210).

Hypophysectomy

In 1953, Luft and Olivecrona (116a) established hypophysectomy as a palliative treatment for painful bone metastases in advanced prostatic carcinoma. Experience proved hypophysectomy to be beneficial in advanced breast carcinoma as well. Talairach (189a) soon thereafter introduced the stereotactic transsphenoidal method of pituitary ablation. Since then, both transfrontal and transsphenoidal stereotactic approaches to the pituitary have been used. Conventional radiography or fluoroscopy without pneumography or angiography have been sufficient, as the sella turcica belongs to the category of "visible targets" by plain x-rays (73). Gland destruction has been accomplished by radioactive isotope implantation, radiofrequency (RF) thermal coagulation, alcohol injection, or cryosurgery.

As experience with the various techniques grew, complications became less frequent and results improved. The extent of destruction necessary to achieve a beneficial result has not been determined. Early open operative series (transcranial or transsphenoidal) accomplished total hypophysectomy with stalk section, resulting in panhypopituitarism, including diabetes insipidus (DI). However, later stereotactic series, with documented preservation of some anterior and/or posterior gland function, achieved good results as well.

The mechanism of pain relief is unknown, as is the mechanism of regression of metastases. The patients who responded best were those who had previously responded to hormonal manipulations, such as oophorectomy or orchiectomy, and would have been candidates for adrenalectomy. Stereotactic hypophysectomy could be accomplished under local or brief general anesthesia with relatively little stress upon severely debilitated patients unable to tolerate prolonged anesthesia or major visceral surgery.

Forrest *et al.* (76) used the transspenoidal approach to implant yttrium-90 (^{90}Yt) in the sella, beginning in 1955. They reviewed the long-term results in a series of 387 patients treated between 1958 and 1970. By the authors' technique, 40% of a small number coming to autopsy had some gland detectable. However, only 20% of those studied endocrinologically had detectable anterior gland function. The metastasis remission rate was <40%, lower than that achieved by contemporary series of oophorectomy or open hypophysectomy. The actual percentage of patients experiencing pain relief, although not specified, has always exceeded the remission rate in hypophysectomy series.

Moser *et al.* (127) reported a series of seven patients operated by the transfrontal route under local anesthesia. Fluoroscopic control, impedance monitoring, and stimulation techniques were employed. RF heating was used to destroy the gland. Although 72% of patients obtained excellent to good pain relief, objective remission occurred in only one patient. A stalk section effect with DI was not seen, suggesting that posterior lobe ablation was not necessary for pain relief.

Zervas and Hamlin (212) employed transsphenoidal RF coagulation of the pituitary in a large series of patients for a variety of indications. Within this group, 186 patients suffered from advanced breast cancer, and 18 had prostate cancer. In the breast cancer group, 63 patients obtained an objective remission, with an additional 41 patients obtaining temporary pain relief for periods up to 6 months. Total anterior hypophysectomy was the goal of surgery, accomplished by making 10 to 20 RF coagulations within the anterior sella. Hypopituitarism was demonstrated in over 90% of patients, with permanent DI in very few.

Levin *et al.* (116) also utilized the transsphenoidal route to accomplish total hypophysectomy by injection of absolute alcohol into the gland. His target, the posterior-superior quadrant of the sella, was deliberately selected to ablate the posterior lobe and to obtain a physiological stalk section. In 17 patients with prostate cancer, 94% good results were obtained with pain relief lasting until death. In a second group of 12 patients suffering from pain due to widespread metastases from an assortment of neoplasms, 10 patients obtained long-term relief. Levin felt that the success of the operation depended upon spread of the alcohol lesion into the inferior hypothalamus.

Avellanosa and West (9) reviewed the results of transsphenoidal cryohypophysectomy in 19 cases of metastatic prostate carcinoma. They felt that posterior lobe ablation or stalk section was not necessary. Dynamic laboratory testing showing early postoperative hypopituitarism was predictive of good pain relief and longer survival due to objective remission of metastases.

The specific complications of stereotactic hypophysectomy include visual or oculomotor deficits, unwanted DI, and CSF leak with meningitis. The incidence of visual deficits due to inadvertant chiasmal damage is lowest in transsphenoidal approaches with anterior-inferior sellar targets not intended to produce stalk section (0.5%). The incidence rises to 10% temporary and 3% permanent deficits in transsphenoidal series with posterior-superior targets. The transfrontal trajectory to the sella in the presence of a prefixed chiasm is also likely to cause visual complications. The occurrence of oculomotor palsies varies from 0 to 10%. The incidence rises with the use of chemical or radiation agents that are not precisely controllable with respect to site and duration of action. Unwanted DI requiring long-term Pitressin administration was seen in <5% of Zervas' series (212) of 400 patients.

CSF leakage occurred in all transsphenoidal series, in 3 to 5% of cases. A number of methods to prevent this complication have been developed. The injection of acrylic cement or the insertion of a small silicone plug into the sellar opening have been successful in preventing or eliminating postoperative rhinorrhea. Meningitis complicating CSF leakage was seen in a relatively high proportion (4.9%) of patients in Forrest's ^{90}Yt implantation series (76). The authors felt that radionecrosis of the sellar floor was responsible. The high incidence of all complications in the ^{90}Yt implant series mitigates against the use of this technique for destruction of nonadenomatous glands.

A number of factors, including improvements in medical oncological treatment and alternative neurosurgical operations to alleviate pain, have greatly reduced the number of hypophysectomies done for the relief of metastatic cancer pain. The operation may still be of benefit in selected cases of hormonally responsive breast or prostatic carcinoma with generalized pain from osseous metastases.

Epilepsy

Stereotactic depth electrode placement has been utilized to determine whether a particular patient is a candidate for seizure surgery and, if so, to outline which areas of the brain should be resected. Depth EEG recordings were applied to the study of epilepsy in the late 1940s. It was not until a decade later, however, that the systematic stereotactic implantation of depth EEG electrodes, with physiological and anatomical correlations, was integrated into comprehensive epilepsy surgery programs (205, 206). The technique is generally used after analysis of scalp EEG recordings suggests that further investigation is likely to make the patient a candidate for surgery. Depth recordings can fill in details poorly seen in scalp recordings, such as mesial hemispheric foci. As a preoperative study, depth EEG can most accurately determine whether a spike focus originates on one or both sides of the brain, thus facilitating rational surgical decision making.

The stereotactic implantation of electrodes is guided by either angiographical, ventriculographical, or CT imaging studies (117). Most stereotactic instruments are suitable for this application. The anatomical position of the electrode wire can be verified by comparison of postoperative stereotactic x-rays with atlas figures. The physiological or electrical responses to stimulation through the electrode provides functional localization.

Most early workers fabricated their own multistrand electrode tresses or multicontact probes. Commercially manufactured multicontact flexible wires are now available. The number of electrode pairs that can be simultaneously monitored is limited only by the number of channels available on the recording equipment. A state-of-the-art monitoring facility should include 24-hr video monitoring of the patient, with continuous EEG readings stored on magnetic tape for later split-screen display. Telemetered EEG can free the patient from the "leash" effect of recording wires.

Numerous deep structures have been the targets of stereotactic ablations in the hope of favorably affecting intractable seizure disorders of various types. The rationale of surgery is to either destroy the epileptogenic focus (83, 103), interrupt the preferential pathways of discharge, or generally reduce cortical irritability. Surgical therapy is currently underutilized in the treatment of medically resistant epilepsy cases.

Psychomotor epilepsy has been the category most successfully treated by conventional or stereotactic surgery. Depth EEG studies in animals and humans have shown that, in many cases, the epileptogenic zone includes the mesial temporal structures: amygdala and hippocampus. In addition, epileptic discharges originating anywhere in the temporal lobe cortex preferentially conduct through the mesial structures. These phenomena explain the generally favorable results of temporal lobectomy in ameliorating intractable psychomotor epilepsy.

A number of surgeons have performed stereotactic amygdalotomy in patients with psychomotor seizures, behavioral disturbance, and mental retardation. In the series reported by Ramamurthi and Kalyarnaraman (155) and Balasubramaniam and Kanaka (18, 19), seizures were reduced or eliminated in 60 to 80% of patients. Good results were obtained after unilateral amygdalotomy if a lateralized discharge was found. A beneficial but incomplete effect from stereotactic amygdalotomy was felt to indicate that an ipsilateral temporal lobectomy might be of further benefit. In contrast to the severe side effects of bilateral temporal lobectomy (recent memory deficit, Kluver-Bucy syndrome) bilateral amygdalotomy usually produces no such sequelae. Reportedly, patients in whom surface and depth EEG readings show bilateral temporal spike foci can be treated surgically with bilateral amygdalotomy. Likewise, a patient who has undergone a temporal lobectomy on one side, then develops recurrent psychomotor seizures due to a focus in the contralateral temporal lobe, can be treated with stereotactic amygdalotomy. To avoid psychic and amnestic complications, care must be taken to keep the stereotactic lesion well anterior within the amygdala, avoiding the more posterior hippocampal structures.

Children with infantile hemiplegia, behavior disorders, and seizures have been considered candidates for hemispherectomy—a major operation with considerable potential morbidity. Balasubramaniam and Kanaka (18, 19) performed unilateral amygdalotomy on 10 such patients, eliminating seizures in three patients and reducing the seizure frequency in five patients. Behavior improved in all 10 patients. They advocated stereotactic amygdalotomy in such patients, reserving hemispherectomy for failures of this operation.

Another operation for the relief of psychomotor seizures was stereotactic fornicotomy, introduced by Hassler and Reichert in 1957 (155) as reviewed by Ramamurthi and Kalyanaraman. This procedure sectioned the fornix at the level of the anterior commissure, interrupting the outflow of epileptic discharges from the hippocampus. The operation was successful in >60% of patients in several European series.

Stereotactic surgery for seizure disorders not originating in the temporal lobes has met with less success. In certain focal seizures with secondary generalization, the preferential pattern of epileptic discharge is felt to be from motor cortex to putamen. From there, discharges travel via the globus pallidus and pallidothalamic connections to the VA and VL nuclei. Lesions at various sites along this putative pathway, including the putamen, globus pallidus, ansa lenticularis, or VA/VL thalamic nuclei, yielded inconsistent results, which were usually poor in the long term. Even in cases with an early postoperative decline in seizure frequency (before recruitment of alternate pathways) the scalp EEG readings remained markedly abnormal. Intralaminar and centromedian thalamotomy, designed to interrupt the nonspecific thalamocortical activating system, has been employed in small numbers of patients with equivocal results. In summary, none of the thalamic operations has acheived the same degree of practical and theoretical acceptance as amygdalotomy or fornicotomy.

One additional operation, capsulotomy, has been performed in selected cases of intractable focal motor seizures or epilepsia partialis continua. Paresis of the involved extremity is a necessary consequence of the capsular lesion, but this may be less disabling to the patient than constant convulsive movements.

The complications of stereotactic epilepsy surgery have been few. Transient Kluver-Bucy-like side effects occurred in less than 1% of patients in a large bilateral amygdalotomy series. Ten percent of patients experienced loss of libido. Thorough preoperative radiological investigation should reduce the possibility of treating seizures in the presence of an undiagnosed neoplasm. Stereotactic biopsy at the lesioning site can be performed if a tumor is suspected on the preoperative imaging studies.

Psychosurgery

Since the early work of Spiegel and Wycis, stereotactic techniques have figured prominently in the development of psychosurgical operations (200). The initial aim of stereoencephalotomy was to perform operations as effective as the then-current prefrontal lobotomy, topectomy, or leukotomy procedures, without the undersirable neuropsychological side effects (181, 182). The introduction of psychoactive drugs led to a drastic reduction in the demand for psychosurgery. In fact, the safety, efficacy, and ethical basis of psychosurgery were investigated by a national commission in the 1970s. The commission's findings, released in 1977, affirmed the benefits and safety of some psychosurgical procedures.

The stereotactic psychosurgical operation most widely accepted in this country is anterior cingulotomy. Stereotactic subcaudate tractotomy has also been widely used in Great Britain. Stereotactic operations to alter the behavior of institutionalized violent persons, although unpopular in this country, have been performed in the United States and elsewhere. The inclusion of dorsomedial thalamotomy (Spiegel's and Wycis' favored psychosurgical target) in thalamotomy operations on certain pain patients has already been discussed. Amygdalotomy for psychomotor seizures and aggressive behavior has also been discussed in the prior section (199).

Introduced as an open operation by Ward in 1948 (207a), bilateral anterior cingulotomy was soon performed stereotactically. The operation has proved useful in cases of severe anxiety and obsessive-compulsive neuroses. Chronic intractable pain with psychic suffering and drug addiction has also been successfully treated by cingulotomy. Ballantine et al. (20-22) reported the results in a continuing series of patients in whom bilateral anterior cingulotomy was performed for either psychiatric illness or pain. The target coordinates and operative technique have evolved over the decades. Through burr holes placed 1.3 cm off the midline and 9 cm behind the nasion, dual-purpose ventricular needle-electrodes were introduced. First, the frontal horns were filled with 5 ml of air. Then RF lesions were made within the cingulum, 3 to 4 cm posterior to the tips of the frontal horns within 5 mm of the midline. The earlier target of Foltz and White (75) had been more anterior (2.5 cm from the tips of the frontal horns) and lateral (1 cm off the midline). As of 1977, Ballantine's series numbered 345 operations performed on 238 patients. A significant number of repeat operations were done. Psychiatric illness, including mood disorder, obsessive-compulsive neurosis, severe anxiety, or life-threatening anorexia nervosa, was present in 204 patients. The remaining 34 patients suffered from chronic intractable pain. The results in 149 psychiatric patients followed long term were analyzed statistically. In summary, 75% of those patients experienced significant overall improvement. There was no surgical mortality; however, seven patients committed suicide during the follow-up period. Three patients developed seizures postoperatively.

Foltz and White (75) introduced pneumographically guided "cingulumotomy" (as they called the operation) for the treatment of chronic pain. In five patients with purely psychogenic pain and in six patients with pain due to invasive cancer, the operative result was good or excellent in nine patients and fair in two patients. In a group of five patients with pain precipitated by emotional factors, including causalgia, dysesthetic pain, and angina, the operation yielded excellent or good results in three patients (60%). One of those patients required reoperation. Two patients with painful paraplegia had fair-to-poor results. None of the 14 patients taking narcotics preoperatively required narcotic analgesics postoperatively.

Brown (46) lesioned the cingulum as one of multiple limbic system targets in a series of 43 patients with intractable pain and drug addiction. In contrast to other workers, Brown used general anesthesia in his patients. Cingulotomy was performed in all patients. Nine patients underwent amygdalotomy, and two underwent additional lesioning of the substantia innominata (subcaudate tractotomy). Thirty-nine patients (90.5%) were improved or "well" at follow up, 1 to 20 yr postoperatively. Four patients (9.5%) received minimal benefit from surgery. There was no operative mortality, and no patients were made worse by surgery.

Cingulotomy appears to have a beneficial effect in a large proportion of carefully selected psychiatric patients suffering from mood disorders or severe anxiety. The operation also blunts the anxiety and suffering associated with chronic pain. Despite the large numbers of patients benefitted by cingulotomy, the mechanism by which the operation works remains unknown. The benefits of including additional limbic system targets in the operation are, so far, unproven.

Based on the production of rage reactions in experimental animals by posterior hypothalamic stimulation, Sano et al. (167) introduced hypothalamotomy for the treatment of violent, aggressive behavior. In humans, he identified the so-called "ergotropic triangle," located 1 to 5 mm lateral to the third ventricle and bounded by the midpoint of the intercommissural line, the rostral end of the aqueduct, and the anterior border of the mammillary bodies. Stimulation within this zone produced desynchrony of the EEG reading, as well as a variety of sympathetic effects. In a series of 51 patients followed for more than 2 yr, the operation had a "marked calming effect" in 95%. Of the patients with seizure disorders, 41% had fewer seizures postoperatively. There were two early reoperations for failed procedures, and a single postoperative death.

Subsequently, Black et al. (31), Dieckmann and Hassler (67, 69), and Schvarcz (173) reported series of stereotactic hypothalamotomies performed upon imprisoned or institutionalized persons with a history of violence, hyperactivity, and, often, sexual criminality. According to the surgeons' criteria, satisfactory or good results were obtained in approximately 80% of these cases. This often meant that the heavy tranquilizer doses necessary to keep the patients under control could be either reduced or eliminated. The complications reported after hypothalamotomy have included transient central fever, incontinence, tachycardia, hypopituitarism, and stupor. One postoperative death due to aspiration pneumonia was reported by Sano et al. (167). Despite the apparent effectiveness of hypothalamotomy (sometimes combined with amygdalotomy) as a method to control behavior in institutionalized patients, moral objections to the operation have been raised.

ANATOMIC STEREOTACTIC SURGERY

Vascular Applications

Stereotactic angiography renders aneurysms and vascular malformations accessible to conventional stereotactic surgery. The target coordinates of an aneurysm neck or sac, or a feeding vessel to an arteriovenous malformation (AVM), can be readily determined on anteroposterior (AP) and lateral angiograms with the patient in a stereotactic frame. Reference to a stereotactic atlas is useful in selecting a trajectory if the target is in or near a sensitive region of the brain.

In cases of aneurysmal subarachnoid hemorrhage, an ideal treatment would permanently prevent rebleeding without aggravating or precipitating vasospasm (157). Even current microsurgical techniques sometimes fall short of this ideal. Alksne et al. (1) developed stereotactic instrumentation to introduce iron powder under magnetic control into aneurysm sacs in order to induce thrombosis. His first trials were in an animal model. In the early operations on patients, a magnetic probe was stereotactically positioned at the aneurysm fundus, while the iron powder was injected into the cervical carotid artery. Initial results were poor. Later modifications of the technique were much more successful. A more powerful magnet was employed, having a hollow core through which a needle was passed, permitting the direct injection of the thrombogenic ferrous mixture into the aneurysm sac. Additionally, acrylic cement was added to the iron powder to hasten thrombosis (3). This permitted removal of the magnetic probe after 1 hr. Previously the probe had to remain in place for 4 to 5 days. Intraoperative serial stereotactic angiography was employed to guide the puncture and, subsequently, to monitor the filling of the sac with the iron-acrylic mixture.

In 1977, Smith and Alksne reported good results in five "inaccessible" aneurysms (2, 179). In 1980, they reported further experience in a consecutive series of 22 anterior communicating artery aneurysms (2). In 16 patients, the approach was transfrontal. In six patients, a sublabial transsphenoidal trajectory was used. In the latter approach, the instrumentation remained extradural with the exception of the needle used to puncture the aneurysm. The results in this series were remarkably good. There was no operative mortality and no rebleeding during follow-up of 0.5 to 4.5 yr. In 17 aneurysms, the sac and neck were totally occluded. Sixteen patients returned to their former occupations. Complications were largely technical, with one failure to obliterate a previously unsuccessful clipped aneurysm and four failures to obliterate the aneurysm neck totally. One CSF leak occurred in a transsphenoidally operated case. The tendancy for distal embolization or irreversible parent vessel occlusion by the iron-acrylic mixture, apparent in the early cases, was eliminated in the later series. Although the results compared favorably with those of conventional management, over a decade of work on the part of the authors was required to perfect the instrumentation and technique.

Mullan (128) reported 61 intracranial aneurysms treated by the introduction of lengths of fine gauge wire followed by the application of a weak direct current to promote intraluminal thrombosis. In two of the cases, a stereotactic technique was used to introduce the wire into aneurysms within the cavernous sinus.

Kandel and Peresedov (104, 105) published their technique of stereotactic aneurysm or AVM vessel clipping. They used the Kandel frame, either local or general anesthesia, and serial angiography. The special vascular clips could be adjusted or repositioned until final detachment from the applicator device. As of 1980, 30 clip applications had been performed on 27 patients. The precise pathology involved and the outcomes of the operations were not described in any detail. Occasional deliberate parent vessel sacrifice, and the use of the technique on uncomplicated posterior communicating artery aneurysms, would not be acceptable to most neurosurgeons. Even with its limitations, the Kandel technique could be useful in obliterating feeding arteries to large AVMs supplied by multiple major vessels. Rand (157) has used a bipolar coagulating probe to eliminate feeding vessels in such situations.

Combined open-stereotactic surgery for deeply situated vascular lesions is described in a separate section. The stereotactic radiosurgical treatment of AVMs is discussed in a following section on stereotactic surgery and radiosurgery. Despite the refinements in microsurgical technique for intracranial vascular surgery, stereotactic and combined open-stereotactical operations offer certain advantages in approaching lesions located deep in the brain, or within important functional areas.

Hydrocephalus and Endoscopy

Radiographical visualization of the ventricular system for localization purposes has been an essential part of most stereotactic operations (45). However, the application of stereotactic techniques to intraventricular surgery for the investigation or treatment of hydrocephalus has been infrequently reported.

Iizuka (103a, 103b) developed instrumentation for stereotactically guiding a fiberoptic endoscope into the ventricular system in cases of hydrocephalus. His "stereoencephaloscope" was only 3 mm in diameter, had end- and side-viewing telescopes, and camera attachments. Iizuka felt that the precise guidance and rigid fixation of the stereotactic method minimized the damage done to cerebral tissue by passage or movement of the endoscope. Pneumography was not always used, as the enlarged ventricles of hydrocephalics were easily entered by reference to external landmarks alone. Direct inspection of the ventricular end of malfunctioning shunts in-situ often disclosed glial scarring as a cause of obstruction.

More recently, Apuzzo et al. (7) utilized CT-guided stereotactic endoscopy to visualize and biopsy or aspirate three selected lesions within the third ventricle. Stereotactic endoscopy offers some of the features of open-stereotactic surgery (manipulations under direct vision) while not requiring as extensive an exposure.

Stereotactic treatments of hydrocephalus include third ventriculostomy and interventriculostomy. Since its introduction by Dandy for the treatment of noncommunicating hydrocephalus in 1922, open-third ventriculostomy has been performed by a number of operative approaches with a success rate between 33 and 80%. Percutaneous free-hand third ventriculostomy, guided by ventriculography or endoscopy, has also been reported by several groups (168).

Poblete and Zambolini (153) reported stereotactic third ventriculostomy using the Riechert-Mundinger frame with intraoperative positive-contrast ventriculography. Their target was the floor of the third ventricle, behind the chiasmatic recess, in the midline. A special end-cutting leukotome was employed to create a 2-mm perforation into the subarachnoid space at the target point. The operation was successful in all of the 10 reported patients with an average follow-up of 10 months. Of the four patients with posterior fossa tumors, two patients eventually died. A third patient died of bacterial endocarditis secondary to a ventriculo-atrial shunt infection despite removal of the shunt. Examination of the fistula site at autopsy revealed patency in those cases.

Hoffman et al. (98) reported 22 cases of stereotactic third ventriculostomy. Their target for puncture was located more posteriorly: in the midline just behind the dorsum sellae. A small amount of pantopaque was introduced through a coronal burr hole and manipulated into the third ventricle under fluoroscopic monitoring. A wire leukotome was then used to perforate the ventricular floor. The free egress of pantopaque into the basal cisterns indicated an adequate opening had been made. Ten of the 22 patients had their hydrocephalus controlled by this operation alone. Patients treated primarily by third ventriculostomy had a significantly higher success rate (60%) than those operated after an unsuccessful or complicated shunting procedure (33%). A temporary third nerve paresis was the only neurological morbidity reported. Of four late postoperative deaths, two were due to uncontrolled hydrocephalus despite ventricular shunting.

The authors concluded that the operation was an "effective method of dealing with obstructive hydrocephalus" provided certain selection criteria were used. Patients with prior meningitis, a small third ventricle, obstruction at sites other than the aqueduct or fourth ventricle, and previous shunt operations had a much lower chance of a successful result from surgery.

Interventriculostomy, the insertion of a cannula between the third and fourth ventricles to relieve aqueductal obstruction, has been occasionally performed since Dandy's first report in 1920. Backlund et al. (15) developed a method for reconstruction of the cerebral aqueduct by means of a stereotactically implanted Teflon prosthesis. Positive-contrast ventriculography and simultaneous pneumography with the patient in the sitting position allowed fluoroscopic visualization of both ends of the occluded aqueduct. The results in seven patients followed 1.5 to 6.5 yr postoperatively were reported. Four of the patients required a total of six stereotactic prosthesis revisions after the initial operation. Three patients ultimately had a good result. One patient remained symptomatic despite a patent aqueduct, and three required shunting. There was no operative mortality. One transient Parinaud's syndrome was the only operative morbidity.

The overall long-term success rate of the various intracranial operations designed to bypass obstructive hydrocephalus has been approximately 50%. Failures were often due to technical factors. Additionally, the presence of unsuspected communicating hydrocephalus in some cases may have prevented intracranial diversion from working effectively. Despite the ease of installation and relative efficacy of shunting devices, the demand continues for an operation to relieve hydrocephalus without depending upon extracranial CSF diversion.

Foreign Bodies

A radiopaque foreign body makes an ideal target for traditional stereotactic surgery. Invasive studies such as ventriculography or angiography are not usually necessary. Fluoroscopy or serial x-rays can adequately localize the target and monitor the progress of surgery. Indications for operation include prevention of late infection or migration of the missile. With CT guidance, even radiolucent fragments can be retrieved. Despite the apparent ease of surgery, very few reports of stereotactic foreign body removal have been published. Hitchcock and Cowie (95) and Sugita et al. (186) removed intracranial air gun pellets from children wounded accidentally. Blacklock and Maxwell (32) removed a retained shunt catheter. Grasping forceps and fluoroscopic monitoring were used in most of these cases.

CT-GUIDED STEREOTACTIC APPLICATIONS

Biopsy and Treatment of Mass Lesions

The stereotactic biopsy and treatment of intracranial masses were all accomplished in the pre-CT era. Likewise, stereotactic radiosurgery and interstitial isotope implantation were also carried out before the advent of CT-guided stereotactic neurosurgery. Mundinger and coworkers (129, 133, 134, 135), Sugita et al. (188), Parker et al. (150, 151), Bosch (37), Edner (72), and others, reported series of stereotactic biopsies guided by ventriculography and/or angiography. A diagnosis was achieved in 55 to 90% of the cases. The neurological morbidity was generally low, comparing favorably with open-biopsy approaches to similar lesions. In some centers, the interstitial implantation of radionuclides into tumors was carried out during the same operation as the biopsy (see below). Later, Mundinger et al. (133), Boethius et al. (33), Ostertag et al. (149), Broggi et al. (44), Edner (72), and other workers integrated CT data into traditional stereotactic systems by either mechanical or computer-assisted methods. The results were encouraging, with a diagnostic rate >90% in most series (50, 64).

The introduction of CT-guided frames led to a substantial increase in the numbers of patients undergoing stereotactic biopsy procedures, especially in the United States. Apuzzo and Gabskin (7, 8), Bouvier et al. (38), Bullard et al. (48, 49), Edner (72), Heilbrun et al. (92), Lunsford et al. (117), Mundinger et al. (133), and others (197) have reported series of patients biopsied using current generation CT-guided instruments. The diagnostic rate in these series varied from 91 to 100%. Therapeutic interventions in the form of cyst aspiration or temporary ventricular drainage were performed in up to 25% of patients in some series. In studies where the issue was addressed, the histological diagnosis obtained by biopsy differed from the initial clinical diagnosis up to 50% of the time. Thus, stereotactic biopsy has led to more appropriate therapy based on tissue diagnosis in patients who would otherwise have been treated empirically. In a number of series, further treatment included craniotomy and resection of benign, encapsulated tumors that had been deemed infiltrative and unresectable on the basis of radiographic studies alone. Sugita, in the pre-CT era, and Apuzzo et al., using the BRW device, each reported several such cases in series of biopsies from the third ventricular region.

Pecker et al. (150, 151) reported their experience with conventional stereotactic biopsy of pineal region tumors. Subsequent CT series have included pineal tumors as well. The variety of pathological entities found there, requiring different therapies, demand accurate histological diagnosis. However, opinions differ as to the value of stereotactic biopsy followed by a secondary resection, if appropriate, versus single-stage open biopsy and tumor resection.

Stereotactic aspiration of colloid cysts, guided by ventriculography, was first reported by Bosch et al. in 1978 (36). Four patients were operated without any complications. One patient required shunting despite successful removal of the cyst. Apuzzo et al. (7), Lunsford (117), and Rivas and Lobato (1985) (164) reported CT-guided colloid cyst aspirations using the Leksell or BRW frames. One patient (164) required shunting after an initially unsuccessful cyst aspiration attempt. Stereotactic aspiration was subsequently successful 4 years later. The stereotactic approach eliminates the need for a formal cortical incision, thus reducing the possibility of postoperative seizures. The operation can be repeated in the event of initial failure or late refilling of the cyst, and does not preclude conventional surgery, if required.

Walsh et al. (207) employed a CT-monitored free-hand technique to aspirate brain abscesses in two patients. A small amount of pantopaque was injected as a radiographic marker at the conclusion of the procedure. Subsequent reaspirations of the original or other abscesses were carried out with conventional stereotactic surgery using the pantopaque as a target and reference marker. More recent CT stereotactic series all include diagnostic and therapeutic aspirations of brain abscesses. Material for culture and microscopic examination was readily obtained. The aspiration and irrigation of abscess cavities with antibiotic solutions was an alternative to open surgery for initial therapy or treatment of cases that had not responded to systemic antibiotics. Stereotactically placed external drainage tubes have been left in the cavity by some surgeons, but are not necessary in many cases. Repuncture can be performed if the abscess does not show satisfactory resolution on follow-up scans.

In 1978, Backlund and von Holst (17) introduced a technique and instrument for the stereotactic evacuation of large intracerebral hematomas. The instrument consisted of a 4-mm blunt-tipped cannula with two small openings near the tip. A spiral drill rotated freely within the length of the cannula. At the outer end of the instrument, a suction port was connected to a collection bottle. The device operated on the Archimedes water-screw principle. Either liquid or solid hematoma was carried up the cannula within the spiral drill grooves, and continuously removed by suction. One early operation, reported in detail, was successful. Higgins and Nashold (93, 94) modified Backlund's instrument by adding an irrigation/ventilation port with a distal aperture near the instrument's tip. The modified instrument was less prone to clog with blood and allowed the introduction of contrast material directly into the hematoma cavity. Of their three patients initially operated, one died, and two were placed in nursing homes. A subsequent report by Broseta et al. (44a), employing the Backlund device, had an 81% mortality.

Kandel and Peresedov (106) introduced their own stereotactic hematoma aspirator, having a much narrower, motor-driven inner screw. They inflated a soft silastic balloon catheter within the hematoma cavity at the conclusion of surgery to tamponade the walls and prevent postoperative rebleeding. The apparatus was used in 32 patients, accomplishing total hematoma removal in 28 cases. All patients were either stuporous or comatose preoperatively. The etiology was hypertension in 30 patients, and ruptured aneurysm or AVM each in two patients. Five patients (16%) developed recurrent hematomas requiring reoperation. Three of these, plus four others, eventually died for a mortalitiy rate of 22%. The completeness of initial hematoma removal was assessed in these series by comparison of the volume of blood aspirated to the volume of the clot calculated from the CT scan. Disagreement remains as to whether complete or subtotal removal should be performed.

Matsomoto and Hondo (120) aspirated deep intracerebral hematomas from 51 patients through a silastic shunt catheter. Although called a stereotactic technique by the authors, no guiding frame was used. Punctures were made free-hand, based on measurements taken from CT scans and drawn on the patient's scalp. Once the maximal amount of liquid blood was aspirated, urokinase (6000 IU/5 ml) was instilled. The catheter was left in place, and the procedure repeated at 6- and 12-hr intervals. Disappearance of the hematoma on serial CT scans was the therapeutic endpoint. Although the mortality in this series was equivalent to historical control patients treated by open surgery, the functional recovery of patients was not good. One explanation was that only limited amounts of hematoma could be aspirated initially in the acute cases. This left many patients with a significant intracranial mass until the urokinase dissolved the clot and a second aspiration could be done.

Since Dandy's report of the first successful removal of an intraaxial brainstem hematoma, other surgeons have reported their experiences with these lesions. A variety of open approaches have been utilized, depending on the location of the clot. Stereotactic aspirations of acute or chronic brainstem hematomas have been reported in the CT era. Due to the relatively small size of these lesions and the compact anatomy of the brainstem, the large water-screw hematoma aspirators could not be used. Standard 1.9 to 2.5 mm stereotactic cannulae with syringe suction have been used in the reported cases.

Beatty and Zervas (24) employed transposed CT data and the Todd-Wells frame to aspirate a chronic pontomesencephalic hematoma, through a frontal burr hole, twice in the same patient. Bosch and Beute (35) performed an emergency CT-guided stereotactic aspiration of a pontomedullary hematoma, also via the transfrontal route. They commented that, when time permits, a suboccipital transcerebellar route is the preferred trajectory to the ventral-lateral pons. Coffey and Lunsford (51) reported the aspiration of two chronic brainstem hematomas among a series of brainstem lesions biopsied or treated by CT-guided stereotactic surgery. A standard transfrontal trajectory was employed in the patient with a mesencephalic hematoma. The chronic pontine hematoma was approached via the suboccipital transcerebellar route. The outcome in these few highly selected cases has been good or excellent. No permanent neurological deficits occurred as a result of surgery. Whether stereotactic aspiration can be of benefit to larger numbers of patients harboring brainstem hematomas remains to be determined.

CT-Guided Functional Stereotactic Surgery

Opinions vary widely as to the suitability of CT-guided stereotactic surgery for functional applications. Some surgeons, employing sophisticated CT-guided systems for anatomical stereotactic surgery, still use traditional ventriculographic localization methods in functional cases. Since coordinates of functional targets are often given relative to the intercommissural line, the radiographic method employed must image both commissures adequately. Some surgeons feel that CT does not display the anterior commissure as reliably as ventriculography. Others feel that late generation, high-resolution CT scanners, when used with an appropriate scanning protocol, can reliably display both commissures.

Both Hadley (87a) and Asakura (8a) recently reported comparisons between functional target coordinates determined by ventriculography versus CT guidance using the BRW system. The two methods differed by 1 mm to greater than 1 cm, depending on the case. In contrast, Laitinen et al. (112) compared CT localization, aided by a head holder of his own design, with air ventriculographic localization. In his detailed study, the two methods varied by only 0.6 to 0.7 mm in the x and y coordinates, respectively. This difference is less than the diameter of many stereotactic probes. The device and CT guidance were successfully employed in functional operations on several patients.

Birg et al. (30) have employed direct CT coordinate determination in large numbers of functional cases. Their original method skirted the anterior commissure visualization issue by utilizing the foramen of Monro-posterior commissure line as their stereotactic reference line. This has always been an acceptable practice, as even traditional ventriculography sometimes failed to image the anterior commissure adequately. These authors have subsequently compared coordinate calculations derived from CT images versus ventriculography. The mean deviation was only 0.6 mm—less than the diameter of the probe used to inflict the lesion. Lunsford et al. (117) have used CT-guided stereotactic surgery to implant electrodes (for DBS or depth EEG) or inflict thalamotomy lesions. Multiplanar reformatted images, based on thin-section, contrast-enhanced axial image data, were employed. The intercommisural line was plotted on the midsagittal reformatted image. Either axial or coronal (reformatted) images could be used to determine the width of the third ventricle and its relation to the internal capsule. For thalamotomy, appropriate corrections of standard atlas coordinates could be made. Physiological control, in the form of impedance monitoring and stimulation or recording at the target point, was also used. In cases of PAG/PVG electrode implantation for DBS, the target coordinates relative to the posterior commissure and aqueduct or third ventricle were determined directly from the CT images.

Although the exclusive use of CT for target localization in functional stereotactic surgery is still controversial, the method has yielded good results with a variety of stereotactic systems. It also appears that MRI, now used by Birg et al. (30), will prove to be superior to all prior imaging modalities for functional stereotaxis. MRI allows direct sagittal imaging of the third ventricle and commissures, as well as direct coronal and axial imaging of the thalamus. One must remember that lesion size is often as great as 1 cm, obviating the importance of small (millimeter) variations in accuracy. In addition, recording and/or stimulation are always necessary (even in the era of ventriculography), as individual differences in anatomy are significant. Further experience with both CT and MRI will probably lead to the abandonment of ventriculography by many stereotacticians.

CNS Transplantation

Developmental biologists have long employed CNS transplantation techniques to study amphibians, fish, and birds. For example, transplantation of an eye primordium from a normal to an eyeless axolotl embryo gives rise to a normal eye in which axons grow from the retina to the tectum in a completely normal manner. Likewise, the goldfish optic nerve regenerates well after crush injury, and a number of avian species can be cross-grafted in the fetal stage. Grafting mammalian tissue is much more difficult, requiring highly developed microsurgery and reimplantation techniques. Few successful experiments occurred prior to 1970. Since then, a number of tremendously exciting advances have occurred.

The vast majority of published studies on neural transplants have employed fetal brain tissue as the donor material. Rat and mouse fetal tissue is relatively easy to obtain and is extremely resistant to hypoxia during transplantation. Such grafts tend to be relatively specific in their ability to reinnervate the CNS. Other sources of grafts include peripheral nervous system tissue (such as sympathetic ganglia) and adrenal medullary grafts. In addition, cultured cell lines, specifically neuroblastoma cells, have recently been used as a graft source. Such cell lines can serve as sources for a variety of neurotransmitters, such as acetylcholine and dopamine. In addition, they may be subject to further manipulation via recombinant DNA techniques.

A number of grafted neurons have been shown to function appropriately within the host brain after transplant. Transplantation of vasopressin neurons and gonadotrophin-releasing neurons into endocrinologically deficient rats can restore normal function. Cognitive defects produced after lesions in the hippocampus have been reversed with fetal septal grafts. Perhaps most exciting is the nigrostriatal lesion model in the rat. Dopaminergic neurons in the substantia nigra can be selectively destroyed by injections of the neurotoxin, 6-hydroxydopamine (6-OHDA). Unilateral 6-OHDA lesions of the nigrostriatal pathway produce slow turning in the direction of the lesion. Dopamine levels are often less than 0.5% of the opposite side. Amphetamine administration increases the imbalance, resulting in increasing rotation. Apomorphine, by acting directly on the supersensitive neurons in the denervated region, causes vigorous rotation away from the lesioned side. In 1979, Perlow (151a) reported that fetal substantia nigra transplants significantly reduced such turning behavior. Subsequent studies have confirmed this functional result and have demonstrated anatomical, neurochemical, and electrophysiological function of the grafted tissue. A recent report documents the transplantation of adrenal medullary tissue into the caudate nucleus of two human patients with severe Parkinson's disease (14). A clear functional improvement was not demonstrated.

In the future, some feel that transplantation of appropriate cell lines to the CNS may be one of the most commonly performed neurosurgical procedures. Many diseases in which neural elements are known to be deficient, including Parkinson's disease, Alzheimer's disease, stroke, etc. are theoretically amenable to neural augmentation by stereotactic implantation.

STEREOTACTIC SURGERY, BRACHYTHERAPY, AND RADIOSURGERY

Interstitial and Intracystic Brachytherapy

In conventional external beam radiation therapy (RT) for cerebral tumors, the total radiation dose is limited by the potential for damage to the overlying brain. The daily dose fraction also must be limited, again to avoid radionecrosis of normal brain. In the interval between daily treatments, tumor cells can repair sublethal damage, leading to reduced tumor destruction per dose fraction. Stereotactic brachytherapy, the temporary or permanent implantation of radioisotopes into brain tumors, is one method of overcoming the limitations of conventional teletherapy (29, 39, 61).

The techniques were pioneered in Europe, beginning in the early part of this century. Depending on the nature of the tumor, various isotopes were employed, including: phosphorous-32 (^{32}P), cobalt-60 (^{60}Co), yttrium-90 (^{90}Yt), iodine-125 (^{125}I), tantalum-182 (^{182}Ta), iridium-192 (^{192}Ir), gold-198 (^{198}Au), and radium-226 (^{226}Ra). Currently, for interstitial therapy of solid tumors, most workers implant either ^{125}I or ^{192}Ir sources. These isotopes are available with gamma energies and tissue penetration characteristics that allow selective tumor destruction and are relatively safe for patient care personnel. ^{192}Ir sources have a half-life of 74.2 days, a gamma energy of 300 to 610 keV, and a half-value for tissue penetration of 5 cm. ^{125}I has a half-life of 60.2 days, a gamma energy of 28 to 35 keV, and a 2 cm half-value for tissue penetration. The half-lives of both isotopes are sufficiently long that only a minor degree of decay occurs during the treatment period. The lower energy radiation of ^{125}I makes the protection of visitors and hospital staff less of a problem than with ^{192}Ir. According to the inverse square law, the radiation dose to surrounding tissue diminishes rapidly as distance increases from the implanted source. The actual dose rate delivered to the target tissue depends upon the number and activity of the sources implanted, and on the geometry of the implanted array of radiation sources. Careful, computer-assisted dosimetry planning must be employed to avoid undertreatment of regions within a tumor, or excessive necrosis of surrounding normal brain. Most workers currently use dose rates on the order of 40 to 60 rad/hr (1000 to 1500 rads/day). At these levels, interstitial irradiation can achieve a therapeutic ratio superior to conventional teletherapy. Destruction of recurrent tumor can be accomplished with relative safety, even in cases where the surrounding brain tissue has already received the maximum tolerated dose of external beam RT.

The advantages of brachytherapy can be explained in terms of the "four Rs" of radiobiology: (a) repair of sublethal damage, (b) redistribution within the cell cycle, (c) reoxygenation of hypoxic cells, and (d) repopulation of the tumor mass. A given dose of radiation kills a larger proportion of cells when delivered as a single dose rather than multiple dose fractions. In the interval between dose fractions, many cells damaged, but not killed by radiation, can repair sublethal damage (SLD). Due to the large volume of overlying brain exposed to conventional teletherapy, the dose must be fractionated, often over several weeks. In contrast, brachytherapy provides continuous irradiation of the tumor volume. At currently employed dose rates, tumor cells do not have the opportunity to repair SLD and are killed by further exposure to the radiation source. Normal cells are more efficient at repair of SLD and are affected to a lesser degree. Certain phases of the cell cycle are more sensitive to radiation (G_2, M), while other phases are more resistant (G_1, S). A single radiation dose fraction leaves surviving cells in G_1 and S phases which continue through the cell cycle to ultimately divide and repopulate the tumor mass. The selective killing of G_2 and M cells produces a synchronizing effect such that a second radiation dose, given at a time when the remaining cells have cycled into G_2 and M, effectively kills the survivors. The continuous dose rate attained in brachytherapy also tends to synchronize cells into the more sensitive phases of the cycle, further enhancing tumor cell killing. Oxygen-free radicals, generated by exposure of molecular oxygen to ionizing radiation, are thought to be an intermediary agent actually causing cellular damage. Hypoxic cells, located in the poorly vascularized core of a tumor, are known to be relatively resistant to single doses of conventional radiation. Low dose rate radiation has been shown to be more effective in killing hypoxic cells. This may be partly due to the fact that radiation can cause hypoxic cells to become reoxygenated, and thus more vulnerable. Continued exposure of tumor cells to radiation causes progressive lengthening of the cell cycle (mitotic delay). Although the dose per unit time remains relatively constant, the dose per cell cycle progressively increases. A critical dose per cycle is achieved with brachytherapy such that tumor cell killing greatly exceeds tumor cell replication. In this manner, repopulation of the tumor can be effectively inhibited.

Mundinger et al. have accumulated a series of over 1200 brain tumor patients treated with stereotactically implanted radionuclides since 1952 (129, 134, 135). They favor permanent implantation of low dose rate ^{192}Ir or ^{125}I sources. This technique minimizes the hazards of delayed radiation necrosis in surrounding tissue. In 108 patients treated with permanent ^{192}Ir implants between 1965 and 1977, the survival rates in patients with gliomas of the hemispheres (grades 1 and 2) were 69.6% at 3 yr and 38.7% at 5 yr. For thalamic, hypothalamic, or midbrain gliomas (grades 1 and 2), survival rates were 63.1% and 45.8% at 3 and 5 yr, respectively. In these deep, midline tumors, the dose rate was calculated to administer 12,000 rad over 7 months. There were two in-hospital deaths due to hemorrhage in this series. Patients with higher grade tumors in these locations did poorly despite treatment.

In cases of larger, histologically malignant intraaxial tumors, Mundinger supplements long-term interstitial radiotherapy with high activity ^{192}Ir treatment using Gamma-Med unit. This device allows the intraoperative application of up to 2500 rads over a period of 1 hr. The isotope, housed in a shielded container, is temporarily inserted by remote control into a stereotactic probe situated within the tumor. During treatment, the operating room staff leaves the immediate vicinity of the patient. At the end of the acute treatment period, the isotope is retracted into its shielded container, and the operating team can return to close the surgical wound. The survival rate in patients with glioblastoma multiforme treated with Gamma-Med and permanent interstitial implants was 30% at 1 yr. In astrocytoma (grade not specified), 60% of patients survived 1 yr; 45% survived 2 yr. These latter figures are not as good as those in more selected series, as many patients with large, recurrent tumors were treated.

Short-term follow-up (<2 yr) in Mundinger's recent series, employing CT localization and ^{125}I permanent implants, showed an overall 80% survival rate for both hemispheric and deep midline gliomas. When analyzed according to histological grade, at the end of the short follow-up period, 92% of patients with grade 2 tumors were alive, 47% of those with grade 3 tumors were alive, and only 22% of patients harboring grade 4 tumors (glioblastoma) were still alive.

Gutin et al. have reported their results with stereotactic implantation of various isotopes into malignant brain tumors (26, 86, 87). The most recent ongoing series has employed the temporary implantation of high activity ^{125}I sources. Using CT-guided stereotaxis and computerized dosimetry planning, catheters are inserted into the tumor and then afterloaded with inner catheters containing the appropriate number and strength of ^{125}I seeds. The catheters are removed after administration of the desired dose of radiation. The results in 34 patients available for follow-up in 1984 were encouraging. All suffered from recurrent primary or metastatic tumors. All had received maximum conventional teletherapy and many had received chemotherapy as well. Twenty-three patients (68%) responded for 4 to 13+ months with documented tumor regression or stabilization of symptoms despite prior deterioration. Eleven patients did not respond to the treatment. Five patients required craniotomy for evacuation of mass-producing focal radionecrosis at 5 to 12 months after implantation. All improved and were alive at follow-up. In a more recent presentation to the Joint Tumor Section of the AANS and CNS, Leibel and Gutin (114) demonstrated remarkably improved survival times in 42 patients with recurrent malignant gliomas. Those patients with grade 4 neoplasms did substantially worse, with a median survival of 9 months from the point of brachytherapy. Those patients with grade 3 neoplasms have not yet reached median survival, with 78% alive at 2 yr after brachytherapy.

Dyck (70, 71) reviewed the short-term results of brachytherapy in 20 patients having recurrent malignant tumors. He used removable, high-activity ^{192}Ir sources implanted into afterloading catheters placed with the Riechert-Mundinger CT-guided frame. There were 13 primary glial tumors and seven metastases distributed in all regions of the brain. Five tumors were at the upper limits of size treatable by brachytherapy—150 g estimated mass. During brief follow-up (<1 yr), all tumors had either disappeared or become smaller on CT exam. Additional brain metastases, or growth of treated tumors, did not occur. One postoperative hematoma caused an increase in a preexisting neurological deficit. Of three deaths during the follow-up, one was due to the intracranial tumor; two others were due to systemic metastases.

Nehls et al. (143) used the BRW frame to implant ^{192}Ir afterloaded catheters into 10 patients with glioblastoma. Prior surgery included debulking operations in six patients and biopsy alone in four patients. All received 5000 rad external beam RT. At the time of implantation, the tumors were all smaller than 6 cm in diameter and the patients were all capable of self care. These selection criteria were felt to predict a favorable response to treatment. Dosimetry was planned to deliver an additional 3000 rad to the tumor and a surrounding margin of 5 to 10 mm. There were no new neurological deficits as a result of surgery. Patients survived for 6 to 24 months postoperatively (average: 14 months). Complications included one case of meningitis, which was successfully treated, and two instances of CSF leak around the catheter insertion site, which were easily stopped with sutures.

The NIH protocol and method of administering ^{125}I intersitial irradiation was recently reported by Findlay et al. (74). Low activity ^{125}I seeds were permanently implanted in a parallel array of silastic catheters loaded in a nonuniform fashion. This allowed tailoring of the approximately 15 rad/hr initial isodose curves to match more closely the contours of the tumor. Parallel trajectory insertion of the catheters was accomplished with the BRW system and a customized intrument block having multiple holes spaced at various radii from the central target aperture. The surgery was performed under general anesthesia through a standard scalp flap and circular bone trephination. The superficial ends of the isotope-bearing catheters were fastened to the dura, after which the bone and scalp flaps were closed over them. Long-term results are not yet available.

The total number of patients treated by the latest protocols of aggressive surgical resection, maximal external beam RT and early implantation with removable high activity sources is still small. However, interstitial brachytherapy appears to offer a significant survival advantage over conventional postoperative radiotherapy either alone or in combination with chemotherapy.

The instillation of radionuclides into cystic tumors (intracystic brachytherapy) was first performed by Leksell (115a) in 1952. He injected a solution containing ^{32}P (NaPO$_4$) into a recurrent craniopharyngioma cyst. The 40-year-old patient had undergone two prior craniotomies and had failing vision. He reportedly improved after treatment. Since that time, others have reported series of patients with craniopharyngioma treated with intracystic ^{90}Yt or ^{32}P. ^{90}Yt is a source of beta particles having an energy of approximately 2.25 MeV and a maximum range in tissue of 11 mm (61). Ninety percent of the energy is deposited within the first 4 mm of tissue. Its half-life (t½) is 2.5 days (64 hr). Thus, >95% of the administered dose is delivered within 12 days (5 t½). This isotope is not available for intracystic brachytherapy in the United States. ^{32}P is a pure beta particle source having an energy of 1.7 MeV and a maximum tissue penetration of 7.9 mm (average 4–5 mm). Its t½ is 14.3 days, requiring 71.5 days to deliver >95% of the administered dose. ^{32}P is currently available in the United States for intracystic brachytherapy.

Backlund and coworkers (11–16) reported 14 cases of cystic craniopharyngioma treated with ^{90}Yt. They delivered the isotope by transfrontal stereotactic cyst puncture. Histological diagnosis was confirmed by analysis of cyst fluid or biopsy of the cyst wall (10). The cyst volume was calculated radiographically, by air cystography, and mathematically by a technetium-99 (^{99}Tc) dilution method (12). Sufficient isotope was injected to deliver 20,000 rad to the cyst wall. Three patients required repeat treatment due to an insufficient initial dose. At 12 days after injection (>95% of calculated dose given), stereotactic cyst aspiration was carried out. In 11 patients (80%) the tumor cyst regressed completely (3 cases) or "considerably" (8 cases). One cyst remained unchanged, two progressed. Symptoms abated in the majority of patients, with 12 fully employed or in school at follow-up. Vision improved in eight patients, remained unchanged in two patients, and deteriorated despite treatment in four patients. Two operative complications in patients excluded from the series were mentioned. One patient suffered a fatal subarachnoid hemorrhage due to injury of the anterior communicating artery by the stereotactic probe. Backlund noted that stereotactic angiography could prevent this complication. In another case, the cyst fluid was so thick that none could be aspirated; no isotope was given. This series, although small, demonstrated the potential effectiveness of intracystic brachytherapy in primary or recurrent cystic craniopharyngioma. Backlund's subsequent cases have been reported in less detail. By 1980, he had operated on a total of 54 patients. Thirty-four primary cases had been treated with no operative mortality and no recurrence. Twenty-nine patients were alive and well. Three patients died due to unrelated causes, and two were lost to follow-up. In the group of 20 patients with recurrent cystic tumors at the time of treatment, 16 (80%) were alive and well at follow-up. The two operative mortalities were in this group. One patient died of unrelated causes, and one patient was lost to follow-up (115).

Sturm et al. (185) reported a series of patients with craniopharyngiomas treated with Backlund's technique. Cyst volume was calculated by ^{99}Tc dilution and CT planimetry. Of their first 10 patients, nine had unilocular cysts. Eight patients (88%) experienced arrest of growth with eventual involution seen on CT. The single patient having a cyst that appeared after external beam RT, developed a second cyst after treatment of the first one. There was one death due to pulmonary complications in a very ill patient presenting with a 200-ml tumor cyst. One intracerebral hematoma occurred that did not require surgical therapy. A single patient developed transient visual deterioration 2 months post-operatively, despite cyst shrinkage on CT exam.

Huk and Mahlstedt (102) used a proprietary CT-guided stereotactic system to implant an intracystic catheter connected to a subcutaneous reservoir in three patients with craniopharyngiomas. They employed a transfrontal route, ^{99}Tc dilution volumetrics, and a dose of 20,000 rad of ^{90}Yt. Retreatment or reaspiration could be carried out without additional surgery. Treatment was a qualified success in all three cases. One patient developed a delayed third nerve paresis which was felt to be a result of traction from the shrinking cyst. Another patient, having a large multilobulated cyst, required multiple aspirations before control of cyst size was achieved.

Stereotactic Radiosurgery

Stereotactic radiosurgery, the controlled destruction of small intracranial targets by irradiation through the intact skull, was introduced by Leksell in 1951 (115). At first using x-rays, then a proton beam, and finally, focused gamma rays, Leksell and his colleagues developed a system to substitute cross-fired beams of radiation for the stereotactic probe in his arc-radius system. This system, called the Gamma Unit, contains ^{60}Co as the gamma source. (Other stereotactic radiosurgical instruments, employing proton or electron beams, have also been developed and are described below.) The first Gamma Unit was installed in Sweden in 1968. It contained 179 ^{60}Co sources collimated to inflict a small disc-shaped lesion 5 mm in diameter. The dose rate was approximately 1000 rad/10 min. The instrument was designed for the functional neurosurgical operations of thalamotomy and capsulotomy. A number of anatomical lesions, including acoustic neuromas, craniopharyngiomas, pineal tumors, and AVMs were also treated with encouraging results. A second Gamma Unit, completed in 1974, provided adjustable, spherical radiation fields more suited to the treatment of intracranial lesions (62, 63, 113). For localization, CT and MRI have recently replaced ventriculography and cisternography. Stereotactic angiography is still required for localization of AVMs.

Backlund (13) reported the results in the first five craniopharyngioma patients to have the solid portion of their tumors treated by the Gamma Unit I. Despite radiographic evidence of tumor necrosis in most patients, there were only two patients clinically improved by the treatment. The results of intracystic brachytherapy in suitable cases were much more striking (see above).

As of 1982, 94 cases of acoustic neuroma had been irradiated with the Gamma Units, either alone or as an adjunct to open surgery. A consecutive series of 14 patients was reviewed by Noren et al. in 1983 (144). The tumors were 7 to 30 mm in diameter. Collimated beams of either 8 or 14 mm were used, depending on the tumor size. The target dose varied from 5,000 to 12,000 rad, also depending on tumor size. Target localization was by means of CT, cisternography, CT-cisternography, and pneumography, with data transposed onto stereotactic plain films. On follow-up exam, eight tumors had decreased in size, two had not changed, and three had grown. No tumor disappeared completely. Five patients with hearing present in the involved ear preoperatively had hearing preserved to a variable degree postoperatively. One patient, previously deaf in one ear, had regained hearing at follow-up. Complications in this series were few. One death occurred 6 months after treatment due to medical causes unrelated to the operation. Transient facial weakness was seen in five patients. Facial numbness occurred in two patients, and was permanent in one. In the entire series of 94 patients, there was no operative mortality and no permanent facial weakness. Since none of the tumors regressed entirely and late recurrences were documented, radiosurgery for acoustic neuroma should probably be considered palliative rather than curative. As the author and reviewer stated, the technique might best be applied to the elderly or other high-risk surgical patients, including those with bilateral tumors wishing to preserve hearing as long as possible.

Significant numbers of pineal region tumors, pituitary adenomas, and other assorted lesions have been treated with the Gamma Units. The role of stereotactic surgery and radiosurgery in these conditions remains controversial. A direct comparison of long-term results between this mode of therapy and open microsurgical methods has not yet been made.

Steiner (184) recently reviewed the Swedish series of 300 AVMs treated by the radiosurgical Gamma Units. Follow-up data, including angiography, were available for 192 patients at 1 yr after treatment, and for 130 patients at 2 to 5 yr after treatment. Patients were grouped according to whether the irradiated field covered the AVM completely or partially or whether the feeding vessels were covered completely or partially. The dose administered at a single session varied between 3,000 to 12,500 rad. Of the AVMs that could be included in the treatment field completely, which were studied 2 yr after treatment, 97.9% showed either partial (11.4%) or complete (86.5%) angiographic obliteration. The results at 2 yr were better than the results at 1 yr, suggesting a delayed but progressive therapeutic effect over time. The number of patients was small in each of the groups having either incompletely treated lesions or irradiation of feeding vessels only. Although only one of these AVMs completely resolved, many showed progressive shrinkage over time (up to 5 yr), suggesting a beneficial effect from radiosurgical "ligation" of feeding vessels. Hemorrhage was the presenting event in 240 patients. Sixty patients had neurological deficits, and 18 patients suffered from seizures at the time of treatment. New neurological deficits resulted from treatment in six patients. One was due to occlusion of a parent vessel. The remaining five deficits were felt to have resulted from radiation necrosis of functional brain tissue included within the 50% isodose volume. Eleven patients (3.7%) rebled during follow-up. The adjusted annual rebleed rate was 6.7%, a figure consistent with the natural history of AVMs. The lack of protection from rebleeding during the first year after radiosurgical treatment has been noted by other workers as well (see below).

Kjellberg et al. (108, 109) has used a proton beam, generated by the Harvard cyclotron, to irradiate pituitary adenomas, AVMs, and other lesions since the mid-1960s. A graphic plot of the dose versus depth of penetration curve for heavy particles (such as protons) shows a steep rise, followed by a sharp drop off to 0, at the end of the particles' course through tissue. This phenomenon, the so-called Bragg peak, concentrates the radiation dose within a small target volume. By adjusting the beam diameter, beam filtration, number and site of entry portals, and exposure time, the dose delivered to the target could be precisely controlled. The collimator was mated to a stereotactic frame having linear adjustments in three dimensions. As in other radiosurgical systems, the radiation beam replaced the stereotactic probe. Local anesthesia was used during application of the frame. Treatment sessions lasted 1 to 2 hr.

By 1968, Kjellberg had performed stereotactic proton beam hypophysectomy in over 150 patients with diabetes mellitus and 44 patients with acromegaly. There was no treatment-related mortality, no diabetes insipidus, and no CSF leak in either group. The results in 14 of the patients with acromegaly were analyzed in detail. A dose of 10,000 to 12,000 rad was administered to the anterior hypophysis. In 12 cases, there was reduction in the fasting growth hormone (HGH) levels after treatment. In many cases, the levels continued to decrease over several months. However, the levels fell below 5 μg/ml (normal level) in only three cases. In this sense, the treatment could not be considered curative in the majority of cases. Three patients presented with chiasmal visual field defects. In the single patient examined postoperatively, the fields had returned to normal. The first patient treated by proton beam hypophysectomy became blind in one eye after treatment, probably due to inclusion of the suprasellar region within the irradiated field. In subsequent cases, the beam was confined to the sella itself. Other complications included transient diplopia in three patients and anterior pituitary insufficiency requiring hormone replacement in one patient. Transsphenoidal microsurgery has become the standard therapy for most endocrinologically active microadenomas as well as the larger tumors with suprasellar extension and chiasmal compression. In patients with recurrent adenomas not amenable to surgical therapy, or in high risk anesthesia patients, stereotactic proton beam therapy is probably superior to conventional external beam RT.

The proton beam instrument has also been used to irradiate more than 200 AVMs since 1965. The results in the first 75 patients, followed up from 2 to 16 yr, were presented in detail by Kjellberg et al. (109). Thirty-three patients presented with hemorrhage, 24 presented with seizures, and eight had progressive neurological deficits. Ten patients had headache or other miscellaneous symptoms. In the group with prior bleeding, seven patients rebled (one rebled four times), one fatally, at 12 months after treatment. Of those with seizures, one had a "minor hemorrhage" 13 months after treatment. In 19 patients (80%) seizures were either reduced or eliminated. Two of eight patients presenting with progressive neurological deficit became either "slightly or moderately worse" during follow-up. At angiography, the AVM was either gone (20%) or reduced to less than half the pretreatment size (56%) in 76% of patients. In 13% the AVM was unchanged; none had enlarged. Craniotomy was subsequently performed in eight patients, in two as an emergency procedure for hemorrhage within 1 yr of treatment. Both of these patients died postoperatively. Other complications included neurological deficits in seven patients. Most occurred early in the series and were related to high doses of radiation given to lesions in sensitive functional areas. Subsequently, changes in the dosimetry protocol were instituted. Ten patients having preexisting seizures suffered a single seizure within days of treatment. Transient fever occurred in some patients having thalamic or hypothalamic lesions. A meaningful comparison of results between the Harvard series (patients analyzed according to clinical presentation) and the Swedish series (patients classified according to treatment strategy), is not possible on the basis of published data. However, in both groups, radiosurgery did not appear to provide protection from hemorrhage during the first year after treatment. The results do appear to justify treatment of lesions deemed inoperable on the basis of large size or location in language areas or the brainstem.

Heifetz *et al.* (91) and Colombo *et al.* (53) reported adaptations of commercially available linear accelerators (LINAC) to perform stereotactic radiosurgery. In the Heifetz instrument, the output beam of the accelerator was collimated to either a 0.5- or 1.0-cm field size. The device was further modified to rotate in a slow, spiral fashion while maintaining the focal point of the beam at the target. Repeating the sequence, with the patient rotated at various angles, would allow even higher doses of radiation to be delivered to the target. The combination of circular and angular rotations caused the incident beam to traverse different regions of overlying brain with each pass. Dosimetry tests in phantoms showed that for the 0.5-cm field size, 90% of a 5000-rad dose was delivered within a 3.8-mm area. The dose at 2 cm from the target was only 150 rad. With the 1.0-cm field, the 90% isodose plot covered a 6.5-cm area, with only 316 rad delivered to tissue 2 cm from the target. The instrument had not been used on patients at the time of the initial report.

Columbo *et al.* (53) performed less extensive modifications on an existing LINAC. The radiation beam was made to traverse an arc defined by the axis of rotation of a proprietary arc-radius frame. The target tissue was placed at the coincident focal point of both the arc and the beam. After each sweep of the arc, the patient was rotated 5 to 10° in an axis through the center of the target and the process repeated. The high dose of radiation reaching the target point was distributed in such a way that each portion of intervening brain received <10% of the total dose. The beam collimation and dose administered were individualized according to the size and histology of the lesion being treated. The system had been used on 22 patients, six of whom were reported. Four tumors regressed to a variable degree; one remained unchanged. One patient deteriorated, requiring craniotomy and internal decompression. The long-term results with this form of treatment are not yet available. The method is similar in principle to the Gamma Unit, but without the large initial expense and the need for periodic reloading of the cobalt sources. Potential advantages over conventional teletherapy are shorter treatment time (hours versus weeks) and less risk of radionecrosis of surrounding brain.

REFERENCES

1. Alksne JF, Fingerhut A, Rand R: Magnetically controlled metallic thrombosis of intracranial aneurysms. *Surgery* 60: 212–218, 1966.
2. Alksne JF, Smith RW: Iron-acrylic compound for stereotaxic aneurysm thrombosis. *J Neurosurg* 47: 137–141, 1977.
3. Alksne JF, Smith RW: Stereotaxic occlusion of 22 consecutive anterior communicating artery aneurysms. *J Neurosurg* 52: 790–793, 1980.
4. Amano K, Kawabatake H, Tanikawa T, *et al.*: Long-term follow up study of stereotactic rostral mesencephalic reticulotomy (RMR) in patients with intractable pain. 9th Meeting of the World Society for Stereotactic and Functional Neurosurgery (WSSFN), Toronto 1985.
5. Andrew J, Edwards JMR, Rudolf N de M: The placement of stereotaxic lesions for involuntary movements other than in Parkinson's disease. *Acta Neurochir Suppl* 21: 39–47, 1974.

6. Andrew J, Fowler CJ, Harrison MJG: Tremor after head injury and its treatment by stereotactic surgery. *J Neurol Neurosurg Psychiat* 45: 815-819, 1982.
7. Apuzzo MLJ, Chandrasoma PT, Zelman V, et al: Computed tomographic guidance stereotaxis in the management of lesions of the third ventricular region. *Neurosurgery* 15: 502-508, 1984.
8. Apuzzo MLJ, Sabshin JK: Computed tomographic guidance stereotaxis in the management of intracranial mass lesions. *Neurosurgery* 12: 277-285, 1983.
8a. Asakura T, Uetsuhara K, Kanamaru R, Hirahara K: An applicability study on a CT-guided stereotactic technique for functional neurosurgery. *Appl Neurophysiol* 48: 73-76, 1985.
9. Avellanosa AM, West CR: Transsphenoidal stereotaxic cryohypophysectomy for the management of pain in disseminated prostatic carcinoma. *J Med* 13: 215-221, 1982.
10. Backlund EO: A new instrument for stereotaxic brain tumor biopsy. Technical note. *Acta Chir Scand* 137: 825-827, 1971.
11. Backlund EO: Studies on craniopharyngiomas. I. Treatment: past and present. *Acta Chir Scand* 138: 743-747, 1972.
12. Backlund EO: Studies on craniopharyngiomas III. Stereotaxic treatment with intracystic yttrium-90. *Acta Chir Scand* 139: 237-247, 1973.
13. Backlund EO: Studies on craniopharyngiomas IV. Treatment with radiosurgery. *Acta Chir Scand* 139: 344-351, 1973.
14. Backlund EO, Granberg PO, Hamberger B, et al: Transplantation of adrenal medullary tissue into striatum in parkinsonism. First clinical trials. *J Neurosurg* 62: 169-173, 1985.
15. Backlund EO, Grepe A, Lunsford D: Stereotactic reconstruction of the aqueduct of sylvius. *J Neurosurg* 55: 800-810, 1981.
16. Backlund EO, Johansson L, Sarby B: Studies on craniopharyngiomas II. Treatment by stereotaxis and radiosurgery. *Acta Chir Scand* 138: 749-759, 1972.
17. Backlund EO, von Holst H: Controlled subtotal evacuation of intracerebral hematomas by stereotactic technique. *Surg Neurol* 9: 99-101, 1978.
18. Balasubramaniam V, Kanaka TS: Amygdalotomy and hypothalamotomy—A comparative study. *Conf Neurol* 37: 195-201, 1975.
19. Balasubramaniam V, Kanaka TS: Why hemispherectomy? *Appl Neurophysiol* 38: 197-205, 1975.
20. Ballantine HT, Cassidy WL, Flanagan NB, et al: Stereotaxic anterior cingulotomy for neurophychiatric illness and chronic pain. *J Neurosurg* 26: 488-495, 1967.
21. Ballantine HT, Giriunas IE: Advances in psychiatric surgery. In Rasmussen T, Marino R (eds): *Functional Neurosurgery.* New York, Raven Press, 1979, pp 155-164.
22. Ballantine HT, Levy BS, Dagi TF, et al: Cingulotomy for psychiatric illness: Report of 13 years' experience. In Sweet WH et al., (ed): *Neurosurgical Treatment in Psychiatry, Pain, and Epilepsy,* Baltimore, University Park Press, 1977, pp 333-353.
23. Barbera J, Barcia-Salorio JL, Broseta J: Stereotaxic pontine spinothalamic tractotomy. *Surg Neurol* 11: 111-114, 1979.
24. Beatty RM, Zervas NT: Stereotactic aspiration of a brain stem hematoma. *Neurosurgery* 13: 204-207, 1983.
25. Bernoulli C, Siegfried J, Baumgartner G, et al: Danger of accidental person-to-person transmission of Creutzfeldt-Jacob disease by surgery. *Lancet* 1: 478-479, 1977.
26. Bernstein M, Gutin PH: Interstitial irradiation of brain tumors: A review. *Neurosurgery* 9: 741-750, 1981.
27. Bertrand G: Computers in functional neurosurgery. In Rasmussen T, Marino R, (eds): *Functional Neurosurgery.* New York, Raven Press, 1979, pp. 75-87.
28. Bertrand G: Computers in stereotaxic surgery. In Schaltenbrand G, Walker AE, (eds): *Stereotaxy of the Human Brain.* New York, Thieme-Stratton, 1982, pp. 364-371.
29. Birg W, Mundinger F, Klar M: A computer programme system for stereotactic neurosurgery. *Acta Neurochir Supp* 24: 99-110, 1977.
30. Birg W, Mundinger F, Mohadjer M, et al: X-ray and MR-stereotaxy for functional and nonfunctional neurosurgery. 9th Meeting of the WSSFN, Toronto, 1985.
31. Black P, Uematsu S, Walker AE: Stereotaxic hypothalamotomy for control of violent, aggressive behavior. (Abstract) *Conf Neurol* 37: 187-188, 1975.
32. Blacklock JB, Maxwell RE: Stereotactic removal of a migrating ventricular catheter. *Neurosurgery* 16:230-231, 1985.
33. Boethius J, Collins VP, Edner G, et al: Stereotactic biopsies and computer tomography in gliomas. *Acta Neurochir* 40: 223-232, 1978.
34. Bohm C, Greitz T, Kingsley D: Adjustable computerized stereotaxic brain atlas for transmission and emission tomography. *AJNR* 4: 731-733, 1983.
35. Bosch DA, Beute GN: Successful stereotaxic evacuation of an acute pontomedullary hematoma. Case report. *J Neurosurg* 62: 153-156, 1985.
36. Bosch DA, Rahn D, Backlund EO: Treatment of colloid cysts of the third ventricle by stereotactic aspiration. *Surg Neurol* 9: 15-18, 1978.
37. Bosch DA: Indications for stereotactic biopsy in brain tumors. *Acta Neurochir* 54: 167-179, 1980.
38. Bouvier G, Couillard P, Leger SL, et al: Stereotactic biopsy of cerebral space-occupying lesions. *Appl Neurophysiol* 46: 227-230, 1983.
39. Bouzaglou A: Radiotherapy of brain tumors. In Dyck P (ed): *Stereotactic Biopsy and Brachytherapy of Brain Tumors.* Baltimore, University Park Press, 1984, pp 87-141.
40. Bravo G, Parera C, Seiquer G: Neurological side-effects in a series of operations on the

basal ganglia. *J Neurosurg* 24: 640–647, 1965.
41. Broggi G, Angelini L, Bono R, et al: Long term results of stereotactic thalamotomy for cerebral palsy. *Neurosurgery* 12: 195–202, 1983.
42. Broggi G, Angelini L, Giorgi C: Neurological and psychological side effects after stereotactic thalamotomy in patients with cerebral palsy. *Neurosurgery* 7: 127–134, 1980.
43. Broggi G, Franzini A: Value of serial stereotactic biopsies and impedence monitoring in the treatment of deep brain tumors. *J Neurol Neurosurg Psychiat* 44: 397–401, 1981.
44. Broggi G, Franzini A, Migliavacca F, et al: Stereotactic biopsy of deep brain tumors in infancy and childhood. *Child's Brain* 10: 92–98, 1983.
44a. Broseta J, Gonzalez-Darder J, Barcia-Salorio JL: Stereotactic evacuation of intracerebral hematomas. *Appl Neurophysiol* 45: 443–448, 1982.
45. Brown FD, Rachlin JR, Rubin JM, et al: Ultrasound-guided periventricular stereotaxis. *Neurosurgery* 15: 162–164, 1984.
46. Brown MH: Limbic target surgery in the treatment of intractable pain with drug addiction. In Sweet WH et al. (eds): *Neurosurgical Treatment in Psychiatry, Pain, and Epilepsy*. Baltimore, University Park Press, 1977, pp 699–706.
47. Bullard DE, Nashold BS: Stereotaxic thalamotomy for treatment of posttraumatic movement disorders. *J Neurosurg* 61: 316–321, 1984.
48. Bullard DE, Nashold BS, Osborne D, et al: CT-guided stereotactic biopsies using a modified frame and Gildenberg technique. *J Neurol Neurosurg Psychiat* 47: 590–595, 1984.
49. Bullard DE, Nashold BS, Osbourne D, et al: Experience using two CT-guided stereotactic biopsy methods. *Appl Neurophysiol* 46: 188–192, 1983.
50. Burger PC: Pathologic anatomy and CT correlations in the glioblastoma multiforme. *Appl Neurophysiol* 46: 180–187, 1983.
51. Coffey RJ, Lunsford LD: CT-guided stereotactic surgery for mass lesions of the midbrain and pons. *Neurosurgery* 17: 12–18, 1985.
52. Colombo F: Somatosensory-evoked potentials after mesencephalic tractotomy for pain syndromes. *Surg Neurol* 21: 453–458, 1984.
53. Colombo F, Benedetti A, Pozza F, et al: External stereotactic irradiation by linear accelerator. *Neurosurgery* 16: 154–160, 1985.
54. Cooper IS: A cryogenic method for physiologic inhibition and production of lesions in the brain. *J Neurosurg* 19: 853–858, 1962.
55. Cooper IS: Dystonia. In Schaltenbrand G, Walker AE (eds): *Stereotaxy of the Human Brain*. New York, Thieme-Stratton, 1982, pp 544–561.
56. Cooper IS: *The Neurosurgical Alleviation of Parkinsonism*. Springfield, Charles C Thomas, 1961.
57. Cooper IS: *Involuntary Movement Disorders*. New York, Hoeber, 1969.
58. Cooper IS: Twenty-five years of experience with physiological neurosurgery. *Neurosurgery* 9: 190–200, 1981.
59. Cosman ER, Nashold BS, Bedenbaugh P: Stereotactic radiofrequency lesion making. *Appl Neurophysiol* 46: 160–166, 1983.
60. Crevier PH: Post-stereotaxic intracranial hematomas. *Acta Neurochir Supp* 21: 71–73, 1974.
61. Csanda E, Joo F, Somogyi I, et al: Structural, ultra structural and functional reactions of the brain after implanting yttrium 90 rods used in stereotactic neurosurgery. *Acta Neurochir Supp* 24: 139–147, 1977.
62. Dahlin H, Larsson B, Leksell L: Influence of absorbed dose and field size on the geometry of the radiation-surgical brain lesion. *Acta Radiol Ther Physiol Biol* 14: 139–144, 1975.
63. Dahlin H, Sarby B: Destruction of small intracranial tumors with ^{60}Co Gamma radiation. *Acta Radiol Ther Physiol Biol* 14: 209–227, 1975.
64. de Divitiis E, Spaziante R, Cappabianca P, et al: Reliability of stereotactic biopsy. A model to test the value of diagnoses obtained from small fragments of nervous system tumors. *Appl Neurophysiol* 46: 295–303, 1983.
65. Delgado JMR: Therapeutic programmed stimulation of the brain in man. In Sweet WH, et al (eds): *Neurosurgical Treatment in Psychiatry, Pain, and Epilepsy*. Baltimore, University Park Press, 1977, pp 615–637.
66. DeSalles AAF, Katamaya Y, Becker DP, et al: Pain suppression induced by electrical stimulation of the pontine parabrachial region. *J Neurosurg* 62: 397–407, 1985.
67. Dieckmann G, Hassler R: Treatment of sexual violence by stereotactic hypothalamotomy. In Sweet WH, et al (eds): *Neurosurgical Treatment in Psychiatry, Pain and Epilepsy*. Baltimore, University Park Press, 1977, pp 451–462.
68. Dieckmann G, Krainick JU, Thoden U: Stereotaxic induction stimulation for pain. In Schaltenbrand G, Walker AE (eds): *Stereotaxy of the Human Brain*. New York, Thieme-Stratton, 1982, pp 498–502.
69. Dieckmann G, Hassler R: Unilateral hypothalamotomy in sexual delinquents. *Conf Neurol* 37: 177–186, 1975.
70. Dyck P: Clinical material. In Dyck P (ed): *Stereotactic Biopsy and Brachytherapy of Brain Tumors*. Baltimore, University Park Press, 1984, pp 77–88.
71. Dyck P: *Stereotactic Biopsy and Brachytherapy of Brain Tumors*. Baltimore, University Park Press, 1984.
72. Edner G: Stereotactic biopsy of intracranial space occupying lesions. *Acta Neurochir* 57: 213–214, 1981.
72a. Eiras J, Garcia J, Gomez J, et al: First results with extralemniscal myelotomy. *Acta Neurochirurgica Suppl* 30: 377–381, 1980.
73. Fairman D, Lavallol MA: New method for stereotactic hypophysectomy with radiological visualization of the lesion size. *Conf Neurol* 37: 172–176, 1975.

74. Findley PA, Wright DC, Rosenow U, Harrington FS, Miller FS, Miller RW: ^{125}I intersitial brachytherapy for primary malignant brain tumors: Technical aspects of treatment planning and implantation methods. *Intl J Radiat Oncol Biol Physiol* 11: 2021-2026, 1985.
75. Foltz EL, White IE: Pain "relief" by frontal cingulotomy. *Neurosurg* 19: 89-100, 1962.
76. Forrest APM, Roberts MM, Stewart HJ: Pituitary ablation by Yttrium-90. *Acta Neurochir Suppl* 21: 137-143, 1974.
77. Fox JL: *Selected Readings in Techniques of Stereotaxic Brain Surgery (a bibliography).* Washington DC, Medical and General Reference Library, Department of Medicine and Surgery, Veterans Administration, 1968.
78. Fraioli B, Guidetti B: Effects of stereotactic lesions of the dentate nucleus of the cerebellum in man. *Appl Neurophysiol* 38: 81-90, 1975.
79. Fujita S, Fujita K, Shirakata S, *et al:* Distribution of evoked potentials on stimulation of the human pulvinar. *Appl Neurophysiol* 39: 158-161, 1976.
80. Gildenberg P: Stereotactic treatment of head and neck pain. *Res Clin Stud Headache* 5: 102-121, 1978.
81. Gildenberg PL: Spinal stereotaxic procedures. In Schaltenbrand G, Walker AE (eds): *Stereotaxy of the Human Brain.* New York, Thieme-Stratton, 1982, pp 469-474.
82. Gildenberg PL: The present role of stereotactic surgery in the management of Parkinson's disease. *Adv Neurol* 40: 447-452, 1984.
83. Gombi R, Velok G, Hullay J: Stereotactic diagnosis of epilepsy by electrical stimulation. *Acta Med Acad Sci Hung* 33: 111-118, 1976.
84. Gornall P, Hitchcock E, Kirkland IS: Stereotaxic neurosurgery in the management of cerebral palsy. *Devel Med Child Neurol* 17: 279-286, 1975.
85. Guidetti B, Fraioli B: Neurosurgical treatment of spasticity and dyskinesias. *Acta Neurochir Suppl* 24: 27-39, 1977.
86. Gutin PH, Phillips PL, Wara WM, *et al:* Brachytherapy of recurrent malignant brain tumors with removable high-activity iodine-125 sources. *J Neurosurg* 60: 61-68, 1984.
87. Gutin PH, Phillips TL, Hosobuchi Y, *et al:* Permanent and removable implants for the brachytherapy of brain tumors. *Int J Radiat Oncol Biol Physiol* 7: 1371-1381, 1981.
87a. Hadley MN, Shetter AG, Rob Amos M: Use of the Brown-Roberts-Wells stereotactic frame for functional neurosurgery. *Appl Neurophysiol* 48: 61-68, 1985.
88. Hassler R, Dieckmann G: Stereotaxic treatment for spasmodic torticollis. In Schaltenbrand G, Walker AE (eds): *Stereotaxy of the Human Brain.* New York, Thieme-Stratton, 1982, pp 522-531.
89. Hassler R, Riechert T: A special method of stereotactic brain operation. *Proc Roy Soc Med* 48: 469-470, 1955.
90. Hawrylyshyn PA, Tasker RR, Organ LW: Third ventricular width and the thalamocapsular border. *Appl Neurophysiol* 39: 34-42, 1976.
91. Heifetz MD, Wexler M, Thompson R: Single-beam radiotherapy knife. A practical model. *J Neurosurg* 60: 814-818, 1984.
92. Heilbrun MP, Roberts TS, Apuzzo MLJ: Preliminary experience with Brown-Roberts-Wells (BRW) computerized tomography stereotaxic guidance system. *J Neurosurg* 59: 217-222, 1983.
93. Higgins AC, Nashold BS: Modification of instrument for stereotactic evacuation of intracerebral hematoma: Technical note. *Neurosurgery* 7: 604-605, 1980.
94. Higgins AC, Nashold BS: Stereotactic evacuation of large intracerebral hematoma. *Appl Neurophysiol* 43: 96-103, 1980.
95. Hitchcock E, Cowie R: Stereotactic removal of intracranial foreign bodies: review and case report. *Injury* 14: 471-475, 1983.
96. Hitchcock E: Dentate lesions for involuntary movement. *Proc Roy Soc Med* 66: 877-879, 1973.
97. Hitchcock ER: Stereotaxic pontine spinothalamic tractotomy. *J Neurosurg* 39: 746-752, 1973.
97a. Hitchcock ER, Schvarcz JR: Stereotaxic trigeminal tractotomy for post-herpetic facial pain. *J Neurosurg* 37: 412-417, 1972.
97b. Hitchcock ER: Stereotactic cervical myelotomy. *J Neurol Neurosurg Psychiat* 33: 224-230, 1970.
98. Hoffman HJ, Harwood-Nash D, Gilday DL: Percutaneous third ventriculostomy in the management of noncommunicating hydrocephalus. *Neurosurgery* 7: 313-321, 1980.
99. Hood TW, Yap JC: A survey of infections in stereotactic surgery. *Appl Neurophysiol* 44: 314-319, 1981.
100. Hosobuchi Y: Chronic brain stimulation for the treatment of intractable pain. *Res Clin Stud Headache* 5: 122-126, 1978.
101. Hosobuchi Y: Combined electrical stimulation of the periaqueductal gray matter and sensory thalamus. *Appl Neurophysiol* 46: 112-115, 1983.
102. Huk WJ, Mahlstedt J: Intracystic radiotherapy (^{90}Y) of craniopharyngiomas: CT-guided stereotaxic implantation of indwelling drainage system. *AJNR* 4: 803-806, 1983.
103. Hullay J, Gombi R, Velok G: Surgical and stereotactic attempts in intractable epilepsy. *Acta Med Acad Sci Hung* 33: 119-124, 1976.
103a. Iizuka J: Development of a stereotactic endoscopy of the ventricular system. *Conf Neurol* 37: 141-149, 1975.
103b. Iizuka J: Stereoencephaloscopic findings in internal hydrocephalus. *Endoscopy* 4: 141-149, 1972.
104. Kandel EI, Peresedov VV: Stereotaxic clipping of arterial aneurysms and arteriovenous malformations. *J Neurosurg* 46: 12-23, 1977.
105. Kandel EI, Peresedov VV: Stereotaxic clipping of arterial and arteriovenous aneurysms of the

brain. *Acta Neurochir Suppl* 30: 405–412, 1980.
106. Kandel EI, Peresedov VV: Stereotaxic evacuation of spontaneous intracerebral hematomas. *J Neurosurg* 62: 206–213, 1985.
107. Kelly PJ: Microelectrode recording for the somatotopic placement of stereotactic thalamic lesions in the treatment of parkinsonism and cerebellar intention tremor. *Appl Neurophysiol* 43: 262–266, 1980.
108. Kjellberg RN, Shintani A, Frantz AG, et al: Proton beam therapy in acromegaly. *N Engl J Med* 278: 689–695, 1968.
109. Kjellberg RN, Hanamura T, Davis KR: Bragg-peak proton therapy for arteriovenous malformations of the brain. *N Eng J Med* 309: 269–274, 1983.
110. Laitinen LV: Anterior pulvinotomy in the treatment of intractable pain. In Sweet WH, *et al* (eds): *Neurosurgical Treatment in Psychiatry, Pain, and Epilepsy.* Baltimore, University Park Press, 1977, pp 669–672.
111. Laitinen LV: Brain targets in surgery for Parkinson's disease. Results of a survey of neurosurgeons. *J Neurosurg* 62: 349–351, 1985.
112. Laitinen LV, Liliequist B, Fagerlund M, *et al:* An adapter for computed tomography-guided stereotaxis. *Surg Neurol* 23: 559–566, 1985.
113. Larsson B, Liden K, Sarby B: Irradiation of small structures through the intact skull. *Acta Radiol Ther Physiol Biol* 13: 512–534, 1974.
114. Leibel SA, Gutin P: Removable implants for brachytherapy. Joint Tumor Section Workshop: Brachytherapy of Malignant Gliomas. Presented at the 1986 American Association of Neurological Surgeons Meeting, Denver, CO. 1986.
115. Leksell L: Stereotactic radiosurgery. *J Neurol Neurosurg Psychiat* 46: 797–803, 1983.
115a. Leksell L, Liden K: A therapeutic trial with radioactive isotopes in cystic brain tumor. In *Radioisotope Techniques, Proc Isotope Technique Conf* Oxford, Her Majesty's Stationary Office, 1953, vol 1 pp 76–78.
116. Levin AB, Katz J, Benson RC, *et al:* Treatment of diffuse metastatic cancer by stereotactic chemical hypophysectomy: Long term results and observations on mechanism of action. *Neurosurgery* 6: 258–262, 1980.
116a. Luft R, Olivecrona H: Experiences with hypophysectomy in man. *J Neurosurg* 10: 301–316, 1953.
117. Lunsford LD, Latchaw RE, Vries JK: Stereotactic implantation of deep brain electrodes using computed tomography. *Neurosurgery* 13: 280–286, 1983.
118. Martin-Rodriguez JG, Obrador S: Evaluation of stereotaxic pulvinar lesions. *Conf Neurol* 37: 56–62, 1975.
119. Matsumoto K, Shichijo F, Fukami T: Long-term follow-up review of cases of Parkinson's disease after unilateral thalamotomy. *J Neurosurg* 60: 1033–1044, 1984.
120. Matsumoto K, Hondo H: CT-guided stereotactic evacuation of hypertensive intracerebral hematomas. *J Neurosurg* 61: 440–448, 1984.
121. Myer CHA: Bilateral improvement in voluntary movement after unilateral diencephalic lesions for parkinsonism. *Appl Neurophysiol* 44: 345–354, 1981.
122. Meyers R: Three cases of myoclonus alleviated by bilateral ansotomy, with a note on postoperative alibido and impotence. *J Neurosurg* 19: 71–81, 1962.
123. Meyers R, Fry WJ, Fry FJ, *et al:* Early experiences with ultrasonic irradiation of the pallidofugal and nigral complexes in hyperkinetic and hypertonic disorders. *J Neurosurg* 16: 32–54, 1959.
124. Mimura Y, Bekku H, Miyamoto T: VL thalamotomy for the treatment of tremor in patients with thalamic syndrome. *Appl Neurophysiol* 39: 199–201, 1976/77.
125. Modesti LM, Van Buren JM: Hemiballismus complicating stereotactic thalamotomy. *Appl Neurophysiol* 42: 267–283, 1979.
126. Mori K, Iwayama K, Ito M, *et al:* Electrical impedance as a locating method in human stereotactic surgery. *Appl Neurophysiol* 39: 216–221, 1976/77.
127. Moser RP, Yap JC, Fraley EE: Stereotactic hypophysectomy for intractable pain secondary to metastatic prostate carcinoma. *Appl Neurophysiol* 43: 145–149, 1980.
128. Mullan S: Experience with surgical thrombosis of intracranial berry aneurysms and carotid cavernous fistulas. *J Neurosurg* 41: 657–670, 1974.
129. Mundinger F: Implantation of radioisotopes (Curie-therapy). In Schaltenbrand G, Walker AE (eds): *Stereotaxy of the Human Brain.* New York, Thieme-Stratton, 1982, pp 410–435.
130. Mundinger F: Postoperative and long term results of 1,561 stereotactic operations in parkinsonism. 9th Meeting of the WSSFN, Toronto, 1985.
131. Mundinger F, Becker P: Late results of central stereotactic interventions for pain. *Acta Neurochir Suppl* 24: 299, 1977.
132. Mundinger F, Becker P: Long-term results of central stereotactic interventions for pain. In Sweet WH *et al*, (ed): *Neurosurgical Treatment in Psychiatry, Pain and Epilepsy,* Baltimore, University Park Press, 1977, pp 685–692.
133. Mundinger F, Birg W, Klar M: Computer-assisted stereotactic brain operations by means including computerized axial tomography. *Appl Neurophysiol* 41: 169–182, 1979.
134. Mundinger F, Hoefer T: Protracted long-term irradiation of inoperable midbrain tumors by stereotactic Curie-therapy using Iridium-192. *Acta Neurochir Suppl* 21: 93–100, 1974.
135. Mundinger F, Metzel E: Interstitial radioisotope therapy of intractable diencephalic tumors by the stereotaxic permanent implantation of iridium 192 including bioptic control. *Conf Neurol* 32: 195–202, 1970.
136. Mundinger F, Neumuller H: Programmed stim-

ulation for control of chronic pain and motor disorders. *Appl Neurophysiol* 45: 102–111, 1982.
137. Mundinger F, Reinke MA, Hoefer TH, et al: Determination of intracerebral structures using osseous reference points for computer-aided stereotactic operations. *Appl Neurophysiol* 38: 3–22, 1975.
138. Narabayashi H: Choreoathetosis and spasticity. In Schaltenbrand G, Walker AE (eds): *Stereotaxy of the Human Brain*. New York, Thieme-Stratton, 1982, pp 532–543.
139. Nashold BS: Brainstem stereotaxic procedures. In Schaltenbrand G, Walker AE (eds): *Stereotaxy of the Human Brain*. New York, Thieme-Stratton, 1982, pp 474–483.
140. Nashold BS, Slaughter DG: Effects of stimulating or destroying the deep cerebellar regions in man. *J Neurosurg* 31: 172–186, 1969.
141. Nashold BS, Wilson WP, Boone E: Depth recordings and stimulation of the human brain: A twenty year experience. In Rasmussen T, Marino R (eds): *Functional Neurosurgery*. New York, Raven Press, 1979, pp 181–195.
142. Nashold BS, Wilson WP, Slaughter DG: Sensations evoked by stimulation of the midbrain in man. *J Neurosurg* 30: 14–24, 1969.
143. Nehls DG, Shetter AG, Rossman KJ, et al: Interstitial irradiation of malignant tumors. *BNI Quart* 1: 34–39, 1985.
144. Noren G, Arndt J, Hindmarsh T: Stereotactic radiosurgery in cases of acoustic neurinoma: Further experiences. *Neurosurgery* 13: 12–22, 1983.
145. Ohye C: Depth microelectrode studies. In Schaltenbrand G, Walker AE (eds): *Stereotaxy of the Human Brain*. New York, Thieme-Stratton, 1982, pp 372–389.
146. Ohye C, Maeda T, Narabayashi H: Physiologically defined VIM nucleus. Its special reference to control of tremor. *Appl Neurophysiol* 39: 285–295, 1976/77.
147. Ohye C, Miyazaki M, Hirai T, et al: Stereotactic selective thalamotomy for the treatment of tremor type cerebral palsy in adolescence. *Child's Brain* 10: 157–167, 1983.
148. Ohye C, Miyazaki M, Hirai T: Primary writing tremor treated by stereotactic selective thalamotomy. *J Neurol Neurosurg Psychiat* 45: 988–997, 1982.
149. Ostertag CB, Mennel HD, Kiessling MK: Stereotactic biopsy of brain tumors. *Surg Neurol* 14: 275–283, 1980.
150. Pecker J, Scarabin JM, Vallee B, et al: Treatment in tumors of the pineal region: Value of stereotaxic biopsy. *Surg Neurol* 12: 341–348, 1979.
151. Pecker J, Scarabin JM, Brucher JM, et al: *Stereotactic Approach to Diagnosis and Treatment of Cerebral Tumors*. Paris, Laboratoires Pierre Fabre, 1979.
151a. Perlow MJ, Freed WJ, Hoffer BJ, et al: Brain grafts reduce motor abnormalities produced by destruction of nigrostriatal dopamine systems. *Science* 204: 643–647, 1979.
152. Plotkin R: Results in 60 cases of deep brain stimulation for chronic intractable pain. *Appl Neurophysiol* 45: 173–178, 1982.
153. Poblete M, Zamboni R: Stereotaxic third ventriculostomy. *Conf Neurol* 37: 150–155, 1975.
154. Ramamurthi B, Davidson A: Central median lesions—analysis of 89 cases. *Conf Neurol* 37: 63–72, 1975.
155. Ramamurthi B, Kalyanaraman S: Stereotaxic targets for epilepsy. In Schaltenbrand G, Walker AE (eds): *Stereotaxy of the Human Brain*. New York, Thieme-Stratton, 1982, pp 563–660.
156. Rand RW: Dystonia musculorum deformans alleviated by chemopallidothalamectomy and substantia nigralysis. *J Neurosurg* 17: 1093–1099, 1960.
157. Rand RW: Stereotaxy for vascular anomalies. In Schaltenbrand G, Walker AE (eds): *Stereotaxy of the Human Brain*. New York, Thieme-Stratton, 1982.
158. Reynolds DV: Surgery in the rat during electrical analgesia induced by focal brain stimulation. *Science* 164: 444–445, 1969.
159. Richardson DE: Thalamotomy for control of chronic pain. *Acta Neurochir Suppl* 21: 77–88, 1974.
160. Richardson DE, Akil H: Pain reduction by electrical brain stimulation in man. Part I: Acute administration in periaqueductal and periventricular sites. *J Neurosurg* 47: 178–183, 1977.
161. Richardson DE, Akil H: Pain reduction by electrical brain stimulation in man. Part 2: Chronic self-administration in the periventricular gray matter. *J Neurosurg* 47: 184–194, 1977.
162. Riechert T: Effect of age on the complications and results of stereotaxic surgery. In Schaltenbrand G, Walker AE (eds): *Stereotaxy of the Human Brain*. New York, Thieme-Stratton, 1982, pp 458–460.
163. Riechert T, Hassler R, Mundinger F, et al: Pathologic-anatomic findings and cerebral localization in stereotactic treatment of extrapyramidal motor disturbances in multiple sclerosis. *Conf Neurol* 37: 24–40, 1975.
164. Rivas JJ, Lobato RD: CT-assisted stereotaxic aspiration of colloid cysts of the third ventricle. *J Neurosurg* 62: 238–242, 1985.
165. Roldan P, Broseta J, Barcia-Salorio JL: Chronic VPM stimulation for anesthesia dolorosa following trigeminal surgery. *Appl Neurophysiol* 45: 112–113, 1982.
166. Ryden SE, Silverman EM: Early and late histologic effects of stereotactic neurosurgery. *Arch Pathol Lab Med* 100: 87–90, 1976.
167. Sano K, Mayanagi Y, Sekino H, et al: Results of stimulation and destruction of the posterior hypothalamus in man. *J Neurosurg* 33: 689–707, 1970.
168. Sayers MP, Kosnick EJ: Percutaneous third ventriculostomy: Experience and technique. *Child's Brain* 2: 24–30, 1976.

169. Schaltenbrand G: The effects on speech and language of stereotactical stimulation in thalamus and corpus callosum. *Brain Lang* 2: 70–77, 1975.
170. Schaltenbrand G, Wahren W: Electroanatomical observations. In Schaltenbrand G, Walker AE (eds): *Stereotaxy of the Human Brain.* New York, Thieme-Stratton, 1982, pp 391–409.
170a. Schvarcz JR: Functional exploration of the spinomedullary junction. *Acta Neurochirurgica Suppl* 24: 179–185, 1977.
171. Schvarcz JR: Paraqueductal mesencephalotomy for facial central pain. In Sweet WH, *et al* (eds): *Neurosurgical Treatment in Psychiatry, Pain and Epilepsy.* Baltimore, University Park Press, 1977, pp 661–667.
172. Schvarcz JR: Stereotactic trigeminal tractotomy. *Conf Neurol* 37: 73–77, 1975.
173. Schvarcz JR: Results of stimulation and destruction of the posterior hypothalamus. In Sweet WH, *et al* (eds): *Neurosurgical Treatment in Psychiatry, Pain, and Epilepsy.* Baltimore, University Park Press, 1977, pp 429–438.
174. Selby G: Stereotactic surgery for the relief of Parkinson's disease. Part I. A critical review. *J Neurol Sci* 5: 315–342, 1967.
175. Selby G: Stereotactic surgery for the relief of Parkinson's disease. Part 2. An analysis of the results in a series of 303 patients (413 operations). *J. Neurol Sci* 5: 343–375, 1967.
176. Siegfried J: Neurosurgical treatment of spasticity. In Rasmusen T, Marino R (eds): *Functional Neurosurgery.* New York, Raven Press, 1979, pp 123–128.
177. Siegfried J: Stereotaxic cerebellar surgery for spasticity. In Schaltenbrand G, Walker AE (eds): *Stereotaxy of the Human Brain.* New York, Thieme-Stratton, 1982, pp 562–564.
178. Siegfried J, Verdie JC: Long-term assessment of stereotactic dentatotomy for spasticity and other disorders. *Acta Neurochir Suppl* 24: 41–48, 1977.
179. Smith RW, Alksne JF: Stereotaxic thrombosis of inaccessible intracranial aneurysms. *J Neurosurg* 57:833–839, 1977.
180. Speelman JD, Van Manen J: Stereotactic thalamotomy for the relief of intention tremor of multiple sclerosis. *J Neurol Neurosurg Psychiatr* 47: 596–599, 1984.
181. Spiegel EA, Wycis HT, Freed H: Stereoencephalotomy. Thalamotomy and related procedures. *JAMA* 148: 446–451, 1952.
182. Spiegel EA, Wycis HT, Marks M, *et al:* Stereotaxic apparatus for operations on the human brain. *Science* 106: 349–350, 1947.
183. Spiegel EA, Wycis HT, Szekely HZ, *et al:* Campotomy in various extrapyramidal disorders. *J Neurosurg* 20: 871–874, 1963.
184. Steiner L: Radiosurgery in cerebral arteriovenous malformations. In Fein JM, Flamm ES (eds): *Cerebrovascular Surgery.* New York, Springer-Verlag, 1985, pp 1161–1215.
185. Sturm V, Rommel TH, Strauss L, *et al:* Preliminary results of intracavitary irradiation of cystic craniopharyngiomas by means of stereotactically applied Yttrium-90. *Adv Neurosurg* 9: 401–4, 1980.
186. Sugita K, Doi T, Sato O, *et al:* Successful removal of intracranial air-gun bullet with stereotaxic apparatus. *J Neurosurg* 30: 177–181, 1969.
187. Sugita K, Kobayashi S: General considerations of pain. In Schaltenbrand G, Walker AE (eds): *Stereotaxy of the Human Brain.* New York, Thieme-Stratton, 1982, pp 462–467.
188. Sugita K, Mutsuga N, Takaoka Y, *et al:* Stereotaxic exploration of para-third ventricle tumors. *Conf Neurol* 37: 156–162, 1975.
189. Sweet WH: Intracerebral electrical stimulation for relief of chronic pain. In Youmans J (ed): *Neurological Surgery 2nd edition.* Philadelphia, Saunders, 1982, pp 3739–3748.
189a. Talairach J, Szikla G, Tournoux P, *et al:* La chirurgie stéréotaxique hypophysaire. *Conf Neurol* 22: 204–213, 1962.
190. Tasker RR: Neurological concepts of pain management in head and neck cancer. *Can J Otol* 4: 480–484, 1975.
191. Tasker RR: Thalamic stereotaxic procedures. In Schaltenbrand G, Walker AE (eds): *Stereotaxy of the Human Brain.* New York, Thieme-Stratton, 1982, pp 484–497.
192. Tasker RR, Hawrylyshyn P, Organ L: *The Thalamus and Midbrain of Man: A physiological atlas using electrical stimulation.* Springfield, Charles C Thomas, 1982.
193. Tasker RR, Hawrylyshyn P, Rowe IH, *et al:* Computerized graphic display of results of subcortical stimulation during stereotactic surgery. *Acta Neurochir Suppl* 24: 85–98, 1977.
194. Tasker RR, Organ LW, Hawrylyshyn P: Sensory organization of the human thalamus. *Appl Neurophys* 39: 139–153, 1976/77.
195. Tasker RR, Rowe IH, Hawrylyshyn P, *et al:* Computer mapping of brain-stem sensory centers in man. *J Neurosurg* 44: 458–464, 1976.
196. Tasker RR, Siqueira J, Hawrylyshyn P, *et al:* What happened to VIM thalamotomy for Parkinson's disease? *Appl Neurophys* 46: 68–83, 1983.
197. Thomas DGT, Anderson RE, du Boulay GH: CT-guided stereotactic neurosurgery: experience in 24 cases with a new stereotactic system. *J Neurol Neurosurg Psychiatr* 47: 9–16, 1984.
198. Toth S, Vajda J: Multitarget technique in parkinson surgery. *Appl Neurophysiol* 43: 109–113, 1980.
199. Vaernet K, Masden A: Stereotaxic amygdalotomy and basofrontal tractotomy in psychotics with aggressive behavior. *J Neurol Neurosurg Psychiatr* 33: 858–863, 1970.
200. van Leeuwen WS: Neuro-physio-surgery in the Netherlands since 1971. *Acta Neurochir* 61: 249–256, 1982.
201. van Manen J: Stereotaxic operation in cases of hereditary and intention tremor. *Acta Neurochir Suppl* 21: 49–55, 1974.
202. von Essen C, Augustinsson L-E, Lindqvist G: VOI thalamotomy in spasmodic torticollis. *Appl Neurophysiol* 43: 159–163, 1980.

203. Voris HC, Whisler WW: Results of stereotaxic surgery for intractable pain. *Conf Neurol* 7: 86–96, 1975.
204. Walker AE: Stereotaxic surgery for tremor. In Schaltenbrand G, Walker AE (eds): *Stereotaxy of the Human Brain.* New York, Thieme-Stratton, 1982, pp 515–521.
205. Walker AE: General principles of stereotactic surgery for epilepsy. In Schaltenbrand G, Walker AE (eds): *Stereotaxy of the Human Brain.* New York, Thieme-Stratton, 1982, pp 645–652.
206. Walker AE, Uematsu S, Niedermeyer E, *et al:* Depth recording. In Schaltenbrand G, Walker AE (eds): *Stereotaxy of the Human Brain.* New York, Thieme-Stratton, 1982, 661–668.
207. Walsh PR, Larson SJ, Rytel MW, *et al:* Stereotactic aspiration of deep cerebral abscesses after CT directed labeling. *Appl Neurophys* 43: 205–209, 1980.
207a. Ward AA Jr: The cingular gyrus: area 24. *J Neurophysiol* 11: 13–23, 1948.
208. Wycis HT, Spiegel EA: Long-range results in the treatment of intractable pain by stereotactic midbrain surgery. *J Neurosurg* 19: 101–107, 1962.
209. Young RE, Feldman RA, Kroening R, *et al:* Electrical stimulation of the brain in the treatment of chronic pain in man. *Adv Pain Res Ther* 6: 289–303, 1984.
210. Young RF, Kroening R, Fulton W, *et al:* Electrical stimulation of the brain in treatment of chronic pain. Experience over 5 years. *J Neurosurg* 62: 389–386, 1985.
211. Zervas NT: Long-term review of dentatectomy in dystonia musculorum deformans and cerebral palsy. *Acta Neurochir Suppl* 24: 49–51, 1977.
212. Zervas NT, Hamlin HH: Technical factors in stereotaxic hypophysectomy. *Acta Neurochir Suppl* 24: 137–138, 1977.

Chapter 3

Stereotactic Surgical Instrumentation

WILLIAM A. FRIEDMAN, M.D. and ROBERT J. COFFEY, M.D.

INTRODUCTION

Stereotaxis is the term coined by Horsley and Clarke (35), to describe their technique of inflicting localized and repeatable lesions within the brains of experimental animals, by means of a precision probe-guiding apparatus keyed to an accompanying brain atlas, also of the inventors' design (Fig. 3.1). Their original device employed many of the principles essential to the later development of stereotactic surgery: rigid cranial fixation, a high degree of accuracy (based on external landmarks), precision (exact repeatability), and flexibility of trajectory selection. Despite the advanced concepts employed in its design and construction, the Horsley-Clarke device was never adapted to human use.

In 19th century Russia, more than a decade before the Horsley-Clarke invention, Zernov, followed by his pupil Rossolimo, developed and used a form of stereotactic device called the "encephalometer" (40). The device, attached to the patient's head by penetrating pins, could locate cortical regions in relation to external cranial landmarks based on an early brain surface map (Fig 3.2). Although the encephalometer and a later model, the "cerebral topograph," did function as intended, the surgical techniques applied to the three patients upon which these devices were used were so poorly developed that the patients succumbed.

Recently, Olivier and coworkers (63, 70) reported a stereotactic device designed by the neuroanatomist-physiologist Aubrey Mussen in 1918. Although intended for human surgery, the device was never actually used. The frame relied on external skull landmarks, and was limited to probe trajectories orthogonal to the sides or top of the device. Kirschner also used a guiding device, based on external landmarks, to coagulate the gasserian ganglion in cases of trigeminal neuralgia (81).

There are numerous geometrical systems upon which stereotactic frame coordinates and guidance devices could have been based (32, 49, 64, 65). However, due to practical constraints, relatively few of the potential systems have actually been utilized. The four main types of stereotactic frames are: polar coordinate, arc-radius, focal point, and phantom target. Some instruments utilize features of more than one type (95).

A typical polar coordinate system (Fig. 3.3) requires that the probe trajectory be described in terms of angles—usually relative to a preselected skull entry point (33). At least two angles are necessary, in planes orthogonal to each other, to describe a unique trajectory. One linear distance, the probe length, must also be determined in order to reach the specific target point along the trajectory.

Arc-radius frames (Fig. 3.4) work on the principle that a probe equal in length to the radius of a semicircular arc, introduced orthogonal to a tangent anywhere along the arc, will reach the center of the system. Linear adjustments of the arc supports, in three dimensions, move the probe impact point to any desired target coordinates. Focal point systems work on the arc-radius

Figure 3.1. Photograph of Horsley-Clarke stereotactic frame, which was utilized in animal research but never in human surgery.

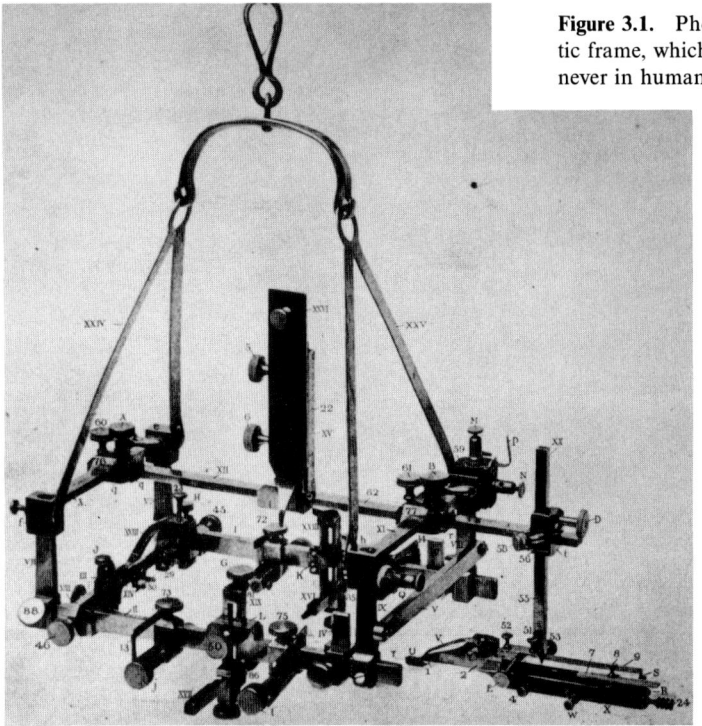

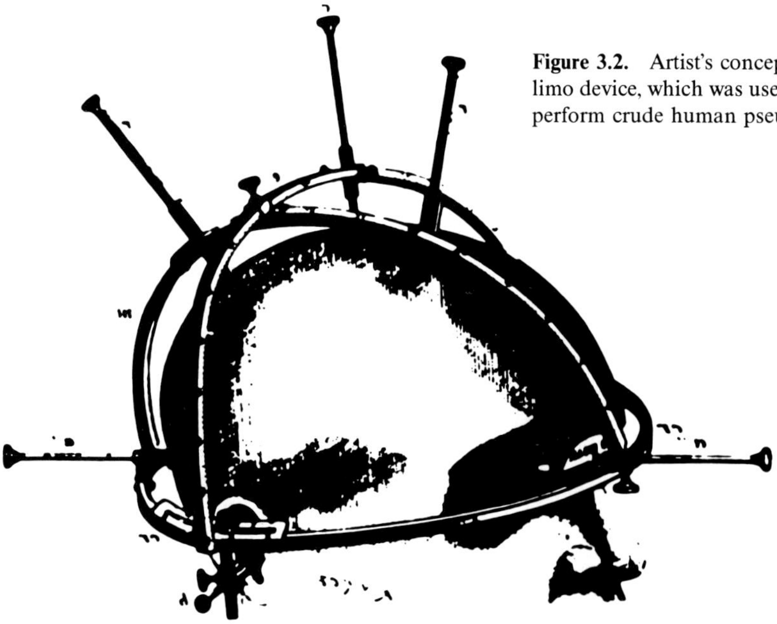

Figure 3.2. Artist's conception of the Zernov-Rossolimo device, which was used in 19th century Russia to perform crude human pseudostereotactic procedures.

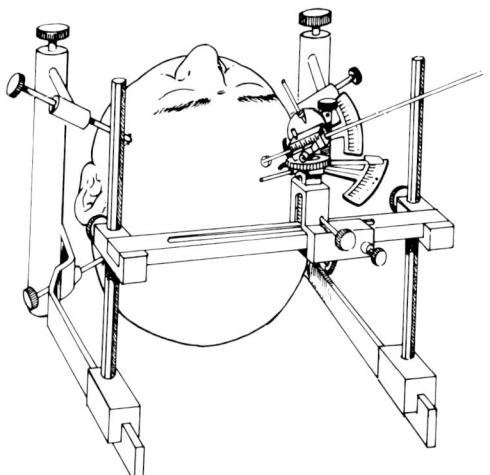

Figure 3.3. Polar coordinate instrument for traditional stereotactic surgery (Cooper's device). Stereotactic ventriculograms were taken to include probe and calibrated protractors. A line was drawn on films to pass through entry point and target. Initial corrections could then be made on the basis of the position of probe relative to the ideal trajectory drawn on films.

principle with one important distinction. The target is brought to the impact point by moving the patient's head, instead of bringing the impact point to the target (Fig. 3.5).

Phantom target devices can theoretically employ any coordinate system, but have been used almost exclusively with polar coordinate frames (Fig. 3.6). The phantom or "dummy" target allows the angles and probe length of complex polar coordinate devices to be determined mechanically instead of trigonometrically. Also, the operation can be rehearsed on the phantom before actual surgery upon the patient begins.

TRADITIONAL SYSTEMS

Spiegel and Wycis first utilized intracranial reference points and radiographical guidance, to perform truly stereotactic operations on the deep structures of the human brain (21, 83, 87). Spiegel proposed and Wycis performed the first dorsomedial thal-

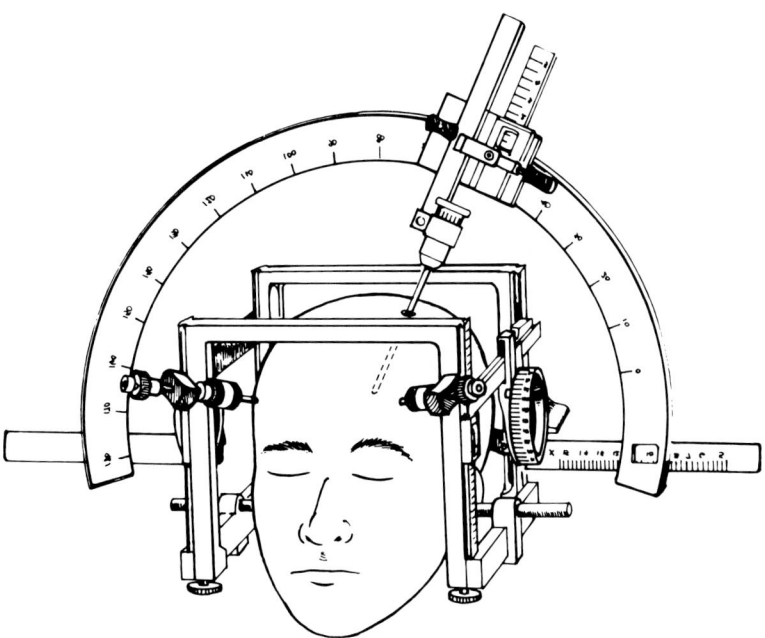

Figure 3.4. Arc-radius stereotactic device (Leksell frame). The probe, equal in length to the radius of the arc, reaches the center of arc regardless of arc rotation around supporting gimbals, or movement of probe carrier along circumference of the arc. Side bars and arc supports, adjustable in three dimensions, move center of arc to coincide with target point.

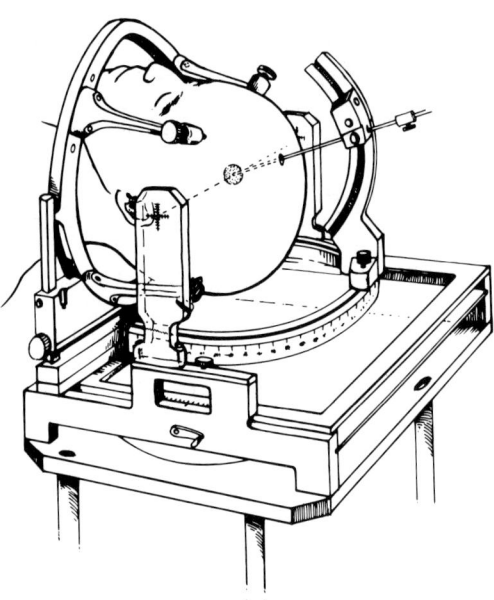

Figure 3.5. Focal-point stereotactic frame (Todd-Wells). Impact point of the probe is always at center of stable probe carrier arc. Fixed reticles, aligned with focal point of frame, appear on stereotactic radiographs. In this variation of the arc-radius principle, the target is brought to probe impact point by movement of head holder.

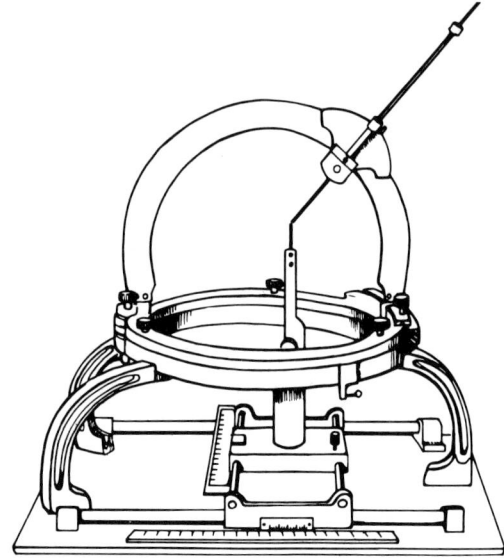

Figure 3.6. Phantom target device (Brown-Roberts-Wells, BRW) allows mechanical determination of probe length and trajectory without complex calculations. Base ring of phantom is identical to head ring on patient. Most importantly, when computations are utilized, phantom device provides a trial run and often detects human errors in setup of the biopsy arc.

amotomy, a psychosurgical operation interrupting the thalamofrontal pathways with less disabling side effects than prefrontal lobotomy (31, 85). Their operative indications and repertoire of targets rapidly expanded, such that by 1952 they reported 90 thalamic operations in 58 psychiatric patients. In addition, 24 cases were operated for medically intractable pain by mesencephalic spinothalamic tractotomy and/or thalamotomy.

The Spiegel and Wycis stereoencephalotome evolved through several models between 1947 and 1956 (84, 86–88) (Fig. 3.7). The initial plaster cast head fixation system was soon supplanted by a device incorporating padded rings and cranial supports. By model V, nonoperative application was abandoned in favor of a system employing hollow screws, threaded internally as well as externally. This allowed secure fixation of the device at initial ventriculography and exact refixation for subsequent surgery.

With each successive model, the stereoencephalotome was made more flexible, allowing a wider choice of trajectories and targets. Although relatively simple in principle, the actual operation of the device was complex. Multiple precisely orthogonal (true anteroposterior [AP] and lateral) teleradiographs, both before and after ventriculography, were required to ensure exact alignment of the frame and electrode carrier in the horizontal, sagittal, and coronal planes. Linear target coordinates were selected from the authors' atlas and plotted on stereotactic ventriculograms. Final transfer of target coordinates to the frame was then carried out, with x-ray distortion compensated by trigonometric calculations. The apparatus, therefore, utilized a combination of linear and polar coordinate systems.

In 1954, Hassler and Riechert (30, 82) established the intercommissural line as the standard reference upon which most subsequent atlases and coordinate systems have been based. Riechert and Wolff (72, 73, 75) and, later, Mundinger (72), developed an elegantly simplified and enduring stereotac-

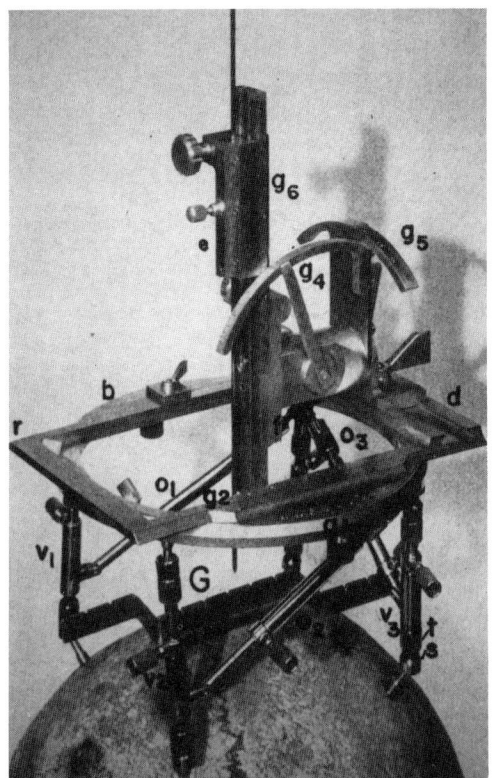

Figure 3.7. Photograph of the Spiegel-Wycis stereoencephalotome, model V. This device was first human stereotactic frame and was utilized extensively in treatment of movement disorders and intractable pain.

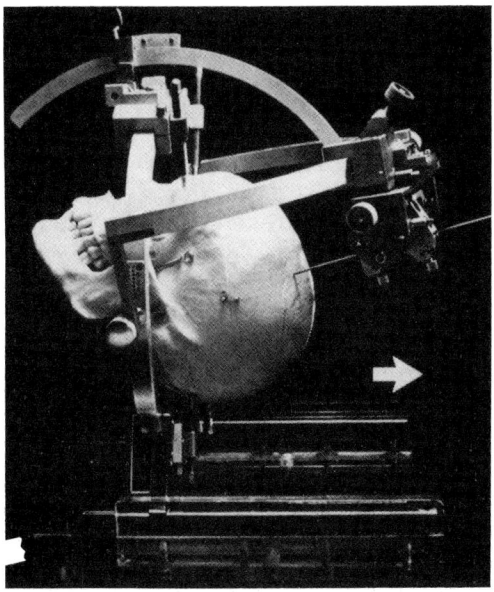

Figure 3.8. A modern version of the Riechert-Mundinger frame is shown. It is a polar coordinate device, now compatible with traditional or image-guided stereotactic neurosurgery.

tic frame design (Fig. 3.8). A base ring, fixed to the patient's head with sharpened pins, supported a removable set of arcs. These consisted of intersecting, calibrated protractors with angular adjustments, establishing a polar coordinate system. The only linear distance that had to be established was the probe depth to target. The arc and its attached instrument block were also mated to a phantom apparatus having a base ring identical to that attached to the patient. Using ventriculographical data relative to a standard brain atlas, target as well as burr hole sites could be simulated on the phantom before the actual operation—both as a check on frame settings, and as a means of directly determining the probe length from burr hole to target. This effectively eliminated the need for cumbersome calculations in the era before microcomputers.

The concept of an intermediary phantom device to mechanically translate linear target and atlas coordinate data to polar stereotactic frame settings represents one of the major contributions of Riechert, Wolff, and Mundinger to stereotactic methodology. Turner and Shaw (93), in 1974, reported their proprietary modification of the Guiot instrument as previously modified by Gillingham. The result was a cylindrical system combining both linear and polar coordinates with an accompanying two-dimensional "mechanical analogue," a phantom-equivalent device. With this instrument, short-distance fluoroscopy was substituted for the more laborious teleroentgenograms. The mechanical analogue plotted necessary corrections for magnification and distortion, giving direct readouts of frame settings. The phantom-target principle, interfaced with a polar-coordinate guidance system, is currently utilized in the Brown-Roberts-Wells (BRW) CT-guided stereotactic instrument.

Numerous less elaborate polar coordinate instruments have been designed and used by their inventors (18). Among them are the instruments of Bradford (8), Cooper (15), Kandel (39), and Walker (95). In all of these, the target point is first plotted on biplane stereotactic radiographs with the device attached such that the probe touches the skull entry point. A line is drawn from the target point through the entry point on both the AP and lateral films. The intersection of this line with the instruments' graduated protractors, also seen on the x-ray films, gives the proper angular settings in each plane. Determination of the depth setting (derived mechanically by the phantom in the Riechert-Mundinger system) is accomplished by inclusion of a radiopaque ruler or markers of known length in the stereotactic x-ray films. Comparison of the marker's size on the x-ray film with its known length gives the correction factor.

In 1949, Leksell (95) introduced the first of a series of instruments based on the three-dimensional arc-radius principle. The probe carrier moves freely along a semicircular arc which is, in turn, mounted by pivoting shafts along its diameter. The shafts, pivoting on gimbals, attach to adjustable graduated bars supported by a frame rigidly fixed to the patient's head. The arc can be moved along its supporting shafts for lateral adjustment, while the graduated side bars and gimbal supports are adjustable in the vertical and AP planes.

The probe is the same length as the radius of the arc. Thus, once the frame has been set to the target coordinates, the probe tip will reach the target regardless of the position of the probe carrier along the arc or of the angle of the arc with respect to the frame. This feature permits the introduction of a probe to the target from any desired entry point or along any selected trajectory. It also allows multiple targets to be approached through one entry point. The flexibility of the arc and probe carrier settings allows transsphenoidal, suboccipital, or straight lateral approaches with equal ease.

Target point determination is by standard ventriculographical technique. Corrections for magnification and rotation of the frame axis off the intercommissural line are calculated with the Leksell spiral diagram, a device included with the frame. Temporary ear plugs employed during frame application eliminate most rotation in the horizontal and frontal planes. In its current form, compatible with x-ray, tomographical, CT, or MRI guidance, the Leksell instrument is one of the most widely used stereotactic systems in the world.

Van Buren (94), in 1960, introduced an instrument incorporating the three-dimensional arc-radius principle of Leksell's device with the calvarial screw fixation and x-ray alignment features of the Spiegel and Wycis model V stereoencephalotome. By placing the radiopaque target alignment scales within the plane of the target, Van Buren was able to reduce the need for magnification and distortion corrections. This was accomplished at the price of flexibility, in that transfacial or suboccipital trajectories were not possible. The instrument was not commercially produced, but has been used effectively by the inventor for more than 20 years.

In 1980, Gouda and Gibson (26) invented an instrument, also based on the three-dimensional arc-radius principle, with one unique feature. After precisely centering the patient's third ventricle in the frame, pillars and bridges on each side of the frame can be exactly superimposed fluoroscopically on the intercommissural line. This feature incorporates the standard stereotactic atlas reference planes into the frame itself. The arc-radius probe guide is fully adjustable in three dimensions with reference to the frame bridges (intercommissural line) and midsagittal plane. The incorporation of atlas references into the frame allows multiple functional targets to be approached without repeat stereotactic radiographs. However, multiple x-rays are necessary during the initial alignment procedure. The Gouda frame has been successfully adapted to CT-guided stereotactic neurosurgery by its inventor (27, 77).

Although different in scale, the elaborate Wurzburg suite designed by Schaltenbrand in 1959 (75) and the semiportable Todd-Wells guide designed by Todd in 1972 (92) represent yet another type of stereotactic instrument. In these devices, the focal point of a stable arc-radius system coincides with intersecting central beams of orthogonal long distance x-ray tubes. The base ring is attached to the patient's head by pin fixation. The target is brought into the coincident-fixed focal point by moving the base ring as needed (61).

In the Wurzburg suite, the x-ray tubes are permanently mounted in the ceiling and wall at a 4 m distance from the target, effectively eliminating parallax and distortion (79). The head ring and operating table are independently adjustable with respect to the arc-guide base. As in other designs, the arc rotates on its horizontal axis, and the probe guide can move along the arc permitting flexibility in selecting an entry point or trajectory to a given target. Another unique feature of the Wurzburg instrument is a photoprojection apparatus that displays, in magnified form, the patient's stereotactic x-rays and ventriculogram overlaid with pertinent atlas sections. All are projected in the appropriate plane, adjusted optically to the patient's ventricular and thalamic dimensions.

The Todd-Wells device, although less elaborate than the Wurzburg instrument, is similar in principle and equivalent in practical accuracy and precision. Transsphenoidal trajectories require reversing the frame to allow access to the facial structures. A suboccipital trajectory is accomplished by the above maneuver plus turning the patient prone. The Todd-Wells guide along with the standard x-ray versions of the Leksell and Riechert-Mundinger instruments are among the most widely used traditional stereotactic devices in the world.

Talairach (68), in 1957, introduced a stereotactic frame aligned by means of parallel beam x-rays projected from a 5-m distance. The exact superimpostion of multiple holes in paired parallel grids in the AP and lateral views indicated frame alignment. The alignment holes also served as probe guides. With Szikla et al. (90), Talairach pioneered stereotactic angiography combined with pneumotomography, in an impressive operative-imaging suite for physiological and electroencephalographical exploration of the cerebral cortex. Pecker et al. accumulated a significant experience in the stereotactic biopsy and treatment of intracranial mass lesions using the Talairach system in the pre-CT era (67, 68).

The Talairach frame in its original form was designed for the placement of multiple electrodes in orthogonal trajectories—an ideal situation for exploration of the cortex, but less suited for reaching deep nuclear targets. A recent modification of the Talairach frame by Scerrati et al. (78) adds a pivoting semicircular arc with probe carrier, thus converting the instrument to an arc-radius device capable of a wider variety of trajectories. The Talairach instrument has been used to a limited extent outside of France.

IMAGE-GUIDED SYSTEMS

Shortly after the introduction of CT scanning, a number of established workers in the field of stereotactic surgery designed new methods for integrating CT data into existing traditional stereotactic systems (1, 3, 22). Others began de novo, constructing theoretical and working models of stereotactic guidance systems based entirely on CT data (i.e., BRW). Numerous other systems, varying in complexity from simple ball-and-socket devices to unique installations, hard wired to powerful computers, have been successful in the hands of their inventors but have not enjoyed widespread use (48).

CT represented a major breakthrough in neuroimaging, in that the normal cerebral structures as well as a wide variety of pathological entities could, at last, be seen and localized directly rather than by inference from displacement of vascular or cerebrospinal fluid containing (CSF-containing) structures. The calculation of instrument and frame settings formerly required reference to an atlas and mathematical corrections for target position relative to standard intracerebral reference points. In CT-guided stereotactic surgery, coordinates in the AP and lateral planes are available directly from the axial slice containing the target. There is no need to correct for magnification, rotation, or parallax (91). The remaining depth coordinate is obtainable by various methods. Ventriculography and angiography with precisely orthogonal projections relative to the frame are usually not needed. Exceptions are certain functional operations in which many experts have been unwilling to abandon standard ventriculography, and selected cases in which stereotactic angiography is helpful. The elimination of invasive radiographical procedures and their attendant morbidity obviates the need to delay surgery while the patient recovers.

Although intraoperative x-rays can confirm accurate probe placement within the coordinate universe of any traditional stereotactic frame, the actual condition of the target cannot be ascertained. Intraoperative or immediate postoperative CT scanning can accomplish both (16, 36, 62). Bleeding or swelling at the target, whether or not clinically detectable, are easily seen with CT. The presence of a small air bubble within a mass lesion, seen by CT after stereotactic biopsy, ensures that the tissue retrieved for pathological examination actually came from the intended target (34). CT is also valuable in cases of interstitial implantation of radioisotopes into tumors—ensuring that an error in trajectory, with potentially harmful consequences, has not occurred.

Maroon et al. (59, 60), in 1977, reported three brain tumor biopsy cases guided and monitored by an early generation CT scanner. Radiodense reference lines were applied to a bathing cap that the patient wore during an initial localizing scan. The resultant marks, appearing on CT images, guided the drawing of reference and trajectory lines directly on the patient's scalp. Freehand puncture was carried out in the CT suite with frequent monitoring of the needle's progress. Although this method was crude, variations in the technique were widely utilized. This "plane of target" trajectory principle has been incorporated into a number of commercially available CT-guided instruments.

In 1982, Gildenberg and coworkers (20, 23) developed a method for transposing CT data onto stereotactic AP and lateral plain films. Using the lateral scoutview capability of the scanner, the angulation of the axial slice series relative to landmarks at the skull base can be determined. A line perpendicular to the longitudinal midpoint of a selected zero slice, transposed onto the stereotactic films, allows calculation of frame coordinates of a target on any slice. As the slice thickness and the distance between slices determines the probe depth to target, the method is dependent upon the accuracy of table registration and movements. It is also important that the patient does not move between the scoutview and any of the successive slices.

Kaufman and Gildenberg (41) also designed a head holder capable of nonoperatively, repeatably fixing the patient's head in precisely the same position on a CT scanner table. The device could potentially be linked to a standard stereotactic frame by scalp marks. Of historical interest now, the Gildenberg method proved accurate to within 3 mm. The drawbacks of this kind of system include imaging without application of the frame and sensitivity to any patient motion during the CT sequence. Dependence of a CT-guided stereotactic method on scanner table readings to determine coordinates in the vertical plane allows for systematic and absolute errors in the calculation of probe length. A number of currently available stereotactic guides suffer this same source of potential inaccuracy. The incorporation of table calibration procedures can minimize these kinds of errors.

Bergstrom and Greitz in 1976 (5), and later Boethius et al. in 1980 (7), developed an entirely CT-guided stereotactic system incorporating the Leksell frame. In early models, a cumbersome thermoplastic cast was applied to the patient's head, upon which a large metal ring was fastened, which mated to the scanner gantry aperture. The head fixation device was reminiscent of the plaster cast originally used by Spiegel and Wycis in 1947, and was abandoned for the same reasons: lack of adequate fixation, time-consuming application, and patient discomfort. A later refinement of the system employed rigid skull fixation and incorporated the Leksell frame into the CT image. Probe depth was still calculated from the relationship of the base plate to the scanner gantry, but could be checked by means of a CT-visible marker adjusted to coincide with the target slice.

Leksell and Jernberg in 1980 (51), introduced the production version of the Leksell model CT frame. It was identical in

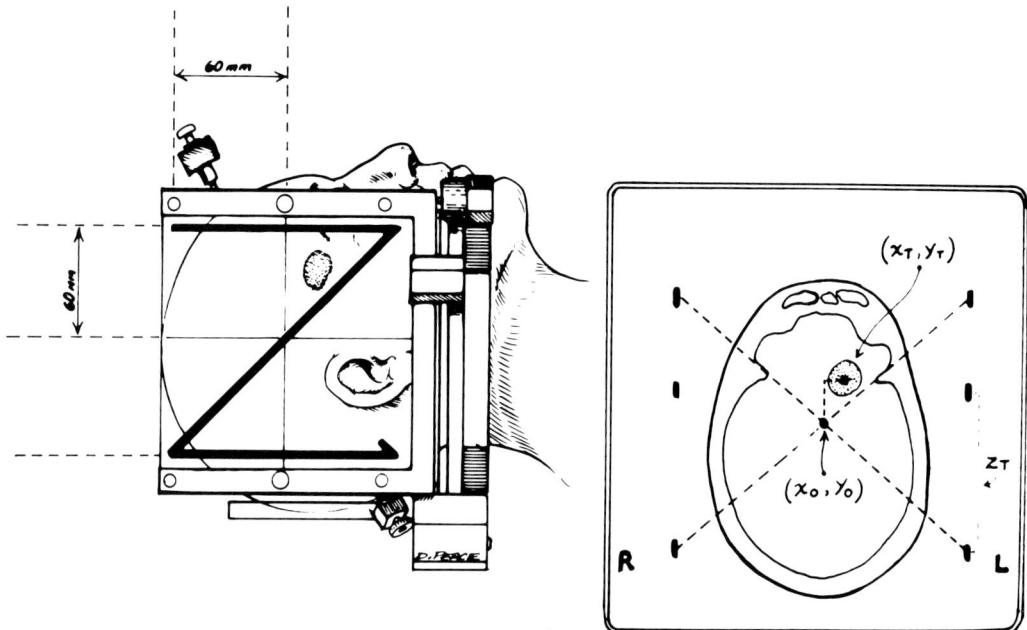

Figure 3.9. Use of CT scanner for direct determination of target frame (Leksell device). "N-shaped" localizer devices (left) produce three fiducial marks on each side of the axial CT image *(right)*. Connecting marks at opposite corners, with CT cursor, determines the center of the frame in the image plane (x_0, y_0). Cursor is also used to find the CT coordinates of the target point (x_t, y_t). Difference between these CT coordinate values (x_t-x_0, y_t-y_0) gives distance of target in millimeters from center of frame in anteroposterior (AP) and lateral planes. Vertical coordinate of target is obtained by subtracting distance z_t from 60 mm. This gives coordinate of target in millimeters above or below the center of frame. Cursor position and distance measurement functions are standard features of current generation CT scanners.

dimensions to earlier Leksell frames, but was constructed of aluminum and other low CT-artifact materials. The base plate of earlier adaptations was eliminated. Steel feet on the frame mate to a magnetic adapter fitted to the CT table. This permits rapid, rigid fixation. Coordinate determination directly from the CT scan is possible by either using the cursor on video display images or by using a transparent ruled grid system on filmed images. Both methods operate upon the same principle. Incorporated into each axial image are small fiducial artifacts produced by thin "N"-shaped aluminum strips set into removable plastic side plates (Fig. 3.9). Connecting the marks at opposite corners of the image to form an "X" defines the center of the frame in the AP and lateral planes. Either of the above localization methods, by giving the distance in millimeters from the frame's origin, gives the actual settings in the AP and lateral planes.

As the diagonal limb of each N is at 45° to each vertical limb, a set of isoceles right triangles is formed. An imaginary line connecting the midpoints of the two diagonals passes through the geometrical center of the frame. The distance between the fiducial artifacts produced by the vertical and diagonal markers on the target slice is subtracted from half the distance between the two vertical markers (60 mm), thus giving the distance in millimeters above or below the frame's origin. In this manner the vertical coordinate is obtained directly from the CT image. The use of N- or V-shaped localizing rods to define either the plane of the target or to simplify determination of the vertical target coordinate in CT-guided stereotactic instruments is a recurring theme. This principle has been employed in unique devices used only by the inventor (4, 69, 71, 94, 95), in commercial or proprietary adaptations of traditional frames (12, 13, 25, 89), and in systems designed initially to use a CT-derived data base (9, 71).

No centering of the frame or other adjustment whatsoever within the CT gantry is necessary with this system, other than placing the steel frame feet into the magnetic table adapter. The operation of the frame is the same as with the preCT units. All of the flexibility inherent in the arc-radius principle is retained in the CT-guided model. Identical localization principles are used in the latest MRI-compatible Leksell frame. Additionally, MRI permits direct multiplanar imaging and coordinate determination without the reformatting steps required in a CT data base (see below).

Birg et al., 1982, (6) described the official form of the CT adaptation of the Riechert-Mundinger frame. A detailed, illustrated account of the actual workings of this system appears in the recent monograph by Dyck (17); only the major features will be outlined here. The Riechert-Mundinger base ring, fixed to the patient's head by low artifact pins, is attached to a special holder on the CT table. By means of fine vernier adjustments, the base ring and scanner gantry are made isocentric. The gantry angle is maintained at 0°, such that the ring and gantry are also coplanar. The origin of the frame (the center of the base ring) then coincides with the center of the scan image. In this system, the position coordinates of the CT cursor become frame coordinates in the AP and lateral planes. Vertical (z plane) coordinates are obtained from CT cursor measurements on sagittal reformatted images.

Entry-point coordinates are obtained from AP and lateral scoutview films, incorporating radiopaque markers along the sagittal and coronal axes of the skull. Considerable ingenuity is sometimes required to attain the flexibility needed for nonstandard trajectories. Important measurements such as the intercommissural line length, width of the third ventricle, and height of the thalamus can be made on appropriate axial or reformatted CT images. The inventors have used this method extensively in cases of biopsy and brachytherapy. They feel that the accuracy achieved (within 0.6 mm in phantom tests) is adequate for functional stereotaxis. Recently, Birg et al. reported that localization in functional stereotaxis guided by MRI, with direct sagittal imaging of the third ventricle and commissures, is superior to all prior methods (6).

The BRW (9–11) stereotactic frame, developed specifically to interface with a CT-derived three-dimensional data base, is unique in this respect among currently marketed systems. The instrument evolved from a Lucite working model initially used with test phantoms before clinical trials of a metal prototype were initiated. The current production model consists of six major components: head ring, CT-localizing system, arc-guidance system, phantom simulator, and programmable calculator or minicomputer. The sixth component, a semipermanent floor stand for use during traditional stereotaxis, is not employed in CT-guided biopsy. It has recently found a new application as an integral part of a stereotactic radiosurgical system employing a linear accelerator.

The head ring, applied with penetrating pins, provides a base for attachment of the CT-localizing system via three indexed ball-and-socket joints. These releasable joints are arranged such that the localizing system fits on the head ring in only one orientation. Once the stereotactic CT scan has been completed and the patient has been prepared for surgery, the localizing system is detached from the ring and the arc-guidance system is applied. The arc-guidance system also mates to the identical base ring of the phantom target apparatus. As in the earlier Riechert-Mundinger system, the phantom can perform the dual function of serving as a check on the accuracy of arc settings, as well as mechanically determining entry-point coordinates and the depth to target. This second function of the phantom can be assumed by the programmable calculator, making the actual operating procedure more efficient by eliminating transfers of the arc, from head ring to phantom and back again.

The arc-guidance system is a polar coordinate instrument with five degrees of freedom: (a) 360° rotation in the plane of the

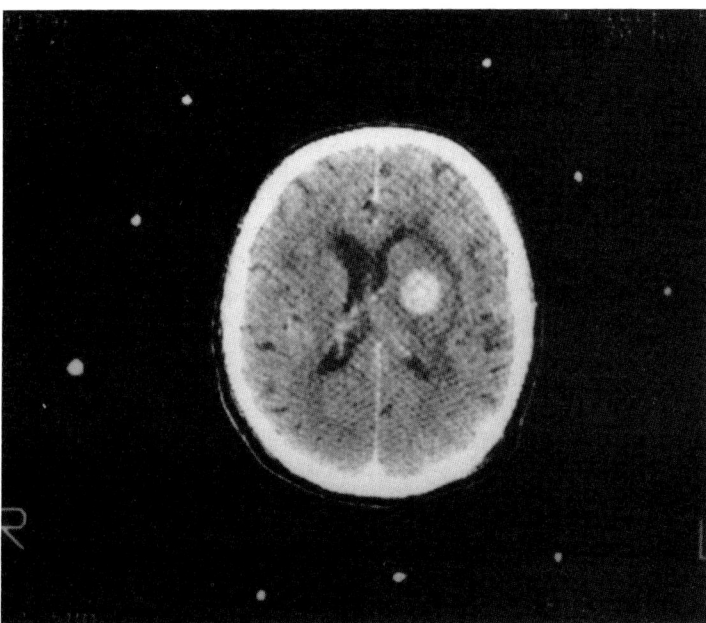

Figure 3.10. BRW localization system. In each axial CT slice taken with localization system in place, nine fiducial marks produced by the three N-shaped sets of carbon fiber rods appear around periphery of image. Once axial image showing the target has been selected, the x, y coordinates of the fiducial marks and the desired target point are determined with the CT screen cursor. These coordinates are entered into the BRW calculator, which then computes linear target coordinates (AP, lateral, and vertical) in relation to the head ring. Once the desired entry point is entered, calculator determines frame settings and depth to target.

base ring (alpha), (b) 30° pivot in the same plane as alpha (beta), (c) 180° radial motion perpendicular to the base ring (gamma), (d) 90° pivot in the same plane as gamma (delta), and (e) probe length. All angular settings are engraved with vernier decimal calibration directly on the frame.

The localizing system consists of six vertical and three diagonal carbon fiber rods which form three N-shaped figures around the circumference of the ring. (In early prototypes, the localizing rods were arranged along only a portion of the ring circumference, with four vertical rods forming overlapping Ns with three diagonal rods.) The rods appear as nine fiducial marks arranged around the periphery of each axial CT image (Fig. 3.10). In each slice, these fiducial points define the vertical coordinate. A series of axial slices forms a three-dimensional data base within which every CT pixel can be described and located mathematically. One feature of the BRW system is that no particular relationship between the patient's head and the scanner gantry is necessary, as long as all nine localizing marks appear on the target slice. The computer software and matrix algebra equations originally developed with the prototype instruments permitted the use of nonparallel CT images containing the entry and target points for a single-probe trajectory. This still applies to routine biopsy operations, however a less random data base makes complex operations considerably easier.

In actual practice, a target point is selected from an axial image. AP and lateral coordinates of that point, as well as of the nine localizer points in the margins of the image, are determined using the position cursor function available on any current generation CT scanner. The coordinate values of these 10 points are then entered in a stereotyped order into the calculator, which outputs linear target coordinates for mechanical duplication on the phantom. As in all polar coordinate systems, the actual angular settings on the frame and determination of probe length require selection and input of entry point coordinates. The BRW system is capable of several alternative approaches to this step of the procedure. Either a mechanical method using the phantom or a mathematical one using the calculator give equivalent accuracy.

The commercial adaptation of the system to use vector addition in the context of a hand-held calculator, and certain practical constraints imposed by CT scanners, allow the BRW system to function more efficiently if the axial CT slices, head ring, and scanner gantry are all coplanar. This is easily accomplished by setting the gantry angle at 0° and fixing the head ring to the CT table with an adapter furnished by the frame's manufacturer. While unnecessary for a routine, single-target biopsy procedure, the more organized data obtained by the above method allow reformation of complex target volumes in multiple planes. The recording of localizer coordinates from multiple slices (for multiple entry and target points), is greatly facilitated by the above arrangement of head ring and gantry in that the coordinates of the six vertical rods do not change in successive slices.

The BRW instrument thus combines the features of CT localization, a polar coordinate guidance frame, and a phantom target to corroborate instrument settings. The calculator software links these elements together in an efficient and versatile manner. The system does have some limitations, however. The dimensions of the base ring and arc system do not permit easy access to the face or occiput in most adults, for transsphenoidal or suboccipital trajectories. Operations involving multiple targets and entry points, in different axial planes, require separate tabulation of localization coordinates and separate calculator runs for each trajectory. Even with the use of the parallel CT scanning protocol outlined above, the calculations can be time consuming.

The BRW system in its current format is not well suited for intraoperative CT scanning, as the arc-guidance system is not artifact-free. There is little to be gained by performing the actual operations in the CT suite with this frame. A CT-lucent arc is now available for performing procedures within the CT scanner. In addition, an MRI localizer device and computer software were recently developed that allow target localization in any plane (axial, coronal, sagittal, or oblique).

A prototype instrument constructed by Rhodes *et al.* in 1982 (71) utilized localizing principles and polar coordinates in a manner remarkably similar to the BRW system. A vector analysis solution was employed for the translation of CT data to polar coordinate frame settings. Subsequently, the software contained in the commercially marketed BRW calculator was also modified to employ vector analysis for the same purpose. The Rhodes-Glenn instrument was constructed entirely of Delrin, a plastic sturdy enough not to deform during surgery, yet CT-artifact free to allow intraoperative scanning. Input of the localizer coordinates from every CT slice into this system's computer was required. The inventors developed an automated computer search program to accomplish this otherwise laborious task. Once the complete scan data was entered, the computer could, on demand, display probe trajectories in multiple planes. This advanced system has not been manufactured or used by other groups to our knowledge.

A number of innovations in the handling and display of CT data, as well as in the application of stereotactic techniques to special surgical situations, cut across proprietary frame boundaries (19, 24). Although the details of various approaches differ, some of the basic principles are shared. Kelly *et al.* used their own CT adaptation of the Todd-Wells guide (employing three N-shaped localizing markers as in the BRW system) as the nucleus of a stereotactic system capable of employing every neuroradiographical modality currently available (46, 47). Data from all stereotactic imaging studies are assembled within an operating room computer system for the on-line video display of three-dimensional reconstructed images. These may be viewed in standard orthogonal projections or along any selected perspective corresponding to a stereotactic trajectory.

This form of advanced image handling was envisioned by Brown in the original software design developed with his stereotactic instrument (9). All highly advanced three-dimensional display programs currently require a dedicated computer, or at least access to the proprietary software of a late generation CT scanner computer. This requirement has limited the use of this technology to a few centers.

Multiplanar display of CT images in the sagittal, coronal, or oblique planes is possible with most CT scanners and applicable to most major CT-guided stereotactic frames. The stereotactic coordinates of a point appearing on axial or reformatted images are readily determined by the use of the scanner's standard software programs. Appropriately selected oblique reformations in the paraxial, parasagittal, or parafrontal planes can display the brain and target in the plane of the stereotactic trajectory. Although not true three-dimensional reconstruction, multiplanar reformation is a widely available and extremely useful tool in complex stereotactic operations.

Kelly et al. have reported two special applications for which the three-dimensional display of volumetric data has proved especially useful: interstitial implantation of tumors with radionuclides (47), and combined open-stereotactic laser surgery of intraaxial neoplasms (2). The display of alternative isodose plots, in three-dimensional space or on multiplanar images, superimposed on a display of the CT or MRI defined tumor volume, is a major advance in dosimetry planning for interstitial irradiation. Irregular tumor volumes and distorted surrounding anatomy can be extremely difficult to visualize without the assistance of computer imaging. Either a three-dimensional display system or careful plotting of dosimetry on standard multiplanar images is helpful in avoiding "hot" or "cold" spots in and around a tumor volume.

Another major application of on-line three-dimensional image handling is the combined open-stereotactic method. An early CT-guided open-stereotactic system was developed by Sheldon and coworkers (37, 38, 80). The apparatus was based on the Riechert-Mundinger head ring adapted to CT. Precise alignment of the ring with the CT gantry was accomplished by imaging a series of incrementally sized pins protruding from the ring in the vertical (z) axis. A highly advanced three-dimensional display program was available, but required transport of the CT data tapes to a computer facility for processing.

The group also invented a microsurgical "resectoscope." This instrument consisted of tandem fiber-optic telescopes focused at the end of a cylindrical guide tube having a blunt conical tip. After the instrument was advanced to a small subcortical target lesion stereotactically, the lesion was exposed by opening the tulip petal-like instrument. Hand-held microsurgical instruments could then be used through the tube under direct binocular vision. The system was used successfully in a number of reported cases. As in the case of laser stereotactic surgery, this mechanical technique might be most useful in approaching small, deep lesions amenable to total removal.

Kelly and coworkers have mounted an operating microscope with CO_2 laser on a specially designed carrier, such that the focal points of laser, microscope, and stereotactic frame coincide (29, 42, 43, 45). The stereotactic technique, based on thorough preoperative imaging studies, allows the safest operative trajectory to be visualized and selected from among various alternatives in advance of the actual operation. A relatively small craniotomy is performed and, after laser corticotomy, special cylindrical stereotactic retractors are employed to maintain the exposure. As dissection proceeds through the tumor volume and the mass is displayed as a series of planes orthogonal to the viewing trajectory. The system automatically advances the image display as the operation progresses. A recent innovation displays the video image in one corner of the microscope eyepiece, eliminating the need for the surgeon to look away from the operative field. The position of the laser beam is also displayed on the serial video images, permitting maximal safe destruction of tumor under direct vision as well as stereotactic guidance.

Even advanced stereotactic systems have limitations. Patient survival after laser surgery of malignant intraaxial neoplasms has not been significantly longer than after conventional surgery. Tumor resection guided by CT images is also limited by the fact that intrinsic glial neoplasms recur despite complete destruction of the CT-visible abnormality. Patients with discrete metastatic nodules or deeply situated but histologically benign masses in important functional areas may benefit most from this technology. Combined open-stereotactic operations are also useful in safely exposing deep-seated vascular malformations (44). Stereotactic angiography can localize major feeding vessels in terms of frame coordinates (97). These vessels can be selectively attacked first while avoiding hemorrhage from the nidus of the malformation.

Open-stereotactic operations do not necessarily require extraordinarily complex equipment (74). Any stereotactic frame, guided by the appropriate imaging modality for the particular lesion, can be used to pass a probe or atraumatic catheter to the target along a selected operative trajectory. According to the individual situation, the probe or catheter left in place can be followed by microsurgical dissection to the target. The growing use of this method promises to reduce negative or harmful explorations for small, deep-seated, space-occupying lesions.

Unless one has a CT scanner in the operating room, intraoperative CT scanning requires that the actual stereotactic operation be performed in the radiology department (56, 57). One must carefully weigh the indications versus the risks in a given case before marshalling the personnel and equipment necessary to temporarily transform a diagnostic radiology suite into an operating room. In addition, not all CT-guided stereotactic frames are well suited to intraoperative CT.

One situation for which intraoperative CT has proved useful is the maximal safe aspiration of deep lesions such as colloid or ependymal cysts (76). Another indication might be to monitor the stereotactic evacuation of a hematoma in the thalamus, basal ganglia, cerebellum, or brainstem. Multiple or multiloculated abscesses which might shift position during the course of aspiration could be serially retargeted to ensure successful puncture. In each of these instances, CT scanning with the probe or other instrument in position allows the condition of the target to be checked during a single probe passage. This use of CT must be distinguished from the necessary serial CT imaging required by some proprietary scanner-linked installations. The requirement for CT monitoring of probe position in a number of simple "plane-of-target" stereotactic devices also does not constitute intraoperative imaging in the sense described above.

Relatively simple and inexpensive stereotactic devices have been introduced by Patil (66), Greenblatt *et al.* (28), Levy (54, 55), and Wester *et al.* (96). All require alignment of the device in the CT scanner such that the entry point is on the same axial slice as the target: hence, plane-of-target approach. This severely restricts trajectory selection such that certain regions of the brain are inaccessible, and no safe trajectory is available to many others. The risk of vascular injury, especially to the middle cerebral artery complex in the sylvian region, is increased. This lack of flexibility in entry point selection limits the utility of these devices. It should be noted that Patil has recently modified his device to include a CT-compatible arc that has effectively converted his plane-of-target device to an arc-radius frame with more flexible entry point selection.

Carol (14) recently introduced a simple skull-mounted stereotactic system (the Pelorus Frame) offering repeat fixation capability. Initial limitations included restriction to a single entry point and restricted aperture for open stereotactic surgery. These drawbacks have been overcome by the incorporation of additional hardware. The system employs an ingenious three-dimensional phantom (the "Gyrantum") which simulates the relationship between the patient's skull, entry point, and target.

None of the "simple" stereotactic devices can achieve the flexibility of the major image-guided systems that are capable of integrating large volumes of brain images into readily accessible, mathematically defined stereotactic space. As stereotactic surgery moves from the treatment of "points in space," such as tumor biopsy or abscess aspiration, to the treatment of "volumes in space," such as interstitial brachytherapy or stereotactic radiosurgery, this distinction will become more and more important.

MAGNETIC RESONANCE IMAGING (MRI) AND STEREOTACTIC SURGERY

The adaptation of nuclear magnetic resonance technology from the field of qualitative analytical chemistry to an imaging modality has generated interest in exploiting both features of MRI for stereotactic surgery. For stereotactic imaging and coordinate determination, direct image acquisition in the axial, coronal, sagittal, and oblique planes is possible without the reformatting steps often employed in CT-guided stereotaxis. Both the Leksell and BRW instruments have been recently modified to make them MRI-compatible. The Leksell frame retained its cubical shape and arc-radius guidance principle. The coordinate indicator slide plates contain N-shaped tubes filled with dilute copper sulfate solution (the protoype used vegetable oil). An additional plate at the top of the frame yields a single set of fiducial marks on sagittal MRI images.

Other engineering details to make the device MRI compatible include magnetic isolation of frame cross members, substitution of plastic for magnetic "feet," and modified adapters for various MRI tables and coils. The target localization and coordinate determination methods are virtually identical to those described for the CT version (53). In fact, substitution of the CT-compatible localized plates allows post-MRI imaging or routine CT-guided stereotactic neurosurgery as desired.

The MRI adaptation of the BRW system employs a smaller magnetically isolated head ring which is applied in the same manner as the standard CT head ring. The MRI localization device consists of an array of N-shaped tubes filled with petroleum jelly producing the nine fiducial marks on the axial images. An additional set of localizer tubes at the "top" of the system, when combined with those around the ring's circumference, supply fiducial marks for use during direct sagittal or coronal imaging. To perform the actual operation, the localizer device must be removed, after which the standard head ring is slipped over the smaller MRI ring and fastened to it. The arc-guidance system then mates to the outer ring as in the performance of CT-guided operations. Target coordinates and trajectories can be simulated on the phantom before actually beginning surgery on the patient. If desired, CT scanning with the CT localizer in place on the outer ring can be performed in addition to the MRI study.

Advantages of MRI-guided stereotactic surgery for the biopsy and/or treatment of mass lesions include lack of image artifact, direct multiplanar imaging, superior differentiation of normal cerebral anatomy (gray versus white structures), and visualization of lesion boundaries appearing as nonenhancing lucencies on CT. Disadvantages include longer imaging times and the current technical impossibility of either intraoperative MRI scanning or the use of general anesthesia for stereotactic MRI scanning in children or uncooperative adults. In addition, some question remains as to the spatial homogeneity of MRI images, especially in high field strength units. That is, the possibility exists that nonlinear distortions of lesion geometry may occur, rendering the MRI-determined target coordinates inaccurate. Further testing will be needed to fully resolve this question. Eventually, linearity testing may become a routine part of MRI-guided stereotactic procedures.

In addition to its use as a stereotactic localization tool, some investigators have begun to examine the correlation between MRI images, relaxation times, and histology of various brain lesions. In one early report, Leksell *et al.* were able to visualize radiosurgical lesions (inflicted with the Gamma Unit) in the anterior limb of the internal capsule as early as 24 hr postoperatively (52). Thus, MRI clearly shows early postirradiation effects at a time when CT scanning would not. Le Bas *et al.* performed extensive physical chemical analyses of 32 glial tumor biopsy specimens (50). Water content, specific gravity, and tissue electrical impedance as well as histological and cytological characteristics were determined. T1 and T2 relaxation times for each specimen were measured with a bench laboratory NMR spectrometer. Their results indicated that T1 values were better than CT in distinguishing solid tumor from peritumoral infiltration. However, MRI was not very helpful in distinguishing peritumoral infiltration from surrounding brain edema. The authors also formulated a malignancy index relating tumor histology to the T1 relaxation time. The validity of these findings awaits confirmation in a larger number of cases.

Lunsford et al., in a preliminary report, also noted difficulty in differentiating brain edema from infiltrating glial tumor on the basis of MR images and serial stereotactic biopsies along one tract (58). Nonetheless, it is hoped that studies comparing CT and MRI images with stereotactic biopsy specimens from known locales within and around tumors and other brain lesions may eventually lead to the ability to accurately predict the histological nature and precise boundaries of such lesions without biopsy.

REFERENCES

1. Alker G, Kelly PJ: An overview of CT based sterotactic systems for the localization of intracranial lesions. *Comput Radiol* 8: 193–196, 1984.
2. Alker G, Kelly PJ, Kall B: Stereotaxic laser ablation of intracranial lesions. *AJNK* 4: 727–730, 1983.
3. Amano K, Iseki H, Kawabatake H: Role of computed transverse axial tomography on stereotactic surgery of the diencephalon. *Appl Neurophysiol* 39: 202–211, 1976.
4. Barcia-Salorio JL, Barbera J, Broseta J, et al: Tomography in stereotaxis. A new stereoencephalotome designed for this purpose. *Acta Neurochir Supp* 24: 77–83, 1977.
5. Bergstrom M, Greitz T: Stereotaxic computed tomography. *AJR* 127: 167–170, 1976.
6. Birg W, Mundinger F, Mohadjer M, et al.: X-ray and MR-stereotaxy for functional and non-functional neurosurgery. 9th Meeting of the World Society for Stereotactic and Functional Neurosurgery (WSSFN), Toronto, 1985.
7. Boethius J, Bergstrom M, Greitz T: Stereotaxic computerized tomography with a GE 8800 scanner. *J Neurosurg* 52: 794–800, 1980.
8. Bradford FK: A simple instrument for use in stereotaxic surgery. *J Neurosurg* 19: 266–267, 1962.
9. Brown RA: A computerized tomography-computer graphics approach to stereotaxic localization. *J Neurosurg* 50: 715–720, 1979.
10. Brown RA: A stereotactic head frame for use with CT body scanners. *Invest Radiol* 14: 300–304, 1979.
11. Brown RA, Roberts TS, Osborn AG: Stereotaxic frame and computer software for CT-directed neurosurgical localization. *Invest Radiol* 15: 308–312, 1980.
12. Bullard DE, Nashold BS, Osborne D, et al: CT-guided stereotactic biopsies using a modified frame and Gildenberg technique. *J Neurol Neurosurg Psychiatr* 47:590–595, 1984.
13. Bullard DE, Nashold BS, Osborne D, et al: Experience using two CT-guided stereotactic biopsy methods. *Appl Neurophysiol* 46: 188–192, 1983.
14. Carol M: A true burr-hole mounted stereotactic device. 9th Meeting of the WSSFN, Toronto, 1985.
15. Cooper IS: *Involuntary Movement Disorders*. New York, Hoeber, 1969.
16. Dettori P, Colombo F, Pinna V, et al: CT control of stereotactic surgery in the diencephalon. *Neuroradiology* 23: 91–94, 1982.
17. Dyck P: *Stereotactic Biopsy and Brachytherapy of Brain Tumors*. Baltimore, University Park Press, 1984.
18. Ehni G: Neurosurgical instrument guide and stereo locator. *J Neurosurg* 19: 353–356, 1962.
19. Gahbauer H, Sturm V, Schlegel W, et al: Combined use of stereotaxic CT and angiography for brain biopsies and stereotaxic irradiation. *AJNR* 4: 715–718, 1983.
20. Gildenberg P: Stereotactic neurosurgery and computerized tomographic scanning. *Appl Neurophysiol* 46: 170–179, 1983.
21. Gildenberg P: Stereotactic treatment of head and neck pain. *Res Clin Stud Headache* 5: 102–121, 1978.
22. Gildenberg PL: Combining CT scanning with stereotactic surgery. *Comput Radiol* 9: 91–100, 1985.
23. Gildenberg PL, Kaufman HH, Murthy KSK: Calculation of stereotactic coordinates from the computed tomographic scan. *Neurosurgery* 10: 580–586, 1982.
24. Giorgi C, Broggi G, Passerini A: Three-dimensional neuroanatomic images in CT-guided stereotaxic neurosurgery. *AJNR* 4: 719–721, 1983.
25. Goerss S, Kelly PJ, Kall B, et al: A computed tomographic stereotactic adaptation system. *Neurosurgery* 10: 375–379, 1982.
26. Gouda K, Gibson RM: New frame for stereotaxic surgery. Technical note. *J Neurosurg* 53: 256–259, 1980.
27. Gouda KI, Freidberg SR, Larsen CR, et al: Modification of the Gouda frame to allow stereotactic biopsy of the brain using the GE 8800 computed tomographic scanner. *Neurosurgery* 13: 176–181, 1983.
28. Greenblatt SH, Rayport M, Savolaine ER, et al: Computed tomography-guided intracranial biopsy and cyst aspiration. *Neurosurgery* 11: 589–598, 1982.
29. Gunby P: Laser-CT scanner-computer linkups

hint of neurosurgery of future. *JAMA* 248: 1545–1551, 1982.
30. Hassler R, Riechert T: A special method of stereotactic brain operation. *Proc Roy Soc Med* 48: 469–470, 1955.
31. Hawrylyshyn PA, Tasker RR, Organ LW: Third ventricular width and the thalamocapsular border. *Appl Neurophysiol* 39: 34–42, 1976.
32. Hayne R, Meyers R: An improved model of a human stereotaxic instrument. *J Neurosurg* 7: 463–466, 1950.
33. Heifetz M: Stereotactic localization. A practical mathematical model. *Appl Neurophysiol* 38: 284–290, 1975.
34. Horner HB, Potts DG: A comparison of CT-stereotaxic brain biopsy techniques. *Invest Radiol* 19: 367–373, 1984.
35. Horsley V, Clarke RH: The structure and functions of the cerebellum examined by a new method. *Brain* 31: 45–124, 1908.
36. Iacono RP, Osborne D, Nashold BS: CT analysis of stereotactic thalamotomy. *Adv Neurol* 40: 453–458, 1984.
37. Jacques S, Shelden CH, McCann GD, et al: Computerized three-dimensional stereotaxic removal of small central nervous system lesions in patients. *J Neurosurg* 53: 816–820, 1980.
38. Jacques S, Shelden CH, McCann GD: A computerized microstereotactic method to approach, 3-dimensionally reconstruct, remove and adjuvantly treat small CNS lesions. *Appl Neurophysiol* 43: 176–182, 1980.
39. Kandel EI: New stereotactic apparatus and cryogenic device for stereotactic surgery. *Conf Neurol* 37: 128–132, 1975.
40. Kandel EI: Stereotaxic apparatus and operations in Russia in the 19th century. *J Neurosurg* 37: 407–411, 1972.
41. Kaufman JJ, Gildenberg PL: New head-positioning system for use with computed tomographic scanning. *Neurosurgery* 7: 147–149, 1980.
42. Kelly PJ, Alker GJ, Kall BA, et al: Method of computed tomography-based stereotactic biopsy with arteriographic control. *Neurosurgery* 14: 172–177, 1984.
43. Kelly PJ, Alker GJ, Goerss S: Computer-assisted stereotactic laser microsurgery for the treatment of intracranial neoplasms. *Neurosurgery* 10: 324–331, 1982.
44. Kelly PJ, Alker GJ, Zoll JG: A microstereotactic approach to deep-seated arteriovenous malformations. *Surg Neurol* 17: 260–262, 1982.
45. Kelly PJ, Kall B, Goerss, et al: Precision resection of intra-axial CNS lesions by CT-based stereotactic craniotomy and computer monitored CO2 laser. *Acta Neurochir* 68: 1–9, 1983.
46. Kelly PJ, Kall BA, Goerss B: Transposition of volumetric information derived from computed tomography scanning into stereotactic space. *Surg Neurol* 21: 465–471, 1984.
47. Kelly PJ, Kall BA, Goerss S: Computer simulation for the stereotactic placement of interstitial radionuclide sources into computed tomography defined tumor volumes. *Neurosurgery* 14: 442–448, 1984.
48. Koslow M, Abele MG, Griffith RC, et al: Stereotactic surgical system controlled by computed tomography. *Neurosurg* 8: 72–82, 1981.
49. Krieg WJS: *Stereotaxy.* Evanston, Brain Books, 1975.
50. Le Bas JF, Leviel JL, Decorps M, Benabid AL: NMR relaxation times from serial stereotactic biopsies in human brain tumors. *JCAT* 8: 1048–1057, 1984.
51. Leksell L, Jernberg B: Stereotaxis and tomography. A Technical Note. *Acta Neurochir* 52: 1–7, 1980.
52. Leksell L, Herner T, Leksell D, Persson B, Lindquist C: Visualisation of stereotactic radiolesions by nuclear magnetic resonance. *J Neurol Neurosurg Psychiatr* 48: 19–20, 1985.
53. Leksell L, Leksell D, Schwebel J: Stereotaxic and nuclear magnetic resonance. *J Neurol Neurosurg Psychiatr* 48: 14–18, 1985.
54. Levy WJ: Simple plastic stereotactic unit for use in the computed tomographic scanner. *Neurosurgery* 13: 182–185, 1983.
55. Levy WJ, Oro JJ: Curved biopsy needle for stereotactic surgery: A technical note. *Neurosurgery* 15: 82–85, 1984.
56. Lunsford LD, Ledsell L, Jernberg B: Probe holder for stereotactic surgery in the CT scanner. A technical note. *Acta Neurochir* 69: 297–304 1983.
57. Lunsford LD, Martinez AJ: Stereotactic exploration of the brain in the era of computed tomography. *Surg Neurol* 22: 222–230, 1984.
58. Lunsford LD, Martinez AJ, Latchaw RE: Stereotaxic surgery with a magnetic resonance and computerized tomography compatible system. *J Neurosurg* 64: 872–878, 1986.
59. Maroon JC, Bank WO, Drayer BP, et al: Intracranial biopsy assisted by computerized tomography. *J Neurosurg* 46: 740–744, 1977.
60. Maroon JC, Sashin D: Electronic radiography in neurosurgery. *Surg Neurol* 8: 187–190, 1977.
61. Nadelhaft I, Morgan C, Herbert L: Stereotactic brain surgery: a method for rapid and precise positioning of a target in the Todd-Wells stereotactic instrument. *Appl Neurophysiol* 40: 13–25, 1977.
62. Ohye C, Kawashima Y, Hirato M: Stereotactic CT scan applied to stereotactic thalamotomy and biopsy. *Acta Neurochir* 71: 55–68, 1984.
63. Olivier A, Bertrand G, Picard C: Discovery of the first human stereotactic instrument. *Appl Neurophys* 46: 84–91, 1983.
64. Olivier A, Bertrand G: A new head clamp for stereotactic and intracranial procedures *Appl Neurophysiol* 46: 272–275, 1983.
65. Olivier A, Bertrand G: Stereotactic device for percutaneous twist-drill of depth electrodes and for brain biopsy. *J Neurosurg* 56: 307–308, 1982.
66. Patil AA: Computed tomography-oriented stereotactic system. *Neurosurgery* 10: 370–374, 1982.
67. Pecker J, Scarabin JM, Vallee B, et al: Treatment in tumors of the pineal region: Value of stereotaxic biopsy. *Surg Neurol* 12: 341–348, 1979.
68. Pecker J, Scarabin JM, Brucher JM, et al: *Stereotactic Approach to Diagnosis and Treatment of Cere-*

bral Tumors. Paris, Laboratoires Pierre Fabre, 1979.
69. Perry JH, Rosenbaum AE, Lunsford LD, et al: Computed tomography-guided stereotactic surgery: Conception and development of a new stereotactic methodology. Neurosurgery 7: 376–381, 1980.
70. Picard C, Olivier A, Bertrand G: The first human stereotaxic apparatus. The contribution of Aubrey Mussen to the field of stereotaxis. J Neurosurg 59: 673–676, 1983.
71. Rhodes ML, Glenn WV, Azzawi Y-M, et al: Stereotactic neurosurgery using 3-D image data from computed tomography. J Med Syst. 6: 105–119, 1982.
72. Riechert T: Development of human stereotactic surgery. Conf. Neurol 37: 399–409, 1975.
73. Riechert T: Stereotactic Brain Operations: Methods, Clinical Aspects, Indications. Bern, Huber, 1980.
74. Riechert T: Combined open-stereotaxic procedures. In Schaltenbrand G, Walker AE (eds): Stereotaxy of the Human Brain. New York, Thieme-Stratton, 1982, pp 449–456.
75. Riechert T, Spuler H: Instrumentation of stereotaxy. In Schaltenbrand G, Walker AE (eds): Stereotaxy of the Human Brain. New York, Thieme-Stratton, 1982, pp 350–360.
76. Rivas JJ, Lobato RD: CT-assisted stereotaxic aspiration of colloid cysts of the third ventricle. J Neurosurg 62: 238–242, 1985.
77. Sabshin JK, Robinson F, Goodrich I, Braune ED: CT-guided stereotactic neurosurgery. A preliminary report using the Gouda frame and stereotactic system. Conn Med 48: 501–503.
78. Scerrati M, Fiorentino A, Fiorentino M, et al: Stereotaxic device for polar approaches in orthogonal systems. J Neurosurg 61: 1146–1147, 1984.
79. Schaltenbrand G: Personal observations on the development of stereotaxy. Conf Neurol 37: 410–416, 1975.
80. Shelden CH, McCann G, Jacques S: Development of a computerized microstereotactic method for localization and removal of minute CNS lesions under direct 3-D vision. J Neurosurg 52: 21–27, 1980.
81. Spiegel EA: History of human stereotaxy (stereoencephalotomy). In Schaltenbrand G, Walker AE (eds): Stereotaxy of the Human Brain. New York Thieme-Stratton, 1982, pp 3–10.
82. Spiegel EA: In memoriam. Traugott Reichert (1905-1983). Appl Neurophysiol 46: 320–322, 1983.
83. Spiegel EA, Gildenberg PL: Guided Brain Operations: Methodological and clinical developments in stereotactic surgery: Contributions to the Physiology of Subcortical Structures. Basel, Karger, 1982.
84. Spiegel EA, Wycis HT, Bross R, et al: A headholder for stereotactic operations. J Neurosurg 19: 606–608, 1962.
85. Spiegel EA, Wycis HT, Freed H: Stereoencephalotomy. Thalamotomy and related procedures. JAMA 148: 446–451, 1952.
86. Spiegel EA, Wycis HT, Goode R: Studies in stereoencephalotomy V. A universal stereoencephalotome (model V) for use in man and experimental animals. J Neurosurg 13: 305–309, 1956.
87. Spiegel EA, Wycis HT, Marks M, et al: Stereotaxic apparatus for operations on the human brain. Science 106: 349–350, 1947.
88. Spiegel EA, Wycis HT, Thur C: The Stereoencephalotome. (Model III of our stereotaxic apparatus for operations on the human brain). J Neurosurg 8: 452–453, 1951.
89. Sturm V, Pastyr O, Schlegel W, et al: Stereotactic computer tomography with a modified Reichert-Mundinger device as the basis for integrated stereotactic neuroradiological investigations. Acta Neurochir 68: 11–17, 1983.
90. Szikla G, Bouvier G, Hori T: In vivo localization of brain sulci by arteriography: A stereotactic and anatomoradiological study. Brain Res 95: 497–502, 1975.
91. Tampieri D, Bergstrand G: Postural displacement of the brain: Feasibility of using CT for determination of stereotactic coordinates. AJNR 4: 725–726, 1983.
92. Todd EM: Stereotaxy. Procedural aspects. Southgate, California, Trent Wells, 1972.
93. Turner JW, Shaw A: A versatile stereotaxic system based on cylindrical coordinates and using absolute measurements. Acta Neurochir Suppl 21: 211–220, 1974.
94. Van Buren JM: A stereotaxic instrument for man. EEG Clin Neurophysiol 19: 398–403, 1965.
95. Van Buren JM, Ratcheson RA: Principles of stereotaxic surgery. In Youmans J (ed): Neurological Surgery, ed 2, Philadelphia, WB Saunders, 1982, pp 3785–3820.
96. Wester K, Sortland O, Haughlie-Hanssen E: A simple and inexpensive method for CT-stereotaxy. Neuroradiol 20: 225–256, 1981.
97. Yamada S, Ritland S, Knierim D: Stereotactic localization of deep seated arteriovenous malformations in the functional area. Appl Neurophys 46: 231–235, 1983.

Chapter 4

Applications of Image-Directed Stereotactic Surgery in the Management of Intracranial Neoplasms

MICHAEL L. J. APUZZO, M.D.,
PARAKRAMA T. CHANDRASOMA, M.D.,
ROBERT E. BREEZE, M.D.,
DEIRDRE M. COHEN, M.D.,
GARY LUXTON, PH.D, and
AMITABHA MAZUMDER, M.D.

INTRODUCTION

The wedding of digitalized imaging data and stereotactic instrumentation has opened an entirely novel perspective to neurosurgery. Nowhere is the current influence more immediately profound or the future more exciting than in the application of this amalgam to intracranial neoplastic disease (3, 7, 12, 37, 38, 44, 47, 53–57, 65, 93). Evaluation and management of intracranial neoplastic disorders are currently facilitated by a number of methods (Table 4.1), which enhance precision, safety, effectiveness and, most importantly, often increase options for the individual patient. This chapter will address limited aspects of this potential and will primarily address issues of universal importance in the evaluation and management of intracranial cerebral structural disease: *biopsy and intralesional therapy*. Although touched upon in this section, a more elaborate discussion of stereotactic radiosurgery is undertaken elsewhere in this volume.

TABLE 4.1.
Imaging-Directed Stereotactic Neurosurgery

Applications to Tumor Evaluation and Management
1. Tissue assay
   a. Diagnosis
   b. Prognosis
   c. Management planning
2. Cyst drainage
   a. Permanent conduit
   b. Therapy
      i. Radiotherapy (colloid)
      ii. Chemotherapy
      iii. Phototherapy (PDT)
3. Endoscopic assessment
   a. Visualization
   b. Biopsy
   c. Aspiration
   d. Excision
4. Computer-assisted laser microsurgery
5. Intralesional therapies
   a. Radiobrachytherapy
      Point source
      Colloid based
   b. Hyperthermia
   c. PDT
   d. Immunotherapy
   e. Pharmacotherapy
6. Intraoperative localization
7. Radiosurgery
8. Radiotherapy

IMAGING-DIRECTED STEREOTACTIC BIOPSY

The development of methodologies of medical imaging over the past decade has expanded the clinician's comprehension of the nature and extent of structural disease processes in many areas. Our appreciation of structural alteration and certain elements of physiological disease has been refined within the intracranial cavity by the modalities of computed tomography (CT), magnetic resonance imaging (MRI), digital subtraction venous angiography (DSVA) and positron emission tomographical scanning (PET). Currently, images, although providing significant structural information, do not present a reliable histological or microbiological assay. This section will discuss methods and applications of imaging-directed stereotactic biopsy from the perspective of the neurosurgical services of the University of Southern California Medical Center, where approximately 1000 such procedures have been undertaken since 1981.

GENERAL METHODOLOGY

As the goal of biopsy technique is rapid and safe point access, with retrieval of tissue from the target point with minimization of risk but maximization of information, our perspective led us to adopt methods that permitted:

1. Rapid translation of accurate imaging data to an operating room setting;
2. Compacted time utilization of imaging areas during the procedure;
3. Performance of all aspects of the procedure using only local anesthesia with neuroanesthesiologists standing by. (This approach was adopted to have insurance of full cooperation of the patient, rapid recognition of complications, and optimization of the period of patient recovery.);
4. Minimization of tissue trauma and handling; and
5. Close interaction with surgical pathologists, cytopathologists, neuropathologists, and microbiologists during the biopsy procedure and tissue processing.

Technical aspects of these goals were achieved employing the Brown-Roberts-Wells (BRW) imaging-directed stereotactic system (47, 48). This system has been used in conjunction with an imaging data base derived from CT technique on various imaging devices including General Electric 8800, Phillips 310 Tomoscan TX-60, and Picker 1200 units and MRI data from a 0.5 tesla Picker Vista MR 0.5 tesla MRI scanner. In addition, it has been necessary to develop a close amalgam with sections of neuroanesthesiology, neuroradiology, and surgical pathology as a composite involved and interested stereotactic team. Without adequate support in these ancillary areas, the capabilities of imaging-directed stereotactic methods cannot be fully or satisfactorily exploited.

ACQUISITION OF THE TARGET POINT

The CT Stereotactic Instrument—BRW System

Point access is consistently and reliably achieved in less than 60 min. The BRW System (CT method) consists of five units:

1. A nickel-plated aluminum *head ring* which is fixed to the skull at four points with plastic and steel set pins. The ring acts as a platform for localization and the secondary application of an arc system during the invasive portion of the procedure;
2. A *localizing unit* which attaches to the head ring and consists of six vertical and three diagonal carbon fiber rods which provide fiducials for establishing the target point in stereotactic space;
3. An *arc guidance system* with four major planes of rotation which allow for an essentially infinite number of settings and transits within the intracranial stereotactic volume;
4. A *phantom base* consisting of a base ring (head ring equivalent) and a movable pointed tip (phantom target) which allow for extracranial determination of intracranial points and trajectories; and
5. An Epson HX-20 *microcomputer* with an associated software package which allows for *simple* and *rapid* calculations of arc settings and target coordinates.

Steps in Point Access

1. Assembly and Application of Base Ring (10 min).—Following preparation of the scalp, the selection of appropriate post and pin positions is made with the patient in the sitting position (Figs. 4.1 and 4.2). This is most easily achieved on an operating room table in an operating area. In most cases, the base ring is positioned in a plane defined by the tip of the nose and the foramen magnum (Fig. 4.3). Not only is the ring secured during placement by a Velcro strap, but observers at the foot of the operating table and lateral to the patient visually monitor ring position (Fig. 4.4). The assistant lateral to the patient assesses ring position and manually maintains the head in a true vertical position. The operator is free to direct the process and, in addition, infiltrate the scalp at the four points of fixation with 1% lidocaine with 1:100,000 epinephrine. He advances the nylon drive pins to the scalp and, adjusting the tracks, advances the four carbon fiber posts to set the pins securely to the peri-

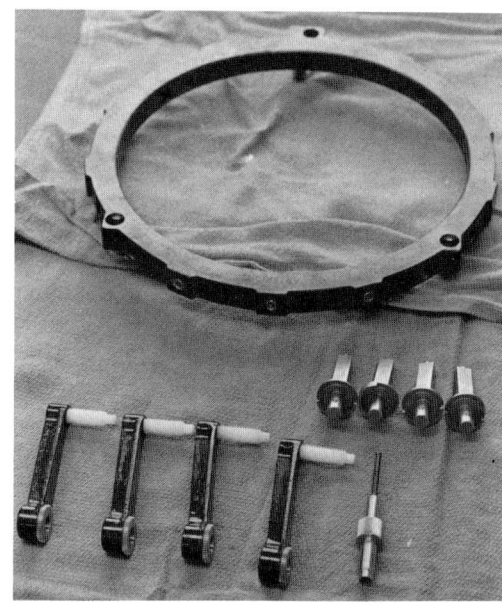

Figure 4.1. Disassembled base ring components of Brown-Roberts-Wells (BRW) system. Carbon fiber rods with nylon set screws in place are in foreground. Tool for assembly to right of rods.

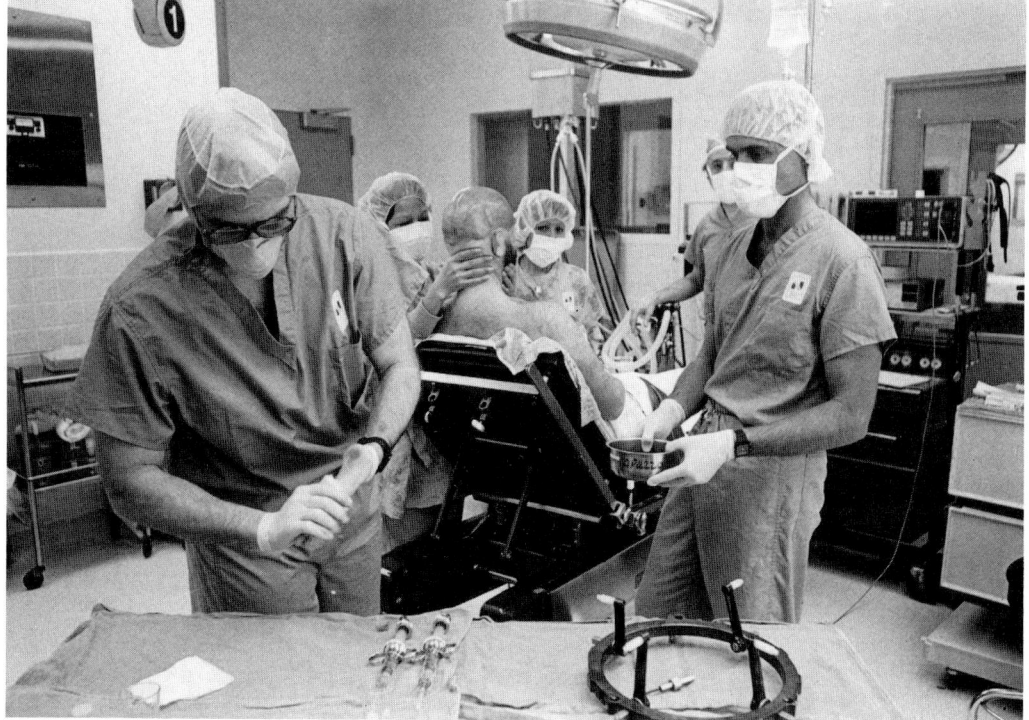

Figure 4.2. Overall operating room perspective prior to placement of base ring, which has been assembled in right foreground. Patient is prepared for controlled placement of base ring in operating room setting.

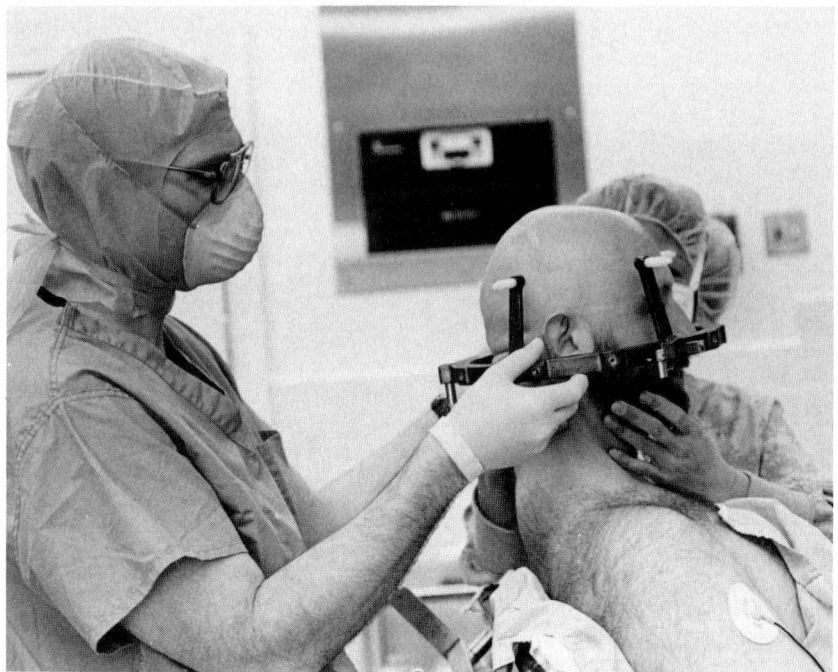

Figure 4.3. Initial positioning of base ring with care being taken to provide access to mouth with anterior plane of ring at tip of nose.

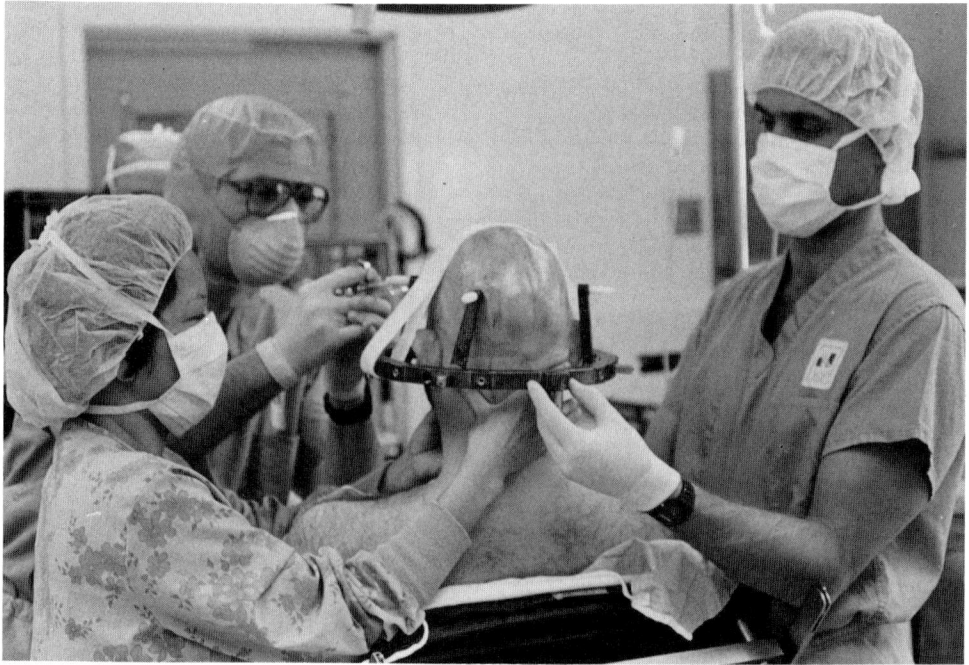

Figure 4.4. Infiltration of pin sites with 0.5% xylocaine with epinephrine. Assistants maintain position of head and base ring in desired relationship during infiltration and placement. Velcro strap provides stability. Note angulation of left posterior fiber rod. Such angulation was required because of previous craniotomy flap.

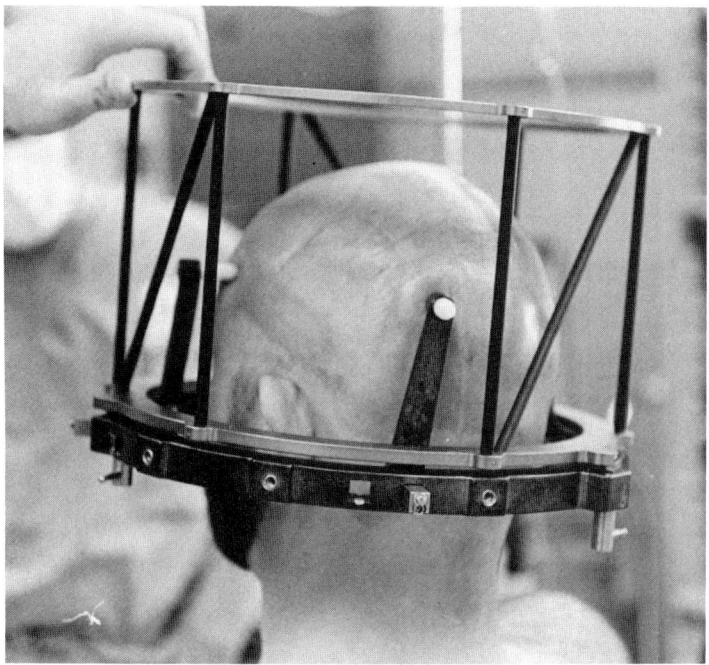

Figure 4.5. Following application of base ring, localizer system is fixed in anchoring sockets.

cranium. (Temporary replacement set pins are available for procedures that require removal and precision repositioning of the ring.) Generally, intravenous contrast medium is being infused during the early stages of this procedure. The patient is transported to the scanner with the anesthesiologist in attendance.

2. **Scan Target (10 min).**—The localizer unit is affixed to the base ring (Fig. 4.5). Since detailed imaging studies have been previously attained, an abbreviated study defining desired aspects of the target region may be obtained (Figs. 4.6 and 4.7). Depending on the number of slices, this generally is accomplished in 10 min. and the patient is returned to the operating room where he is prepared for the formal surgical aspect of the procedure where the base ring is fixed to a Mayfield adaptor and secured to the operating table. The surgeons then study the scan slices, select a slice for targeting and derive and record pixel coordinates for the nine localizer rods and the targets (Figs. 4.8 and 4.9). These steps require 10 min.

3. **Entry Point Selection (5 min).**—Entry point and transit trajectory are not standardized, but are individually selected. Entry points are selected according to the target position and may vary according to special elements of the lesion, its disposition, and extent. Entry point selection is critical for the safety of transit to individual target points. A number of points must be considered in its selection: (a) lesion location, size, and suspected composition; (b) any intervening neural and vascular structures; and (3) the objectives of the procedure.

Once a scalp point is selected, the arc system is affixed to the base ring and the entry point is marked in position by a probe placed to the point and rigidly fixed in the arc system. The arc is then detached from the head ring and applied to the phantom base where the x, y, and z coordinates are derived from the three appropriate scales (AP, lateral, and vertical) and recorded (Fig. 4.10).

Optimal entry point selection may be attained within the scanning unit. In the event

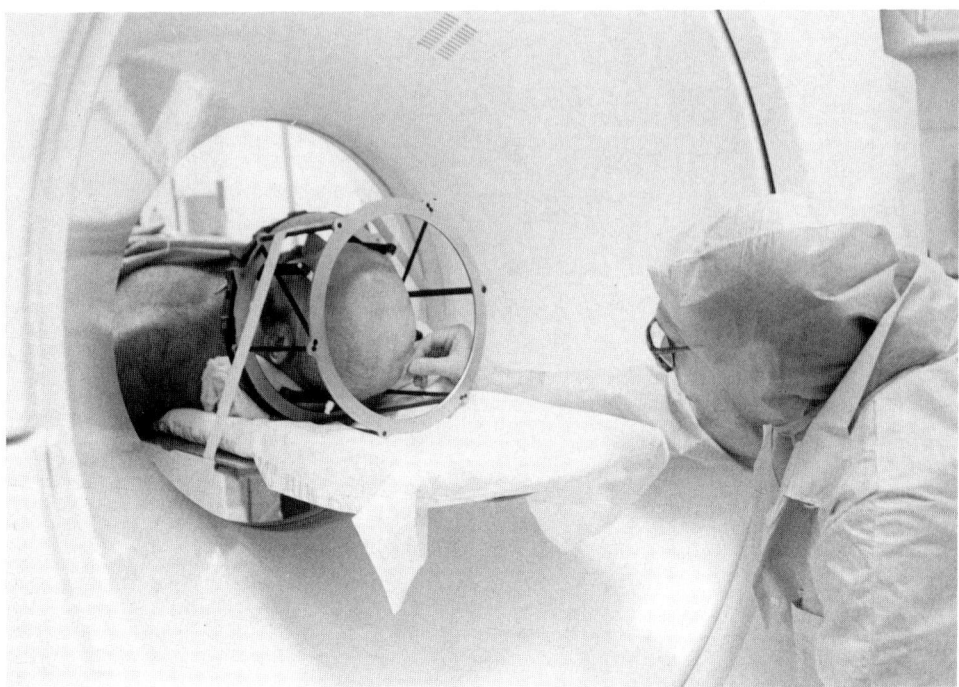

Figure 4.6. Patient positioned in scanner. Surgeon applies lead marker for approximation of entry site for transit, which serves as reference during imaging study evaluation.

that scanner software is appropriate, an entry site may be marked during the imaging and planes of transit reconstructed to the target point. This technique, used concurrently with rapid bolus contrast infusion to define vascular structures, will increase the safety and control of the entry-to-target transit.

4. **Data Processing (10 min).**—All reference localization values taken from the nine localizer rods, the target values, and, finally, the entry point coordinates are entered on the Epson HX-20 microcomputer and appropriate alpha, beta, gamma, and delta settings are derived for the arc system along with data describing the *depth* of the target from the arc slide bushing. In addition, coordinates for localization of the target within the phantom base system are calculated (Fig. 4.11).

5. **Arc Settings and Phantom (10 min).**—The settings for the arc are entered and initially checked on the phantom base with the phantom entry point which has been previously set (Fig. 4.12). The target coordinates in the vertical, lateral, and AP planes (x, y, z) are then placed on the phantom, defining the phantom target. Using the probe, the arc coordinates and depth of transit are checked to the phantom target point, thus providing the extracranial assessment of the arc setting and transit trajectories and distances. Additionally, instrumentation to be introduced to the true target point may be precisely calibrated to the phantom target.

In general, these preparations are usually completed in 45 min with additional time for transportation to and from the scanner to be considered.

6. **Final Access to Instrumentation at Target Point (10 min).**—Depending on the type of procedure being done, a number of options are available at this point. These will be discussed in the following section.

INSTRUMENTATION

A number of instruments are available and will produce satisfactory specimens for closed biopsy. The major types of instrumentation include (Fig. 4.13): (a) needle-

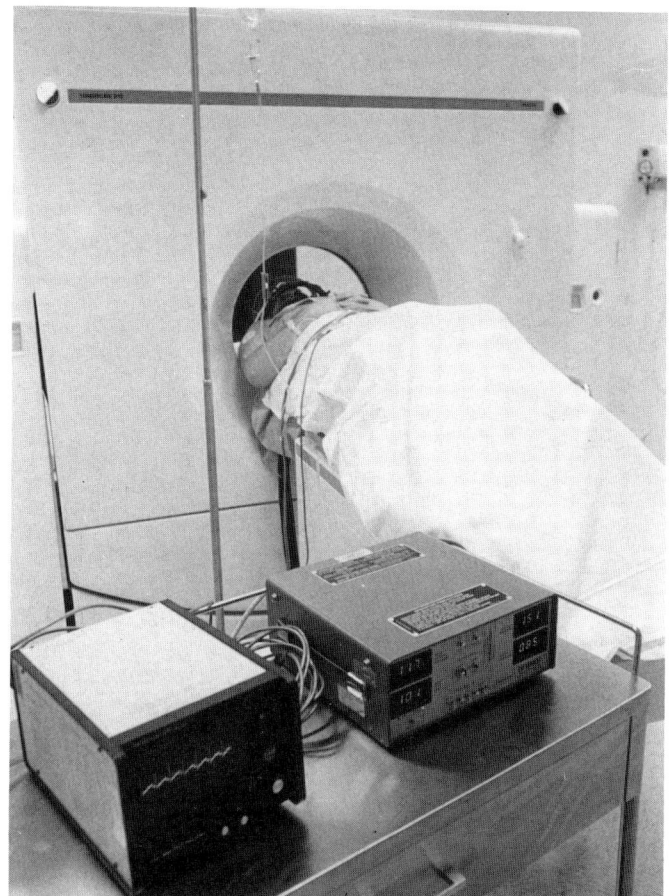

Figure 4.7. Rapid limited scan with patient monitored.

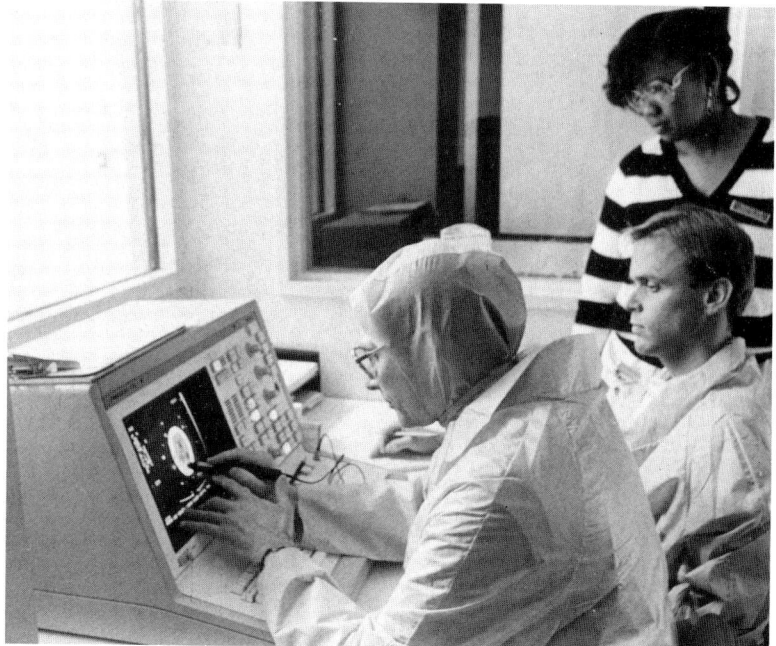

Figure 4.8. Surgeons review scans, select targets, and plan transit trajectories on scanner console.

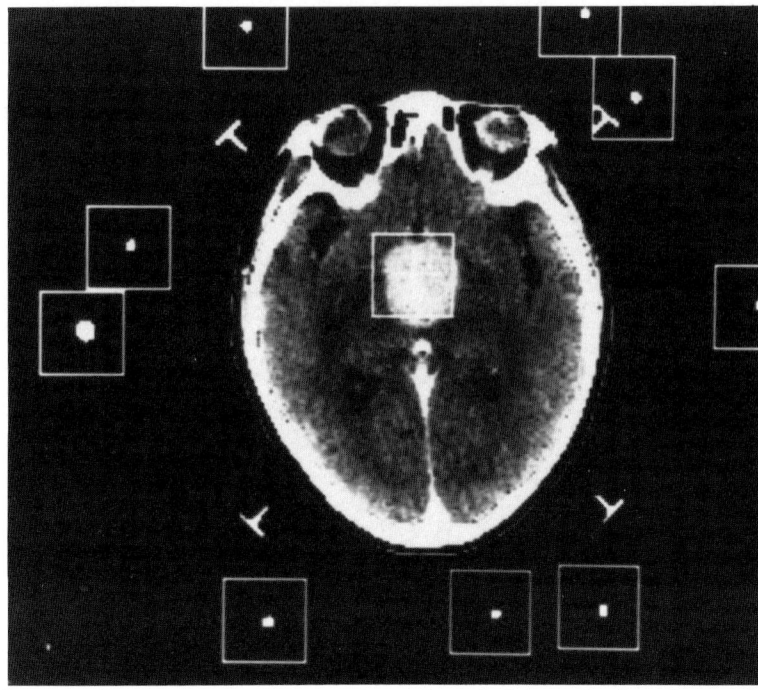

Figure 4.9. Scanner monitor demonstrating target slice in case of hypothalamic primary lymphoma. Position of nine carbon fiber localizer rods, which act as references for mathematical determination of x, y, and z coordinates of intracranial target, are apparent on this slice.

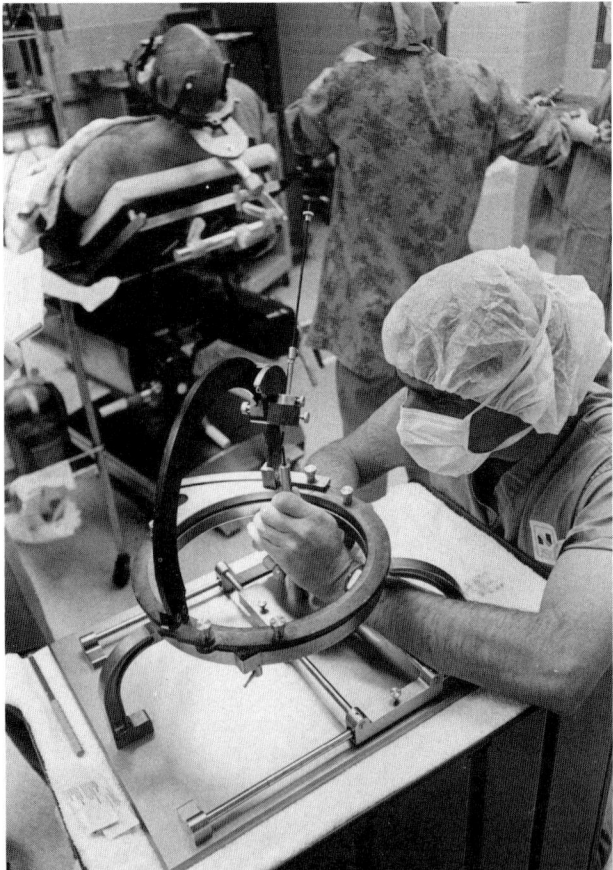

Figure 4.10. Patient being prepared for surgical aspect of procedure with base ring fixed to Mayfield adapter for head stability. In foreground, assistant employs phantom base simulator to determine x, y, and z coordinates of entry sites.

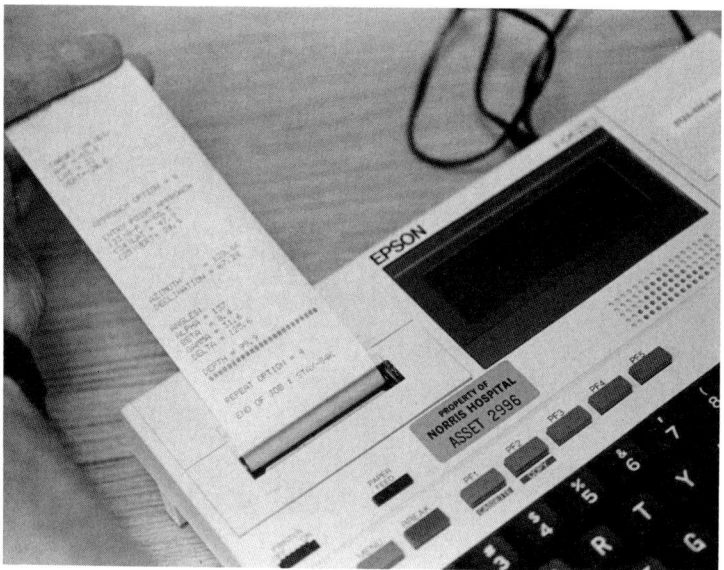

Figure 4.11. Epson HX-20 programmable calculator is used to process all data rendering x, y, and z coordinates of intracranial target, angle settings for arc system to assure proper trajectory in relation to determined entry point and depth of target.

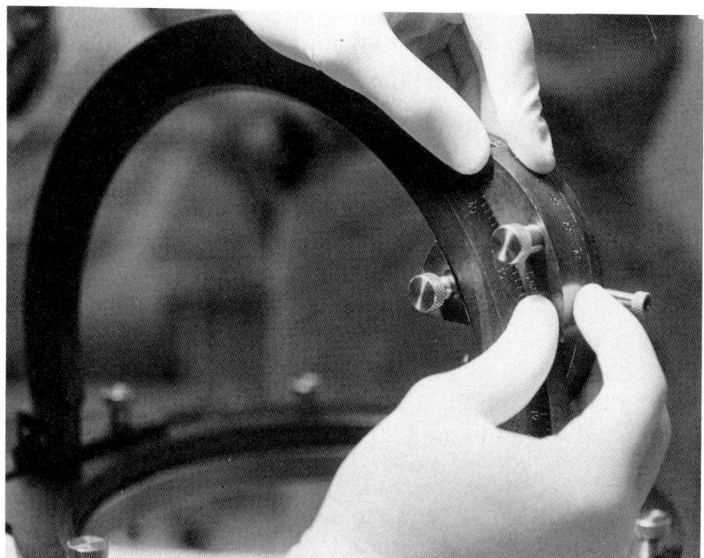

Figure 4.12. Alpha, beta, gamma, and delta settings are adjusted on arc system and checked in relation to entry and target points on phantom simulator.

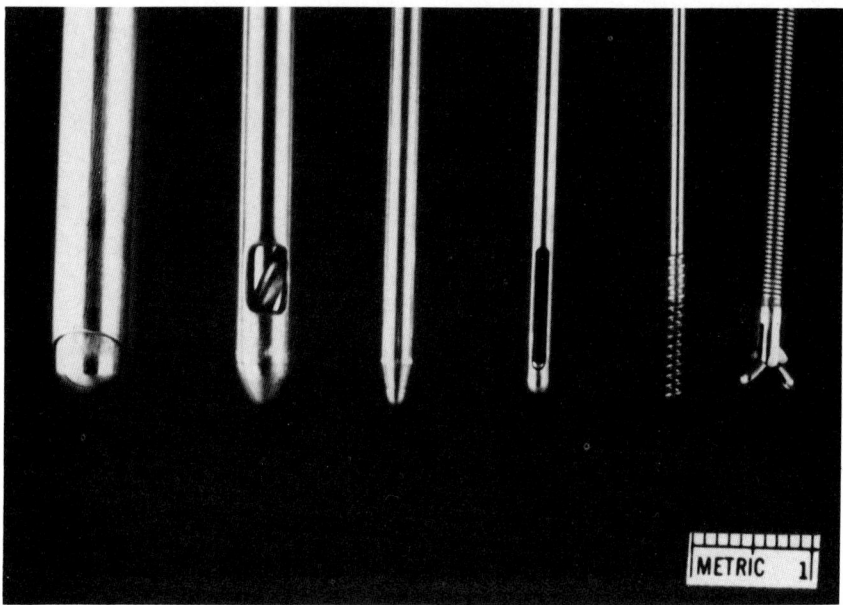

Figure 4.13. Biopsy and aspiration devices from reader's right to left. Flexible cup forceps, spiral needle, side-cutting aspirator, 14-gauge cannula (needle core device), Archimedes screw-type hematoma aspirator, 6.2-mm endoscope sheath.

core device, (b) side-cutting aspirator, (c) spiral needle, and (d) cup forceps.

The *needle core* device is a 14-gauge or smaller cannula with a stylet for entry. A core may be aspirated at the target site. Retrieval of tissue is greatly dependent on lesion texture and, in our hands, is unreliable.

The *side-cutting aspirator* can be considered a refinement of the needle-coring device. In soft tissue, it provides an excellent 1.0 x 10-mm cylindrical sample, but is largely dependent on tissue texture for satisfactory retrieval. It has proved to be unsatisfactory in our hands for firm or varigated tissues.

The *spiral needle* has likewise been inconsistent in allowing satisfactory and reliable tissue sampling.

For these reasons, we have largely relied upon *flexible cup forceps* (1.5-mm cups) for tissue sampling. These produce a reliable 1.5-mm$_3$ sampling, which is less dependent on tissue texture than the other devices. In addition, better assessment of tissue texture and resistance is possible during the procedure.

Within the ventricle, direct visualization during tissue manipulation may be preferred, especially with cystic structures that may be excised or aspirated.

Biopsy Technique
Biopsy

For purposes of closed biopsy, a 14-gauge cannula with a blunt stylet is introduced to the target site as a conduit (Fig. 4.14). In preparation for the introduction of this instrument to the target point, a flexible bronchoscopy cup biopsy forceps is advanced through the cannula and the distance to the emergence of the cups is carefully marked with a 3-M Steristrip (Fig. 4.15). The cup closure and length of introduction is determined on the phantom base target point and marked with an adjustable sleeve in reference to the rigid bushing and guide tube fixation of the arc system (Fig. 4.16).

The scalp entry point is infiltrated with 1% lidocaine with 1:100,000 epinephrine, and a 7-mm incision is made. The arc system is now affixed to the base ring, and a guide tube appropriate for fixation of a long

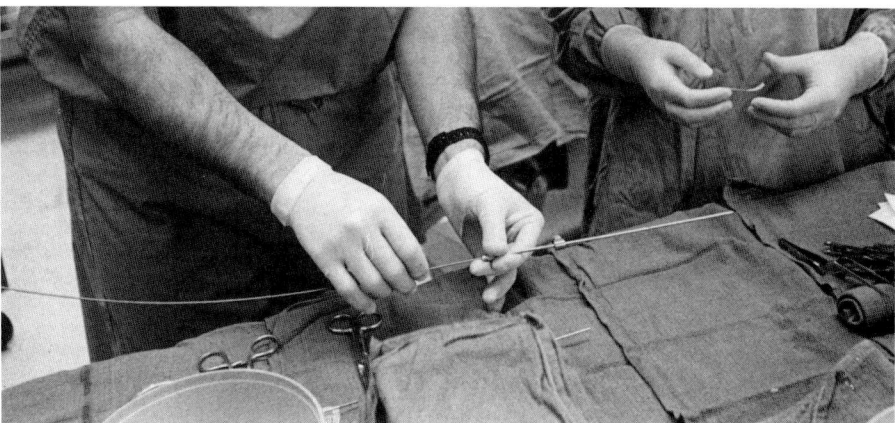

Figure 4.14. Surgeon introduces flexible bronchoscopy forceps shaft into 14-gauge cannula, which will act as conduit to target site.

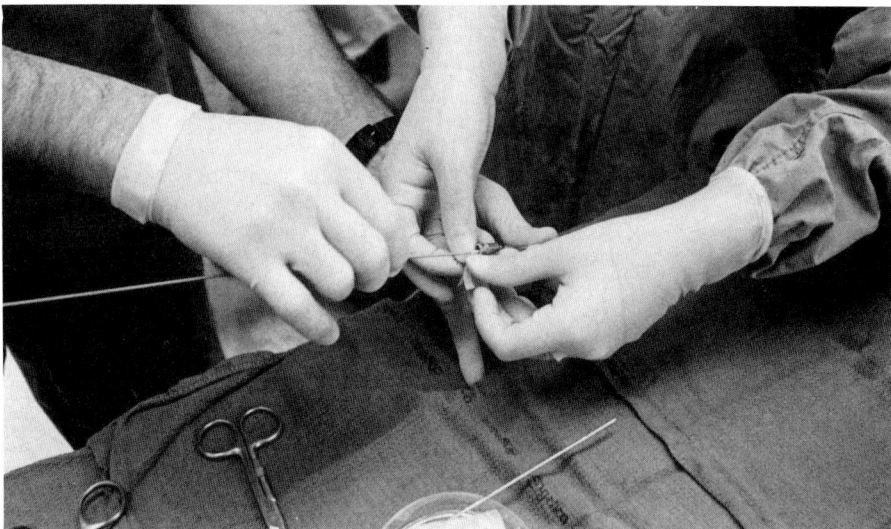

Figure 4.15. Nurse applies Steristrip marker to shaft of bronchoscopy forceps at point where forceps cups emerge from cannula.

4.5-mm twist drill is passed and secured within the arc slide bushing (Fig. 4.17). The twist drill is then employed to penetrate through the skull; the inner table is recognized by a catch of the drill, and minimal discomfort is appreciated by the patient as the dura is encountered. A sharp probe is used to penetrate the dura after the drill guide tube is exchanged for a 2.7-mm guide tube in the slide bushing. The 14-gauge cannula is then advanced to the target site (along the trajectory of the drill hole) in rigid fixation (Fig. 4.18). The blunt stylet is removed and the biopsy forceps is advanced to the Steristrip marker, opened, and used to obtain tissue samples at various vectors and, if appropriate, at various depths (Fig. 4.19). An assistant opens and closes the cups of the instrument, while the operator manipulates the forceps, appreciating resistance and tissue texture changes (Figs. 4.20–4.22). Aspiration for drainage and fluid analysis may be undertaken.

The assistant remains in the operating room while the surgeon and pathologist process the tissue (Figs. 4.23–4.27).

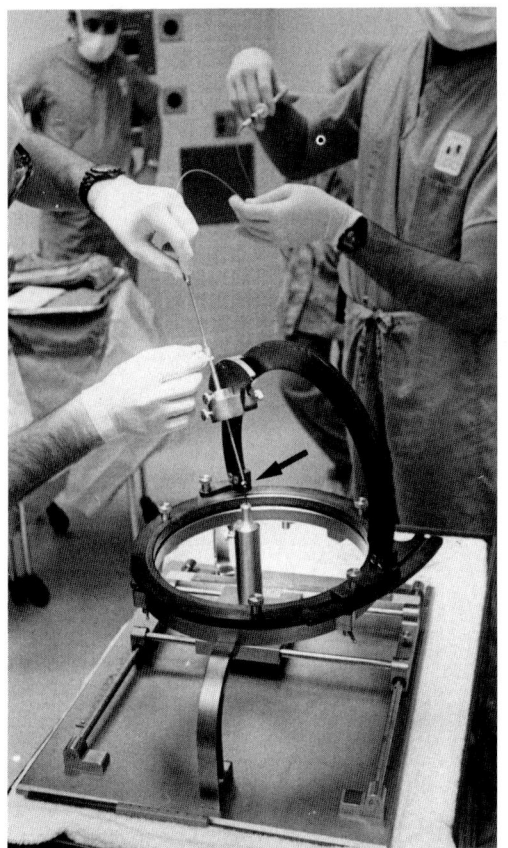

Figure 4.16. Cannula forceps complex is adjusted in relation to true target (*arrow*) on phantom base simulator.

Endoscopy Technique

A 6.2-mm diameter endoscope with a 20-cm length barrell has been employed for both cerebroscopy and ventriculoscopy (Fig. 4.28*A*) (5, 6, 8). The instrument produced by Karl Storz Endoscopy (Tuttlingen, West Germany) provides capabilities of *visualization, irrigation,* and a port for introduction of point instrumentation for *biopsy* with either flexible or rigid-cupped forceps. In addition, specialized cannulae for *cyst wall puncture* and *aspiration* are readily accepted. Submersible quartz fibers for transmission of laser energy may likewise be introduced for applications of *hemostasis* or lesion *coagulation*.

These procedures are undertaken with local anesthesia with a neuroanesthesiologist in attendance (Fig. 4.28*B*). For visualization of the foramen of Monro, a scan slice through the structure is obtained and the target point selected at the orifice. An 18-mm burr hole is then made 1 cm anterior to the coronal suture in the right pupillary line and the entry point coordinate selected from

Figure 4.17. With arc system anchored in base ring, 4.25-mm twist drill is utilized to perforate the bony calvarium in the line of transit as established by drill guide in arc system bushing.

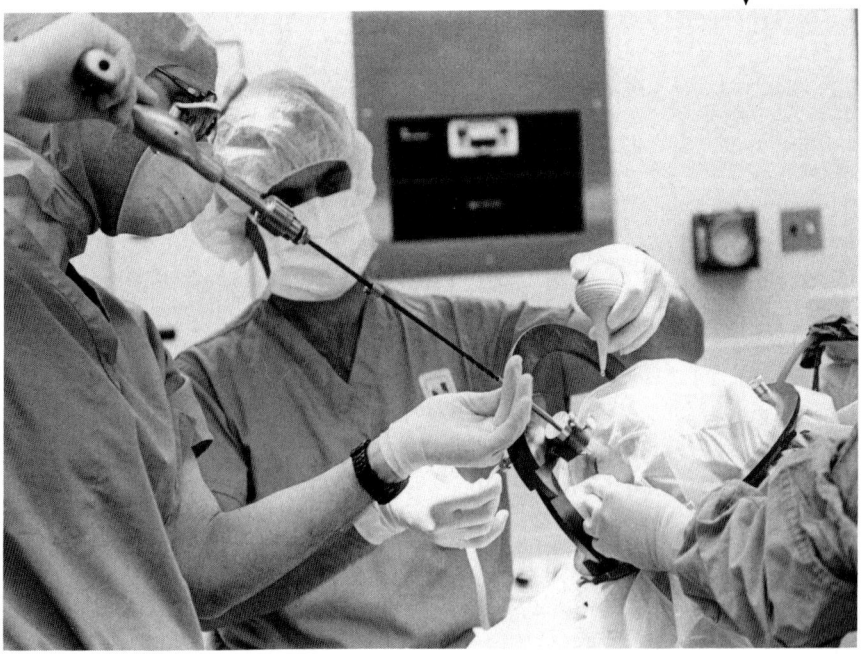

IMAGE-DIRECTED STEREOTACTIC SURGERY FOR INTRACRANIAL NEOPLASMS

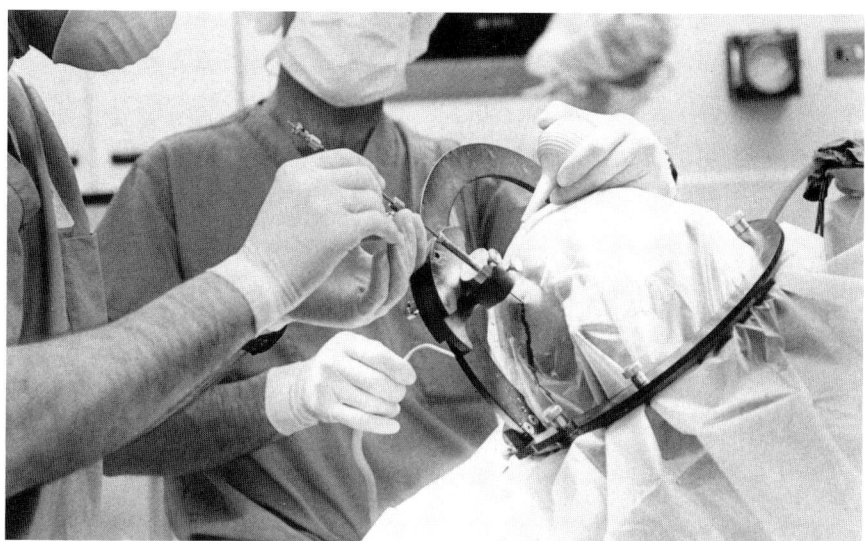

Figure 4.18. After perforation of dura with a sharp probe, the 14-gauge cannula is introduced to target region.

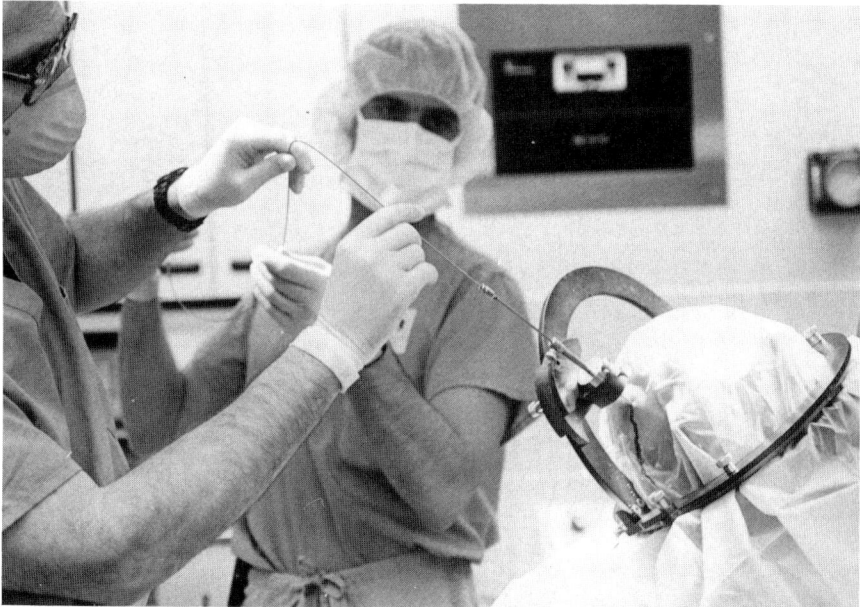

Figure 4.19. Flexible forceps are introduced through cannula, which acts as a conduit. Surgeon palpates tissue while assistant controls cup opening and closure.

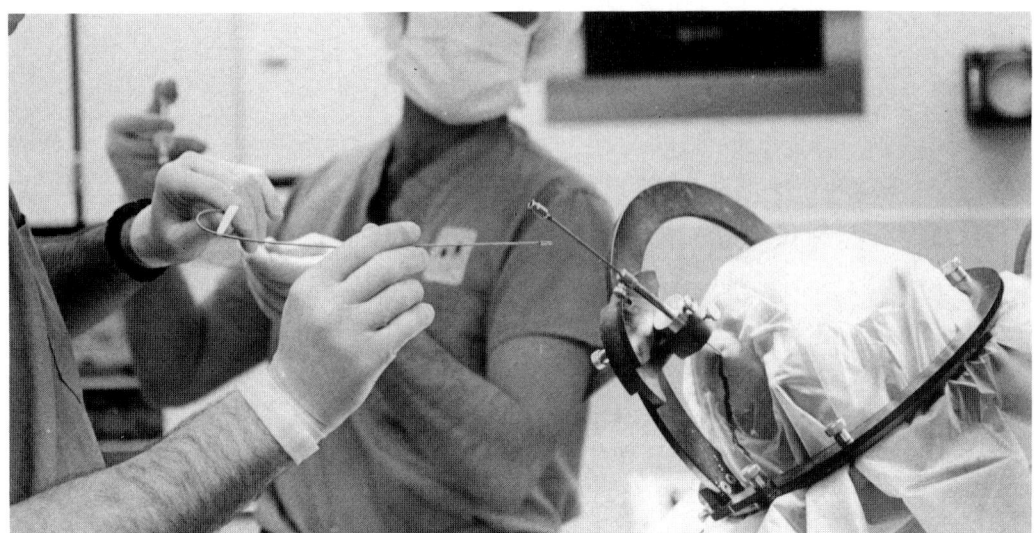

Figure 4.20. Tissue specimen is withdrawn from cannula.

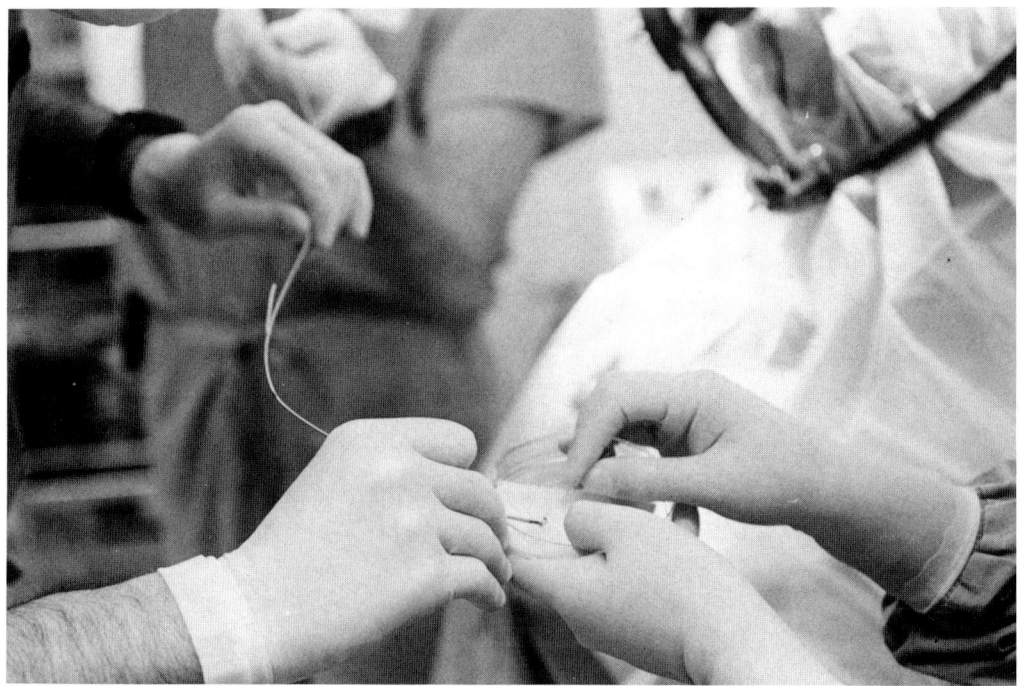

Figure 4.21. Nurse accepts specimen in Telfa- or Gelfoam-lined Petri dish. A long 25-gauge needle is used to separate the specimen from the forceps cups.

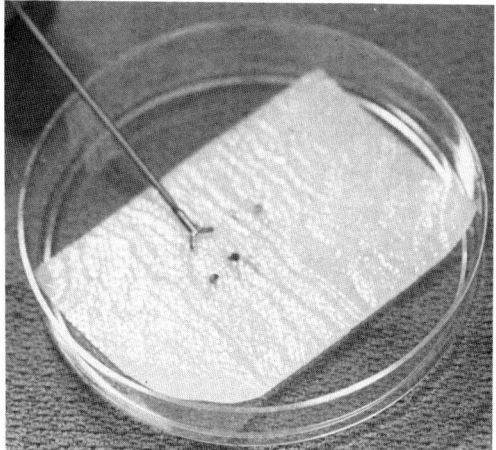

Figure 4.22. Two 1.5-mm specimens are placed on Telfa bed.

the center of the exposed dura. After checking the arc coordinate settings on the phantom base, the dura is opened and a 5-mm corticopial window is fashioned with bipolar coagulating forceps. The endoscope sheath with a blunt stylet in place is then introduced through the rigid bushing (with a Teflon sleeve for ease of passage) to the target point. The stylet is then removed and the fiberoptic visualization package is introduced, sealing the system to the target point. Irrigating fluid (Ringer's lactate), at body temperature, is then introduced intermittently through adjustable side ports. Visualization may be enhanced in both clarity and scope by minor alterations of depth and angulation within the arc system as well as employment of irrigating fluid and instrumentation through the central point.

Colloid cyst puncture and aspiration may be undertaken under direct visualization at the foramen of Monro (5, 89, 92). A 13-gauge cannula with a blunt stylet is introduced to the cyst wall. Next, a sharp-tipped stylet replaces the blunt stylet and puncture of the cyst wall is undertaken. The cannula is then advanced into the cystic cavity and aspiration is undertaken.

Cyst Puncture

Puncture of a cyst abscess is usually possible with the 14-gauge blunt-tipped cannula. However, the shape of the cavity and

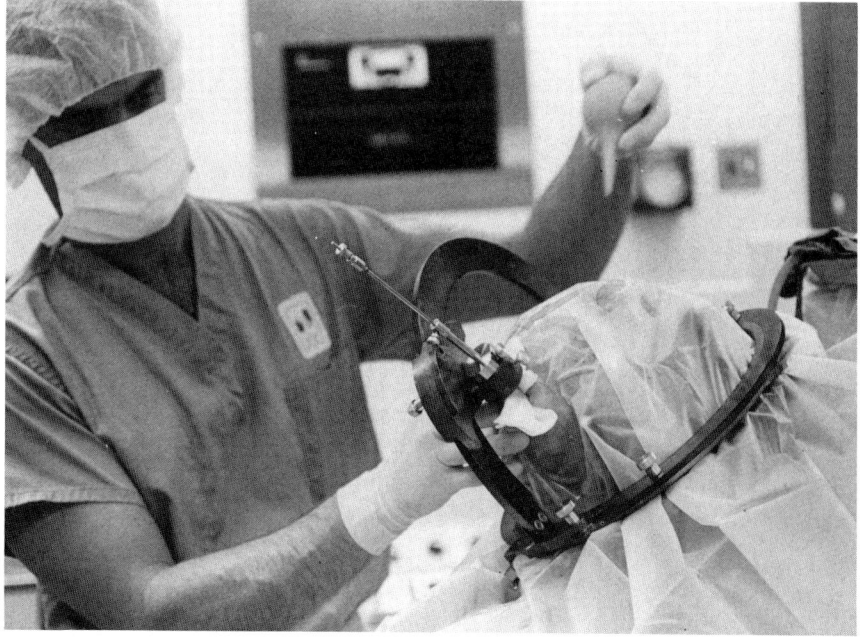

Figure 4.23. With stylet in place and entry site wrapped in cottonoid, assistant irrigates wound while the surgeon and anesthesiologist assess patient status.

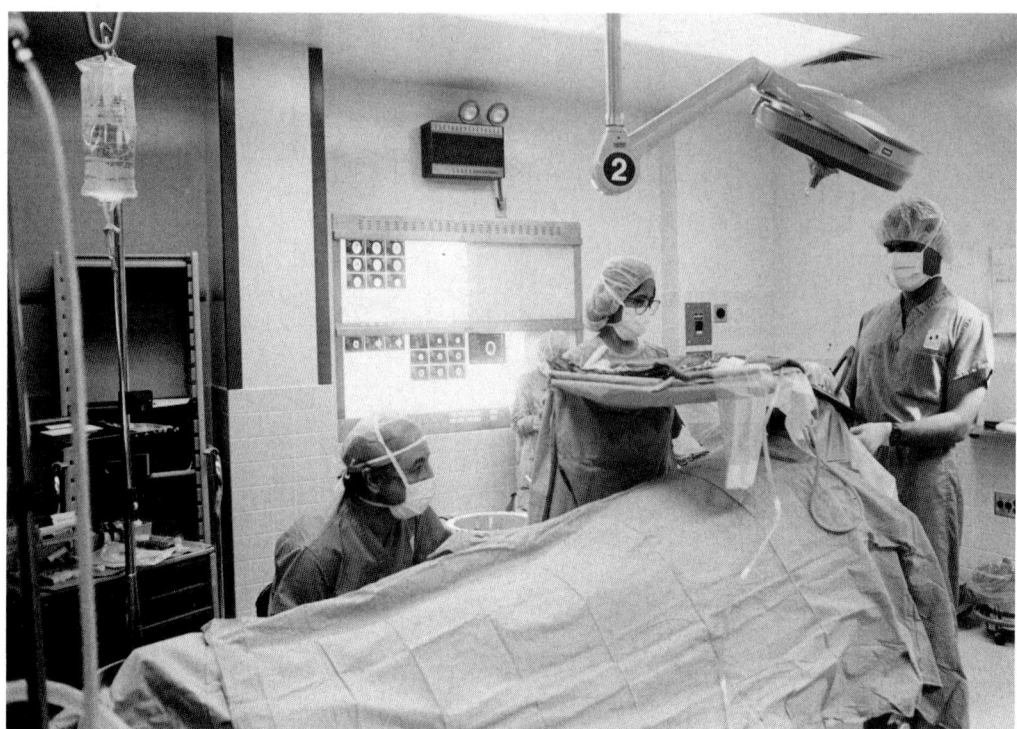

Figure 4.24. Operating room setup. Picture taken following tissue retrieval.

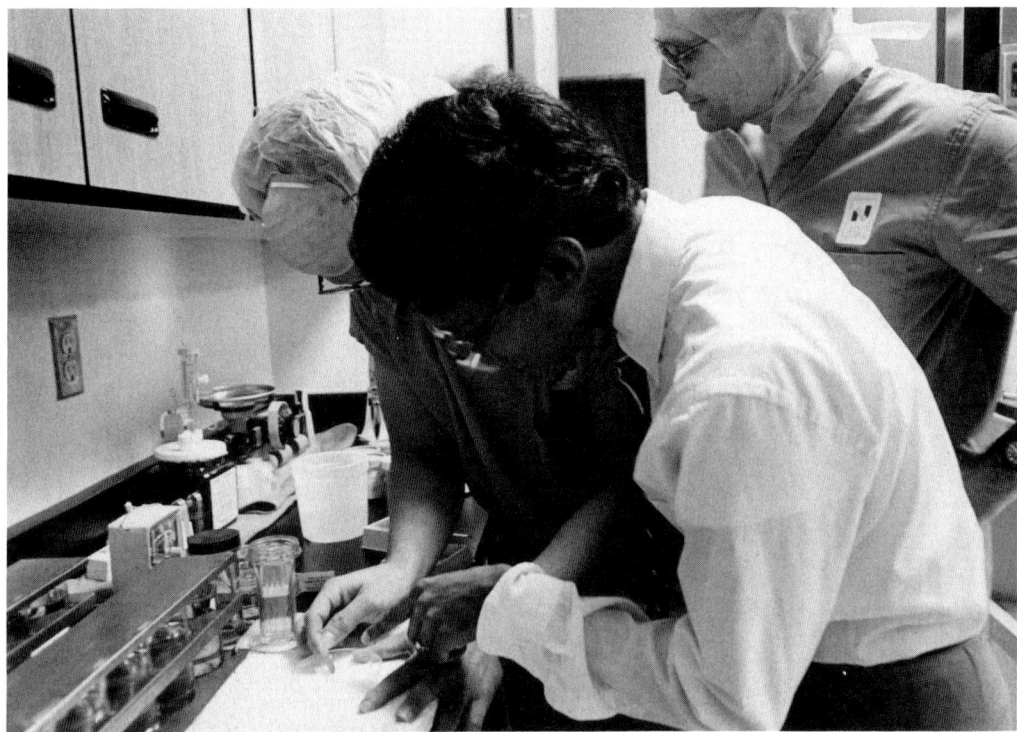

Figure 4.25. Surgical pathology area adjacent to operating room. Pathologists inspect specimens both grossly and with dissecting microscopes.

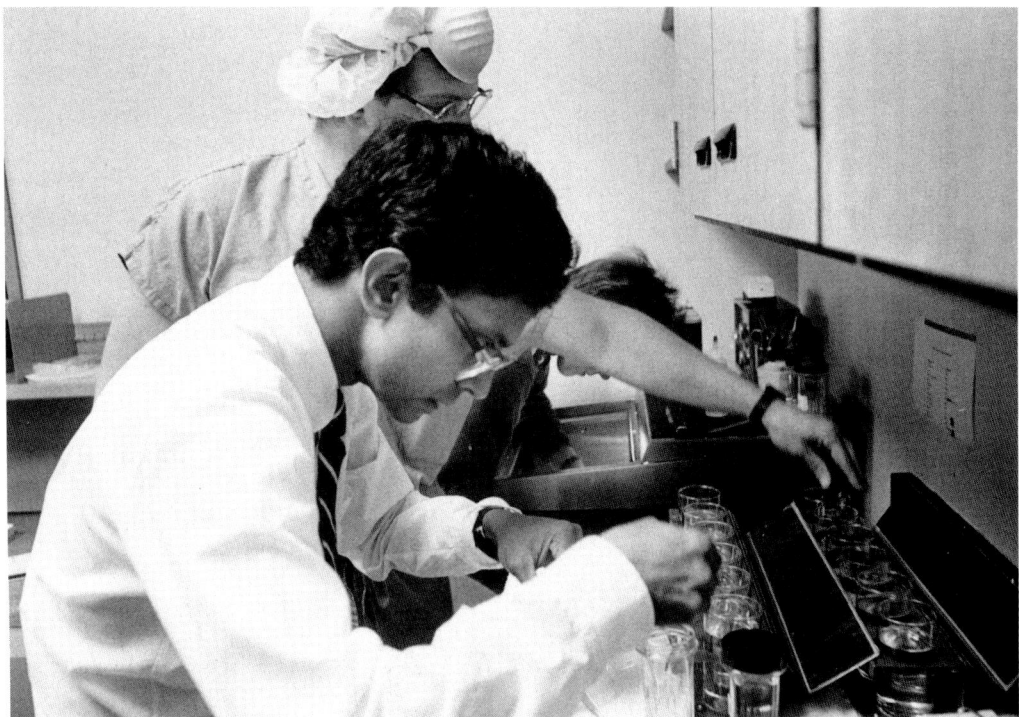

Figure 4.26. Following subsampling of tissue and smear technique, rapid staining is undertaken. Technician in rear prepares frozen section.

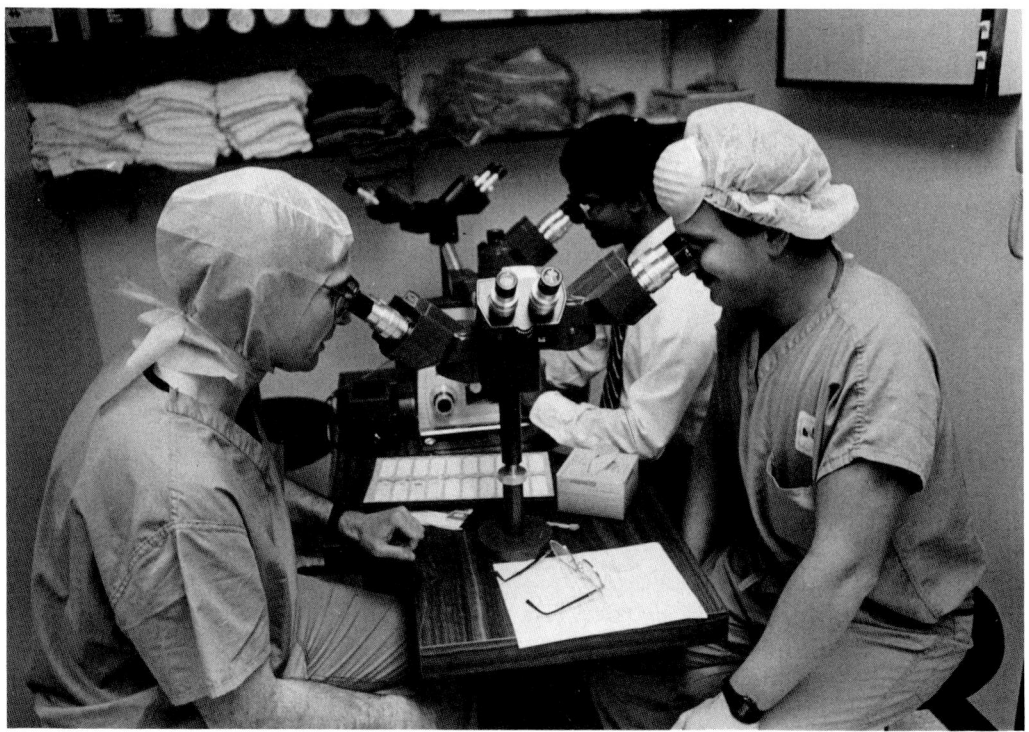

Figure 4.27. Pathologists and surgeon review histological preparations of tissue assay prior to termination of procedure.

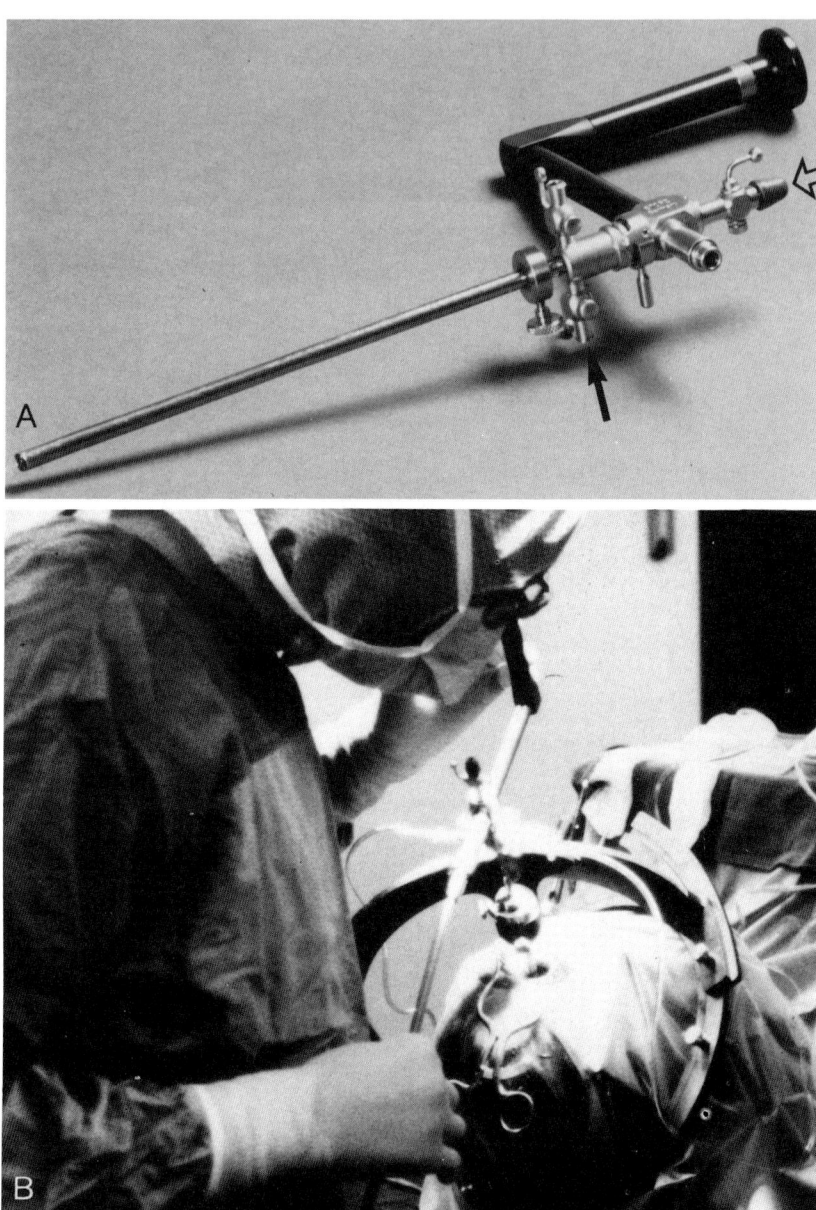

Figure 4.28. *A.*) Illumination and visual package of endoscopy system used for both cerebroscopy and ventriculoscopy. *Open arrow* indicates entry port for introduction of straight instrumentation through shaft of visual package. *Solid arrow* indicates irrigation port. *B.*) Intraoperative utilization of endoscopy unit for ventriculostomy in third ventricular tumor. An 18-mm burr hole is used for cranial entry; the endoscope's tip is stereotactically placed at the foramen of Monro. Fluid entry and exit (Ringer's lactate solution) insures excellent visualization.

thickness of the wall may make puncture and aspiration difficult with this instrumentation. For such cases, we have designed a number of cannulae with various gauge lumens and sharp, but short, beveled tips to permit cavity access (Radionics, Inc). Catheters appropriate for temporary or permanent drainage are likewise available and offer routes for radiotherapy or chemotherapy (Figs. 4.29 and 4.30*A–C*).

TISSUE EVALUATION

Stereotactic brain biopsy must be looked upon as a clinicopathological procedure performed by a team that includes the neuroradiologist, neurosurgeon, and pathologist. In a patient with a mass lesion, the objective of stereotactic biopsy is usually to obtain a tissue diagnosis so that appropriate treatment can be planned. The pathological evaluation of a biopsy is always accompanied by discussion of the clinical features, imaging findings, and specific target point in the lesions. If the location of the lesion, its rate of growth clinically, and its radiographical appearance do not conform to the pathological diagnosis, the case is reevaluated. For example, a biopsy showing only astrocytoma may be deemed insufficient and a request is made for additional sampling if the imaging findings or clinical history suggests a more malignant neoplasm.

In our institutions, the neurosurgeon carries the specimen with the CT/MRI scan to the Pathology frozen section area. For transport from the operating room, the specimen is placed on a saline-soaked piece of gelfoam in a Petri dish. In rare cases where there is difficulty obtaining a solid specimen, the pathologist comes to the operating room with fixative, stain, and microscope.

The pathologist that interprets the stereotactic biopsy may be either a neuropathologist with experience and interest in cytology and in handling small specimens, or a general surgical pathologist with experience and interest in surgical neuropathology and in aspiration cytology. The pathologist should train himself by familiarizing himself with the appearance of smears of normal brain from various sites obtained at routine autopsies. The ap-

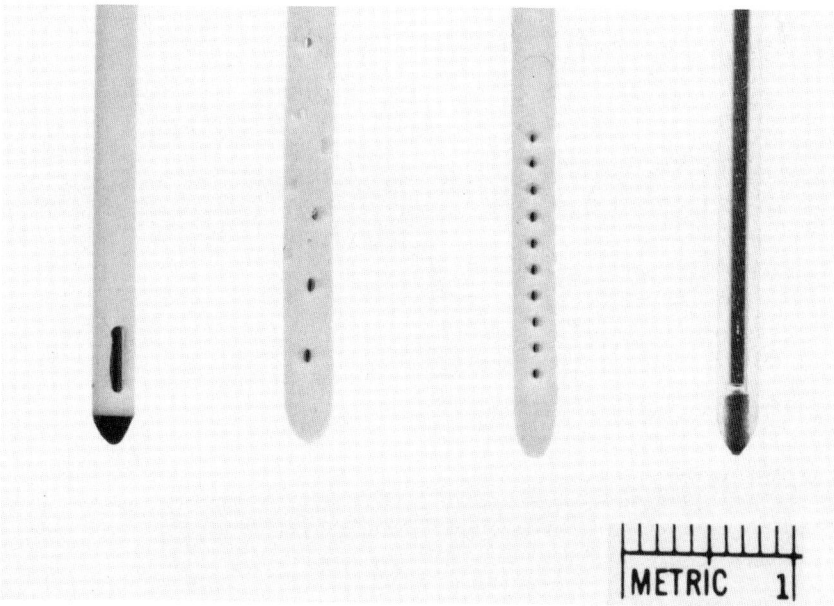

Figure 4.29. Silastic catheters employed for therapy or drainage procedures from reader's right to left. ^{192}Ir brachytherapy catheter (dark line indicates stylet in place); next two catheters are standard ventriculostomy catheters which can be stereotactically placed in cyst structures. At reader's left is a large slotted catheter designed for temporary or intermittent drainage of viscous cyst contents.

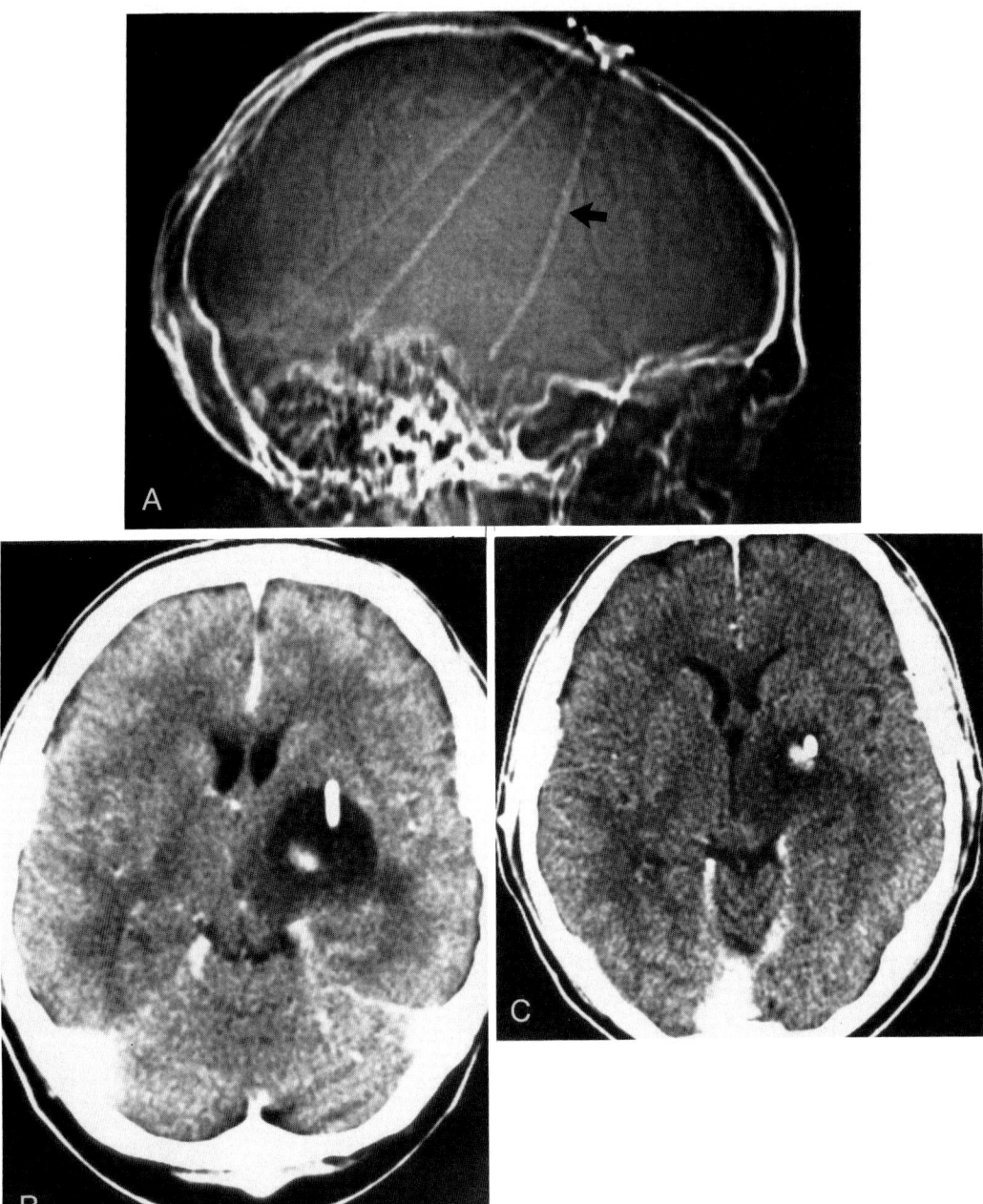

Figure 4.30. *A*) Lateral CT scanogram indicates Silastic catheter (*arrow*). Rickham reservoir complex placed for recurrent drainage of thalamomesencephalic cyst. *B*) CT scan showing a left thalmomesencephalic cyst with catheter in place prior to drainage. *C*) CT scan following transcutaneous aspiration of cyst contents via Rickham device.

pearance of smears with meningothelium, cerebral cortex, deep white matter, basal ganglia, cerebellum, and choroid plexus are different and must be recognized if encountered at stereotactic biopsy. The range of cellularity of normal brain varies with different locations and the manner in which the smear is made, and the pathologist must develop a feel for this variation.

The stereotactic biopsy specimen differs from open-brain biopsy specimens in two ways, one of which is a disadvantage and the other an advantage. The major disadvantage with the specimen is its size. The usual specimen in our institution consists of one to three pieces which are 1 to 2 mm in diameter. While the small size tends to intimidate the pathologist initially, as experience with the technique increases, he will come to recognize that the biopsy represents an adequate sample in the majority of cases. A more serious limitation is the potential sampling error resulting from the small specimen. When a neoplasm has different appearances in different areas, errors may result. Differences in degree of malignancy in astrocytomas, and variations in appearance of pineal neoplasms in different areas are obvious examples of such sampling problems. The major advantage with the specimen is that it is obtained from a predetermined CT scan target point in the lesion. With little exception, this provides a more representative specimen than an open-brain biopsy at the edge of the lesion where the greatest difficulty exists with regard to establishing a diagnosis or from a region that is nebulous in location with respect to the imaging study.

A *smear* is almost invariably the first step in processing the specimen (1, 26, 32, 52, 71, 78, 95, 113). The only exception to this is if the neurosurgeon reports an unusually firm consistency of the lesion at the time of biopsy. Very firm lesions tend to smear poorly, and we proceed directly to frozen section in this circumstance. This happens very rarely. In most cases, the smear provides a diagnosis.

To make the smear, a small piece (approximately 30% of total volume) is taken from each biopsy specimen with a sharp scalpel blade. These pieces are then laid out in a horizontal row on a glass slide and smeared using a second glass slide. The best method of smearing is to first crush the tissue between the flat surfaces of the two slides and then draw the slides apart. With experience, the amount of pressure needed to make the optimum smear can be assessed by the way in which the specimen crushes between the slides. All pieces are sampled. When the biopsies are very small, the entire specimen is used to make the smear. Both slides used to make the smear are stained.

The smear or crush preparation is immediately fixed in 100% methanol and stained by a rapid hematoxylin and eosin (H & E) (or phloxine-eosin) technique. This takes 1 min to perform, provides a permanent smear that can be stored indefinitely, and gives excellent cytological detail. We have discarded the routine use of Romanowsky stain and Papanicalaou stain, as they provide less information than H & E stain. Currently, we use Romanowsky stains in addition to H & E stain only if a diagnosis of malignant lymphoma is suspected.

Microscopic examination of the smear determines the further processing of the specimen. If the initial smear is diagnostic, the remainder of the material is placed in 10% formalin for permanent paraffin-embedded sections. If the smear is not diagnostic, the rest of the material is processed, either by repeat smear or frozen section. If a diagnosis is still not reached, additional biopsy material from a slightly different target point is requested. It has never been necessary to request more than one additional series of biopsies, and we have been successful in providing diagnostic information in over 90% of cases. Where necessary, specimens may be taken for electron microscopy, snap frozen for immunoperoxidase studies, or sent for culture if an infectious etiology seems possible.

DIAGNOSIS OF INTRACEREBRAL NEOPLASMS

Astrocytic Neoplasms

Glial neoplasms constitute the most common type of neoplasm encountered at stereotactic biopsy, and enter into the differential diagnosis of almost all biopsies. We use a three-tiered grading system for astrocytomas recognizing well-differentiated *astrocytoma* as a neoplasm with mild hypercellularity, mild pleomorphism, and absence of mitotic activity; *anaplastic astrocytoma* as a neoplasm of greater than mild cellularity and pleomorphism, mitotic activity, and the presence of gemistocytic astrocytes or endothelial proliferation; and *glioblastoma multiforme* as necrosis in addition to the features of anaplastic astrocytoma (34).

The differentiation of well-differentiated astrocytoma from reactive gliosis presents fewer problems on stereotactic biopsy than on open biopsy. Delineation of such low-grade astrocytomas at surgery is difficult and open-biopsy specimens are frequently from the periphery where normal brain is infiltrated by astrocytoma. We have great difficulty interpreting such open-biopsy specimens where infiltration of brain by neoplastic astrocytes is very difficult to differentiate from reactive gliosis. The stereotactic biopsy specimen is from a selected region of the much more accurately delineated CT/MRI lesion and presents an appearance that is usually diagnostic.

The majority of well-differentiated astrocytomas smear poorly, the cells tending to remain in fibrillar masses. The masses show a network of coarse fibrillary processes within which are uniformly scattered fibrillary astrocytes. The cells are slightly larger than normal glial cells and have short spindle-shaped, often angulated, nuclei with blunted ends. More rounded cells may also be present. There may be considerable cytological distortion. On frozen and permanent section, the cellularity is only slightly increased, and the diagnosis is more difficult to establish with confidence than in the smear. A minority of astrocytomas smear easily. The increased cellularity, enlargement of nuclei, and the presence of coarse fibrillar processes distinguishes these from normal brain. Astrocytomas tend to be more uniform for their degree of hypercellularity than reactive gliosis, where the cell population appears to consist of a heterogeneous cell population that includes fibrillary, protoplasmic and gemistocytic astrocytes, microglial cells, and oligodendroglial cells. Inflammatory cells, such as neutrophils, lymphocytes, and foamy macrophages and degenerative features such as hemosiderin pigment, calcification, and fibrosis may be present. These changes of reactive gliosis may occur in a background that may have the fine granularity of normal brain or be composed of coarse fibers. The presence of more than mild hypercellularity, significant cytological atypia, pleomorphism, endothelial proliferation, mitotic activity, or necrosis, even in a small area of the smear, suggests the probability of a more malignant astrocytoma.

The diagnosis of malignant (or anaplastic) astrocytoma and glioblastoma multiforme is usually not difficult. Both commonly present highly cellular smears in the characteristic fibrillary background of astrocytic neoplasms. There is cytological pleomorphism, nuclear enlargement, and abnormal chromatic distribution in nuclei. These features are very prominent in glioblastoma multiforme. The presence of numerous gemistocytic astrocytes is also a common feature in high-grade astrocytomas. Gemistocytic astrocytes are recognizable as large cells with homogenous eosinophilic cytoplasm and a small, often eccentric nucleus. Neovascular endothelial proliferation is recognizable as collections of cohesive, plump spindle cells arranged in cohesive masses. Sometimes these demonstrate a linear arrangement recognizable as an abnormal blood vessel. Endothelial proliferation in an astrocytic neoplasm is a criterion for the diagnosis of anaplastic astrocytoma.

Differentiation between malignant (anaplastic) astrocytoma and glioblastoma multiforme is possible when there is evidence of necrosis on the smear. Necrosis is recognizable as either coagulated pink-purple debris or, better, as individual cells that have undergone coagulative necrosis. We make a diagnosis of glioblastoma multiforme only when necrosis is present. Sampling is an important factor here, particularly because the target point of an enhancing lesion is often chosen to avoid areas that may be necrotic. As such, a report of malignant astrocytoma is always accompanied by a comment that glioblastoma multiforme cannot be excluded.

The differentiation of glioblastoma multiforme from metastic carcinoma can be made, usually without much difficulty, by the lack of cohesiveness of the malignant astrocytes, presence of numerous gemistocytes, and most importantly, by identifying the fibrillary processes of neoplastic astrocytic cells. The presence of extensive necrosis presents problems at stereotactic biopsy. A specimen composed of necrotic tissue is inadequate and necessitates further sampling.

Nonastrocytic Glial Neoplasms

Nonastrocytic glial neoplasms present as cellular smears easily recognizable as neoplasms, without the typical fibrillary background and cell processes that characterize astrocytomas. *Oligodendroglioma,* which is the most common in the group, presents a highly cellular smear with small, discohesive cells that have uniform round nuclei with a delicate chromatic distribution. The cytoplasm and cell membranes cannot usually be seen on smears, and a halo-like appearance is seen only rarely around cells. The cells are usually separated by numerous small blood vessels recognizable as endothelial-lined linear structures containing erythrocytes. We have not yet encountered endothelial proliferation, although this may occur in oligodendroglioma. Calcospherites are commonly found and are helpful in diagnosis.

Oligodendroglioma frequently occurs as a component of a mixed glioma and is then associated with a neoplastic astrocytic component. In such a case, it is frequently the degree of malignancy of the astrocytic component that determines prognosis. The limitation of the small stereotactic sample must be recognized as being potentially misleading in cases diagnosed as oligodendroglioma. Where imaging features or follow-up indicates that the diagnosis of oligodendroglioma is not likely, sampling of multiple target sites is recommended.

Oligodendroglioma must also be distinguished from other neoplasms such as ependymoma, malignant lymphoma, and primitive neuroectodermal tumors that present broadly similar features.

Ependymoma frequently enters into the differential diagnosis of third ventricular neoplasms. On smear, they present a fairly uniform population of small, round to polygonal cells presenting as lightly cohesive groupings and single cells. The cells have somewhat hyperchromatic nuclei and scanty cytoplasm. The smear is highly cellular and the background lacks astrocytic processes. Mild cellular atypia is commonly present. The tendency to form rosettes varies. In one of our cases, the smear was composed almost entirely of rosette-like cell clusters. These had a central mass of fibrillar material surrounded by ependymal cells. In other cases, rosettes could not be identified on smears except for a tendency for the cells to group around vascular structures.

Primitive neuroectodermal tumors occur mainly in children and appear as a highly cellular, anaplastic, small-cell neoplasm on smears. We process these neoplasms for immunohistochemistry and electron microscopy to increase the likelihood of a more specific diagnosis, and use the term primitive neuroectodermal tumor only when these diagnostic modalities have produced nonspecific results.

Metastatic Neoplasms

Stereotactic biopsy finds a major application in establishing a histological diagnosis of a brain lesion in a patient with a known primary malignancy elsewhere. In these cases, the diagnosis of metastatic carcinoma presents few problems. Two types of smears may be seen. The first is a highly cellular smear composed of cohesive, malignant epithelial cells without a fibrillary background from an area where the neoplasm has replaced normal brain. The cells vary in their differentiation. Melanin pigment of malignant melanoma is more clearly seen in smears than in frozen or permanent sections. The second type of smear shows a small number of cohesive cell groups in a background of necrosis or normal brain. In this type of specimen, the smear represents a much more sensitive method of establishing a diagnosis than does a frozen section.

When a patient is not known to have a primary malignancy elsewhere, the diagnosis of metastatic neoplasm enters into the differential diagnosis with glioma. Carcinomas show cohesive groups of round or oval malignant epithelial cells without fibrilary processes. The diagnosis of specific sites is possible for a few distinctive tumors like oat-cell carcinoma of the lung and renal adenocarcinoma. In most cases, however, the carcinoma is too poorly differentiated to indicate the primary site. The presence of multiple CT/MRI lesions in the brain is usually taken as favoring metastatic carcinoma, but we have encountered cases of "multifocal" anaplastic astrocytoma, lymphoma, and various inflammatory processes.

Malignant neoplasms composed of noncohesive spindle cells are very difficult to diagnose specifically. Metastatic sarcoma, sarcomas of the brain including meningeal sarcoma, and gliosarcoma are all possibilities.

Malignant Lymphoma

Primary lymphomas of the brain are more frequently encountered since the onset of the current epidemic of Acquired Immunodeficiency Syndrome (AIDS). In these patients, the neurological mass lesion is frequently the first manifestation of AIDS. Rarely does primary malignant lymphoma of the brain occur in patients without AIDS.

Smears from lymphomas show a monomorphous population of transformed lymphocytes. The most common subtype is β-*immunoblastic sarcoma*, the immunoblasts appearing as round, large cells with large nuclei, showing prominent nucleoli and abundant cytoplasm. The lymphoid origin of these cells must be established by demonstrating lymphoid markers such as common leukocyte antigen. More rarely, the lymphoma is composed of small lympocytes, frequently showing plasmacytoid features. These cases are unusual and difficult to differentiate from a reactive lymphocytic infiltrate associated with an inflammatory process. Smears or frozen sections to establish monoclonal staining for immunoglobulin markers are essential for diagnosis in these cases.

In patients with AIDS who present with an acute onset of cerebral symptoms and a mass lesion in the cerebrum, toxoplasmosis represents the main alternate diagnosis to malignant lymphoma. The lesions of toxoplasmosis are difficult to distinguish from malignant lymphoma clinically and, on imaging, both may show multiple lesions. Stereotactic biopsy is the method of choice in most cases to establish a tissue diagnosis. Toxoplasmosis is usually characterized by a necrotizing encephalitis in which toxoplasmosis psuedocysts can be identified. We have successfully indentified pseudocysts on both frozen sections and smears. Pseudocysts of toxoplasmosis appear as large, rounded structures containing numerous trophozoites. A polymorphous inflammatory infiltrate containing lymphocytes, plasma cells, numerous foamy histiocytes, and necrosis is often present. If no trophozoites are identified on smear, serial sections must be performed on the permanent sections and a search for the organisms is made.

Choroid Plexus Neoplasms

Normal choroid plexus is very distinctive, appearing as a highly cellular cohesive mass of cuboidal to columnar cells with a central fibrovascular stroma. It normally has a distinct papillary appearance. Cytological differentiation of papillomas from normal choroid plexus is very difficult and requires extreme confidence in the accurate CT/MRI localization of the target point. Choroid plexus carcinoma presents with the features of a mucinous adenocarcinoma.

Pineal Neoplasms

Pineal neoplasms represent a very important group of neoplasms in the region of the third ventricle. They may be troublesome because of their frequent polymorphism and may cause sampling errors (98).

Germinomas show a typical dual population of germ cells and lymphocytes on smears. The germ cells appear as highly active-looking, large, round cells with central nuclei. Cytological atypia and mitotic activity are present. While not appearing cohesive, the cells tend not to separate extensively. Interspersed among these large cells are numerous small lymphocytes and collagenous bands of varying thickness. One germinoma in our series presented the greatest difficulty among all our cases. Two separate stereotactic biopsies showed chronic inflammatory cells on smear and epithelioid granulomas on sections. Although the culture was negative, the patient had an unsuccessful trial of antituberculous therapy before the diagnosis was made on open biopsy. The germinoma had areas of extensive granulomatous inflammation leading to a sampling error at stereotactic biopsy.

Pineal germ cell tumors are frequently mixed, with *teratoma, embryonal carcinoma, choriocarcinoma, and yolk sac carcinoma* present in varying amounts. This presents obvious sampling problems. It must be noted that germinomas and other germ cell tumors can occur in the floor of the third ventricle ("ectopic pinealoma"). Serum and cerebrospinal fluid (CSF) assays for β-*human chorionic gonadotrophin (β-HCG) and alphafetoprotein* should be performed in all pineal neoplasms (2, 10, 19, 29, 45, 58). We recently encountered a case of a pineal germ cell neoplasm that had elevated levels of β-HCG in both serum and CSF. On stereotactic biopsy, which was accompanied by minor hemorrhage, there were primitive large cells resembling embryonal carcinoma and large syncytiotrophoblastic giant cells.

Pineal parenchymal neoplasms also present problems. *Pineocytomas* are characterized by a uniform population of round, discohesive cells with scant cytoplasm arranged around masses of collagen. On sections, the uniform round cells are separated into nests by fibrovascular structures.

Pineoblastomas are neoplasms mainly in children and composed of very primitive, intermediate-sized cells that tend to form cohesive groups. The cells have hyperchromatic nuclei, scanty cytoplasm, and tend to show nuclear molding. Extensive necrosis and a high mitotic rate is common. We have encountered neoplasms of pineal parenchymal cells in adults that demonstrate features of both pineocytoma and pineoblastoma on smear. We use the term *malignant pineocytoma* for these adult neoplasms that present cytological evidence of anaplasia.

Meningioma

Meningioma is rarely encountered at stereotactic biopsy, because the diagnosis is usually apparent by clinical and imaging studies, and the patient proceeds directly to craniotomy. Meningioma may rarely be encountered as an intraventricular neoplasm.

On smear, meningiomas are highly cellular and composed of meningothelial cells. These are easily recognizable as plump spindle cells with central nuclei and abundant pink cytoplasm. The cells present as cohesive groups with numerous single cells. While they usually present a very regular cytological appearance, considerable cytological atypia is not uncommon. Enlargement of cells, pleomorphism, nuclear chromatic abnormalities, and rare mitotic figures may be seen. Tight whorls are seen in most cases. Psammoma bodies are seen in a few cases. Foamy histiocytes are common and correlate well with xanthomatous degeneration. The background material is usually scant. While we evaluate cytological atypia in meningiomas and include these in our report, we do not attempt to predict biological behavior on the basis of smears. In a few cases, extreme atypia on smear has correlated with malignancy. We also do not attempt to classify meningiomas according to histological subtypes on the small stereotactic sample.

Pituitary Adenoma

Such tumors are usually obvious on imaging studies and stereotactic biopsy is rarely undertaken. On smears, cells from pituitary adenomas appear as small, discohesive round cells with delicate nuclei and a variable amount of cytoplasm. Those lesions that are invasive tend to have greater degrees of cytological atypia.

Craniopharyngioma

The cytological identification of craniopharyngioma depends on the presence of squamous epithelial elements. Tissue from solid areas shows large cohesive sheets of benign squamous epithelium. Considerable cytological atypia may be present. Smears from cystic areas show anucleate squames. Examination of fresh smears made from the oily fluid under polarized light for the presence of cholesterol crystals is a useful diagnostic maneuver. Calcification is very common, both on smears and permanent sections, and is helpful in making a diagnosis in a cystic lesion of the third ventricle. Correlation of CT scan and clinical features precludes confusion with well-differentiated metastatic squamous carcinoma, which may be suggested when cytological atypia is present. Distinction from an epidermoid or dermoid cyst is impossible on the smear, although the CT appearance of a solid component to the mass would suggest craniopharyngioma.

Colloid Cyst

Colloid cysts of the third ventricle enter into the differential diagnosis of a cystic lesion, which also includes cystic craniopharyngioma, epidermoid and dermoid cysts, and cysticercosis. Colloid cysts are characterized by their epithelial lining, which is usually cuboidal or columnar and may be ciliated, and their gelatinous contents. Smears from the cyst wall show columnar epithelium that resembles choroid plexus epithelium. In one of our cases, there was marked cytological atypia and increased mitotic activity. Histological examination of this case showed the epithelial lining to be three to four layers thick without any invasive tendency. Smears of cyst contents do not have any diagnostic characteristics.

Immunohistochemistry in Diagnosis

The availability of numerous tumor markers has facilitated specific diagnosis in many cases, and it is important to use this tool whenever it increases diagnostic certainty (Table 4.2). While a large number of tumor markers has become available, relatively few of them are sufficiently reliable for routine clinical use. We rarely use glial-fibrillary acidic protein (GFAP) to confirm the diagnosis of an astrocytoma because the smear features of most of these are diagnostic. We use lymphoid markers routinely to establish the lymphoid nature of a malignant lymphoma, and process tissue for monoclonal light-chain studies when we encounter any atypical lymphoid proliferation. Keratin is useful in those cases in which there is any doubt as to the epithelial nature of a metastasis and we employ it frequently. Alpha-fetoprotein and β-HCG are useful in pineal germ cell neoplasms. S100 protein is a very nonspecific antigen present in a variety of cell types. Its greatest use is in the diagnosis of a metastatic neoplasm, such as malignant melanoma as most melanomas will stain positively for S100 protein and negatively for keratin.

TABLE 4.2.
Immunohistochemical Markers in Diagnosis of Brain Tumors

Marker	Neoplasm	Material Required
Gliofibrillary acidic protein	Astrocyte	Smears, frozen, or paraffin sections
Common leukocyte antigen, other lymphoid markers	Lymphoid cells	Smears, paraffin sections (B_5-fixation)
Kappa, lambda chain (monoclonality)	β-lymphocyte	Smears and frozen section
Keratin intermediate filaments	Carcinomas	Smears and paraffin sections
S_{100} protein	Neuroectodermal cells, melanoma	Paraffin sections
Alphafetoprotein	Embryonal carcinoma and yolk sac carcinoma	Paraffin sections
β-HCG	Choriocarcinoma	Paraffin sections

When it is decided that immunohistochemical studies are necessary at the time of stereotactic biopsy interpretation, we process the tissue accordingly. B5 fixation and frozen sections are necessary for lymphoid markers. For other markers, paraffin sections are adequate, but we instruct the histopathology department to serial section the tissue at the time of cutting to make maximum use of the small amount of tissue that is available. In cases where immunohistochemistry is thought to be vital for diagnosis, the procurement of more tissue may be requested.

EXPECTATIONS AND PROBLEMS

As noted, diagnostic material should be expected in greater than 90% of samplings, in a detailed review of our first 500 cases (95.6%). This rate was achieved with a mortality rate of 0.2%, 741 targets, greater than 2000 specimens, and a complication rate of 1%. These data approximate the experience of other groups with extensive experience and serious interest in developing expertise in these methods.

Failed diagnosis has occurred in less than 5% of cases. Normal tissue indicating a targeting error was never encountered. Of the nondiagnostic retrievals, *necrosis* was evident in 45%. This problem can be avoided if targets are selected within regions of contrast enhancement. However, secondary targets have yielded reactive tissue or nuclei without sufficient cytoplasmic detail to allow specific diagnosis.

Inflammatory response of a nonspecific nature was encountered in 41% of the nondiagnostic group of cases. In each of these, the tissue demonstrated regions of infiltration with combinations of inflammatory cells without associated architectural alteration or agent identification with exhaustive staining, culture, or electron microscopy techniques. These processes were most often multifocal on imaging studies and most often involved both gray and white regions.

Remaining problems were related to failures to identify specific agents in *granulomas,* failures to satisfactorily perforate *cystic lesions,* and inadequacy of sampling in a *pineal region tumor* (98). In the case of an intraaxial pineal region germ cell tumor, mixed components were not specifically identified with precision in the circumstance of normal biochemical markers. Multiple-target biopsy is recommended for all potential germ cell tumors even in the presence of normal serum and CSF markers.

CASE EVALUATION AND SELECTION

Important considerations in selection of patients for biopsy procedures include *lesion location, size,* and *vascularity.* Neurorad-*iological* support in assessment, selection, and planning is essential. Detailed studies with strict three-dimensional comprehension of the structural alterations and regional anatomy of instrument transit is imperative. Invasive studies, however, are not usually required. Preoperative angiography was obtained in 10% of our patients. For individuals considered candidates for CT guided stereotactic surgery, MRI studies were obtained in 60%, while all cases undergoing biopsy procedures with MRI guidance had prior CT studies. The techniques should not be employed with lesions indicating extensive vascularity, and proximity to a major vascular trunk or channel should cause concern. This consideration is particularly important in firm lesions which lie adjacent to or incorporate complex vascular structures such as the cavernous sinus or periinsular region. During detailed appraisal of 500 cases for such procedures, 5% have been managed by more "traditional" neurosurgical methods or observation because of such presentations. Care is required in approaching structural targets immediately adjacent to *polar, corticopial,* and *ependymal* surfaces.

Lesions of <1 cm in size and rubbery in consistency may resist efforts at cannula penetration or tissue retrieval, migrating through the softer brain stroma.

Lesions in the deep midline and brainstem *do not* pose a problem by virtue of their location alone and, in fact, are not technically difficult transits. In our experience and that of others, transits are generally uneventful, with complications manifested in relation to manipulation at the target point. The method of a single pass to the target with a blunt-tip cannula (14-gauge) provides minimal trauma and virtually no opportunity for vascular injury within the brain parenchyma. Calvarial and dural penetration is uneventful provided strict techniques related to instrumentation, stop utilization, and omission of dural dissection are followed.

TARGET SELECTION

Safe target selection at the scanner console relies upon optimization of the image and thorough evaluation of preprocedural images with the neuroradiologist. Definition may be refined by methods of *double-dose contrast* enhancement with a *delay* to maximize contrast and puddling of dye within the lesion. This is particularly of value in *low density* lesions suggestive of low grade glial tumors where regions of maximum cellular activity and alteration of blood-brain barrier are indicated by contrast presence. A biopsy of such regions will usually yield a higher grade of tumor than unenhanced regions.

Bolus infusion of contrast media shortly prior to scanning may be helpful in defining vascular elements at the time of the targeting scan. In general, the target should be well within the lesion, particularly if major vascular elements are adjacent (i.e., pineal regional mass) and preferably within an enhancing region. Study at the console should define the anticipated trajectory tract throughout its course to allow for sampling above and below the designated target point if indicated at the time of tissue analysis.

Targeting at the rim of an *enhancing margin* should be selected toward a pole if possible with transit into the nonenhancing component of the lesion. Care is indicated in *large cystic lesions* where biopsy of the wall could precipitate hemorrhage into a fluid-filled cavity with little opportunity for tamponade. In such a case, we have occasionally targeted the central cyst, retrieved and analyzed fluid, installed a permanent intermittent drainage system (Rickham reservoir with catheter), and followed the patient with imaging to monitor reduction of mass and cyst collapse. Wall biopsy, if necessary, has been performed when intracranial dynamics are more stable and less cyst void is present.

Tract biopsy with slotted instrumentation is of value in defining the extent of glial tumor presence in relation to imaging findings. In this case, targeting and sampling will proceed in the order of the surgeons' preference. This technique requires unusually refined neuropathological support, but is an important method of definition of intracerebral and invasive neoplasms (27, 28).

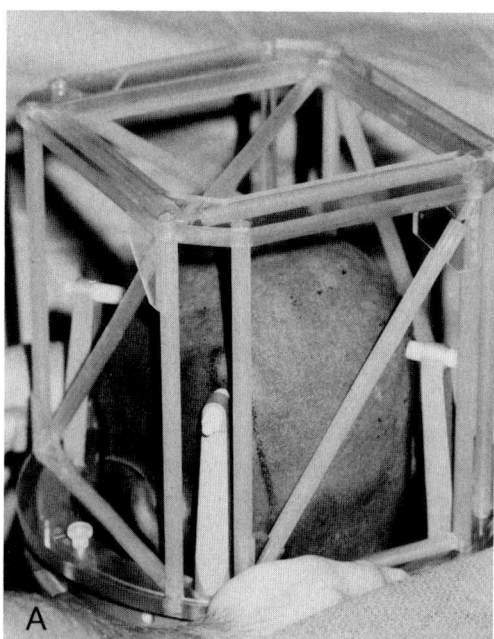
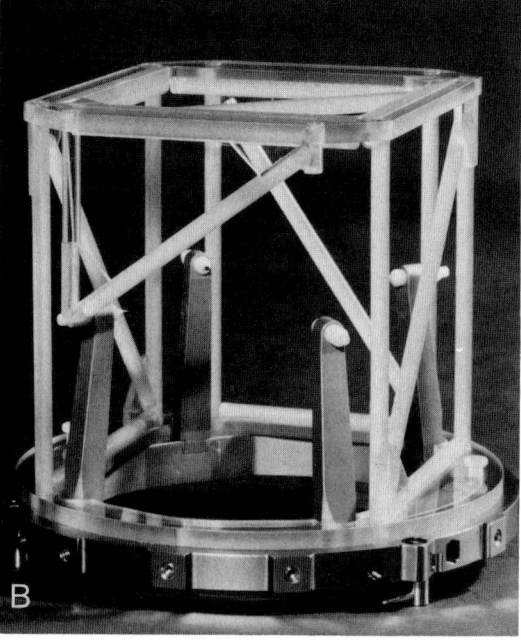

Figure 4.31. *A*) MRI localization device in place following application of special base ring adaptor. Structure of localizer system permits retrieval of information in three planes of reference. *B*) Magnetic resonance localizing device interfaces with base ring of CT-compatible BRW system. This amalgam is established following data collection in magnetic resonance scanner.

MRI METHODOLOGY

As MRI is complementary and, at times, superior in defining structure and extent of intracranial process, methodology is evolving to permit rapid MRI localization in relation to stereotactic space. These devices employ localizing systems that take advantage of the MRI instrumentation's ability to yield coronal and sagittal images quickly as well as those in axial planes (69, 72). No ferromagnetic materials are employed and a variety of compounds have been used as fiducial markers (Fig. 4.31A and B).

Experience with this method of targeting is in its early stages, but it promises to be a valuable adjunctive method of structural definition in biopsy and therapeutic operative guidance.

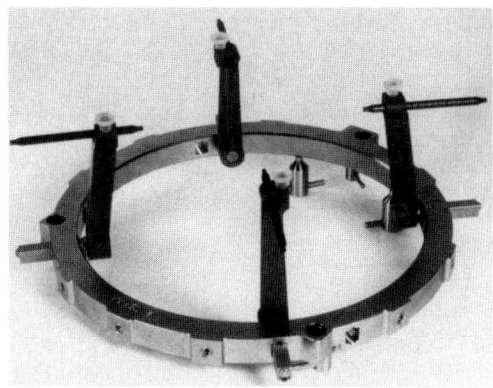

Figure 4.32. Base ring with replaceable fixation system which permits imaging data retrieval and exhaustive processing in timeframes remote to actual surgical procedure.

DIGITALIZED DATA MANAGEMENT

A composite data base consisting of digitalized computer-processed images from CT, MRI, digital subtraction venous angiography, and PET allows for development of a complete profile of the intracranial volume. This volume is precise and unique to the individual patient and his pathology. Software graphics packages such as the LUCASFILM product PIXAR promise to further revolutionize preoperative and intraoperative planning by elaborate graphic displays.

Utilization of this composite as a stereotactic data base for planning and alteration of transits and biopsy sites will no doubt increase the precision and safety of biopsy procedures in the future. In addition, using a base ring system with replaceable pins (drill holes in outer table) (Fig. 4.32), such data may be gathered, stored, and processed prior to the day of a procedure. A *stereotactic work station* combining hardware, software, and monitor capability is feasible for transport of all information to the operating room setting for graphic displays of transit design and intraoperative treatment planning and modifications. Such a system would be particularly useful in intralesional therapies and other intraoperative therapeutic alternatives.

INDICATIONS

In consideration of these methods, the indications for "open" biopsy are rare (4, 20). Stereotactic methodology should be considered for the following types of patient groupings: (a) Those with deep, intrinsic cerebral lesions that can be approached by open surgery only with risk of adverse functional sequellae; (b) Those with any lesion poorly defined on imaging studies in whom alternate considerations of surgical or nonsurgical management exists; or (c) Those who apparently harbor a lesion in which the value of open surgery is debatable.

INTRALESIONAL THERAPIES (SOLID TUMORS)

Precision localization of structural intracranial processes in relation to stereotactic space allows the introduction of physical, biological, chemical, and other therapeutic modalities within this defined region. With localization of the treatment envelope, impact of modalities may be restricted to regions of pathological involvement in solid tumors. The most commonly utilized technique for tumor control is radiobrachytherapy. However, experimental and innovative biological and physical methodologies are currently being investigated and promise to evolve as substantive additions to the armamentarium. The rationale and technique for placement of *multiple catheter arrays* in creating the proper biophysical impact in brachytherapy is relevant to emerging adjuvant treatment and therefore will be discussed in some detail. These methods described for management of solid tumors are applicable with modification, and at times with greater ease, to cystic lesions.

Radiobrachytherapy

The local employment of radionuclides in the management of neoplastic processes was initially considered more than 80 years ago and has enjoyed increasing enthusiasm in somatic and CNS tumors over the past 30 years (17, 80). Major practical considerations have related to *radionuclide selection, localization of tumor margin or target volume, dose delivery, geometry* (or spatial relationship of source placement within the tumor mass), *source drift, patient selection, and scheduling* (the consideration of the relation of this treatment to other therapeutic modes). Developments in computer science concurrently initiating improvement in neuroradiographical imaging and the recent availability of precise imaging-direct guidance stereotactic systems have instigated an impetus to redefine the role of this therapeutic concept, especially in malignant intrinsic cerebral neoplasms (13, 15, 37, 38, 62, 80–88, 91, 104–107, 112).

General Logic of Employment

Until recently, standard radiotherapy for malignant gliomas, the most common of malignant cerebral neoplasms, had consisted of 50 to 65 Gy (SI unit of absorbed dose, equal to 1 j/kg or 100 rad) given over a 6 to 8 week period by teletherapy, frequently with the final 10 to 15 Gy given as a boost to the tumor bed. However, it is now clear that recurrence found at autopsy is most frequently within the treatment field, indicating the inadequacy of the total tumor dose and the persistence of relatively resistant hypoxic cells (41, 49). Additionally, the impact on unaffected cerebral tissue and mentation may be striking, initiating a trend toward regional rather than whole brain radiation. Tolerance of the normal brain to radiation has been considered to be within the range of 55 to 60 Gy. Above 60 Gy, the incidence of brain necrosis increases sharply.

Since it appears that larger total doses are required to enhance cell kill, an approach that is directed toward increasing the dose to the tumor bed while sparing surrounding nervous tissue is logical. Interstitial implantation of radionuclides conceptually accomplishes this goal. Current technique employs the placement of radionuclide sources encased in silastic catheters which are directed into the tumor bed in a precise *geometrical* manner in order to provide a *homogeneous distribution of radiation* (Fig. 4.33). The number of sources, their intensity, the distribution in each catheter, and the number of catheters are selected to deliver as uniform a dose as possible in an effort to avoid "cold spots" within the tumor mass and simultaneously to reduce the incidence of induced necrosis associated with volumes of excessive dose (7, 17, 40, 42, 86).

From the radiobiological perspective, delivering a constant protracted dose of radiation will destroy radiosensitive cells in the primary *cell cycle-sensitive phases* (M, G_2), arresting cells in mitosis. As these cells are destroyed, cells in the radioresistant phase of the cell cycle will traverse the more sensitive phases during continued irradiation and will in turn be destroyed.

With interstitial radiation at the dose rates employed in clinical medicine, *mitotic delay* progressively lengthens the cell cycle so that dose per cell cycle increases rapidly, cell division becomes totally inhibited, and the tumor cell population declines as a result of mitotic death.

Delivering constant radiation over a period of time generally results in greater damage to tumor cells while maintaining the same level of normal tissue tolerance. Further, hypoxic cells may become oxygenated during this extended radiation exposure thus enhancing the radiation impact. In this situation, the decrease in biological effect which could occur due to repair of sublethal damage is balanced by the increased biological effect due to reoxygenation. Compared with a single acute radiation exposure, protracion of the exposure with the use of the lower dose rates employed (200 cGy/min with teletherapy versus 50 cGy/hr with interstitial brachytherapy) leads to differential sparing of nor-

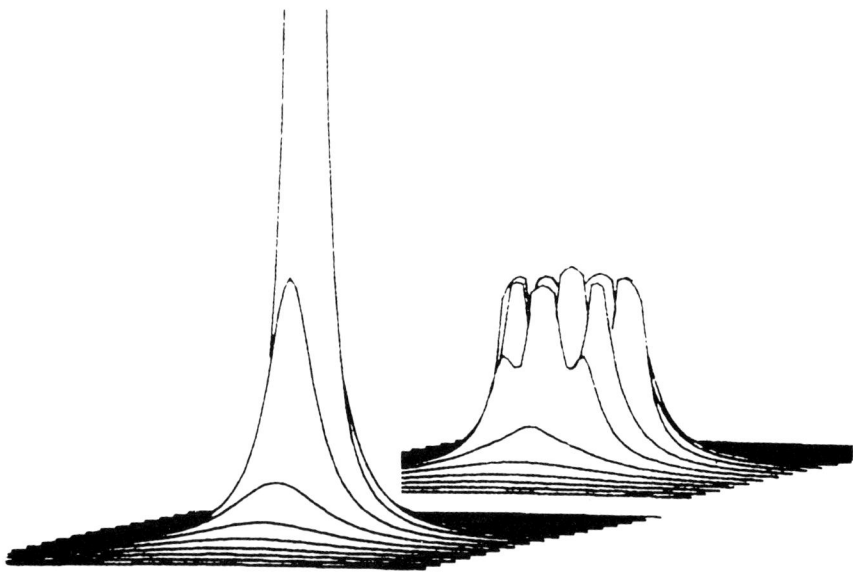

Figure 4.33. Graphic schematic represents idealization of a multisource homogeneous area brachytherapy on reader's right versus similar volume coverage with single source high-intensity method on left.

mal tissues since they can undergo repair of sublethal damage during irradiation. At the same time, tumor cells are continually entering radiosensitive phases of the cell cycle.

Dose per cell cycle becomes more relevent than the dose rate in terms of hours. In consideration of malignant gliomas, at dose rates in the range of 50 to 60 cGy/hr and a cell cycle time of 24 to 120 hr, the dose per cell cycle will be in the range of 12 to 16 Gy. At such protracted dose rates, mitotic delay induced by irradiation progressively lengthens the cycle so that the dose per cycle increases rapidly and cell division is inhibited. The cell population declines as a result of cell death. Recurrence, therefore, will occur in those areas which have not received a sufficient dose, i.e., a geographic miss or an underdosed area secondary to cold spots due to poor geometry. The latter occurs when an insufficient number of catheters is employed, when there is inadequate spacing of isotope sources within the catheters, and/or the dose rate is too low. The *dose rate* is a function of the number of radioactive sources used, their geometrical distribution, and the specific activity of each seed. The maximum dose that can be delivered without unacceptable damage to normal tissue depends on the *volume irradiated* and the dose rate. When iridium-192 (^{192}Ir) is employed at 64 cGy/hr to a total dose of 46 Gy in 3 days the effect produced is approximately the same as that from a dose rate of 36 cGy/hr to a total of 60 Gy delivered in 7 days.

The biological effect of gamma emitters is oxygen dependent (17). Californium-252 (^{252}Cf), a man-made radionuclide, emits both gamma rays and fast neutrons in a fission process. The killing effect of fast neutrons at low dose rates is less dependent on oxygen. However, personnel exposure presents a significant hazard.

Radionuclide Selection

Although numerous radionuclides are available, ^{192}Ir and iodine-125 (^{125}) are the most commonly employed in efforts directed toward adjuvant therapy of invasive or malignant cerebral neoplasms.

The selection of a radionuclide for a procedure is determined by a therapeutic goal of a particular dose rate and treatment time. If one considers that the desired dose rate to encompass the entire volume of interest is generally in the range of 40 to 60 cGy/hr, several days are needed to reach therapeutic dose levels of 50 to 60 Gy at the periphery of the tumor. For this reason, it is preferable to use a radionuclide with a sufficiently long *half-life* so that the dose rate does not diminish appreciably during the time of the implant. Both ^{192}Ir (74 days) and ^{125}I (60 days) have adequately long half-life.

The *energy* of the radionuclide will determine the protective methods employed for keeping the exposure of personnel to a minimum. Iodine-125, with an average photon energy of only 28 keV, is particularly easy to manage. The tumor dose rate will depend on the *activity* of each seed and on the *number* and *distribution* of the seeds employed. The dose distribution within the tumor volume depends upon the geometry and intensity factors rather than upon the particular radionuclide employed. The very rapid (inverse square) fall-off of the dose rate from an individual source makes placement of the source extremely important.

Iodine-125 has the advantage of reduced exposure with just a small thickness of lead (0.25 mm) being sufficient. These patients do not present a radiation hazard to those around them. Iodine-125 radiation has a lower absorption of energy in fat, a tissue which is more like the composition of brain than either muscle or bone. The absorbed dose in bone, on the other hand, reaches a maximum value of 4.4 cGy/rad of exposure at the wavelength of ^{125}I energy. This high absorption in bone could be a problem at the skull base. The more rapid dose fall-off at the periphery would appear to be ideal when considering the protection of surrounding normal brain tissue. It may, however, have a disadvantage resulting in a geographical miss of tumor cells when located further from the periphery of the target area. When used in small numbers not placed geometrically to account for its rapid fall-off, cold spots within the tumor mass may lead to recurrence. Iodine-125 has predominantly a photoelectric interaction governed by attenuation for distances greater than 1.5 cm from the seed. Within that range, it follows the inverse square law. In tissue, the half-value layer (HVL) is approximately 2 cm, although the attenuation is less severe in the first few centimeters due to the buildup of scatter dose. Beyond 2 cm, the dose falls off rapidly; consequently a larger tumor mass may be underdosed. For very small lesions located in inaccessible areas, this isotope may be valuable when the specific activity of the seeds is high.

Iridium-192, on the other hand, has an average gamma energy of 0.38 MeV (380 keV). The absorbed dose in centigray per roentgen exposure for ^{192}Ir is approximately the same for soft tissues, bones, and fat. Its fall-off essentially follows the inverse square law with attenuation balanced by scatter. Soft tissue absorption for this radionuclide is by Compton interaction. While the HVL for ^{125}I is 2 cm in soft tissue, the HVL for ^{192}Ir in tissue is approximately 7 cm and the attenuation in the first 10 cm of tissue tends to be balanced by the build up of scatter dose. At a distance of 10 cm, there is an effective dose of only about 10%. Thus, for all practical purposes, the dose fall off in tissue from an ^{192}Ir seed follows the inverse square law. Thus, with proper catheter placement, surrounding normal tissues are effectively protected.

Theory, Issues of Practicality, and Technique of Employment

In spite of periodic and recent intense interest in application of interstitial brachytherapy, there is no clear definition of optimum technique or overall factors related to protocol design in the therapy of invasive cerebral neoplasms. Current reported results, although promising, do not allow precise definition of treatment factors or expectations in relation to patient stratification. However, in consideration of the theoretical factors related to brachytherapy and radionuclide selection, including the characteristics of various nuclides to be employed, the radiobiological effects of low-dose continous radiation, and and neuroglial tissue tolerance, the authors have designed a program for interstitial implantation of brain neoplasms attempting to minimize injury to normal tissues by appraisal of technical factors related to an adequate implant adjusted to the locale of the disease and to patient tolerance. Iridium-192 was selected because of institutional familiarity with the radionuclide, cost, and availability.

To achieve ideal dose distribution, ribbons containing multiple sources of ^{192}Ir were designed to encompass the imaging-defined tumor target region, with the ribbons positioned near the target volume margin and separated around the periphery by no more than 2.5 cm in order to obtain the most homogeneous distribution of radiation within the target volume (7, 9). The extensive and irregular nature of the majority of malignant gliomas dictates the use of multiple catheters which contain these radionuclide sources spaced at 3-mm intervals to produce a grid effect. When the target diameter exceeds 5 cm, it is necessary to add additional catheters in the central region to supplement those placed around the periphery in order to avoid cold spots in the central area.

When possible, maximum effort to reduce brain distortion by the mass should be undertaken surgically. In the event that a large percentage of hypoxic, nonproliferating cells can be excised, it is possible that the chance of controlling residual disease is enhanced. Increase in the growth fraction of the tumor by volume reduction and recruiting cells into the proliferative compartment as well as reducing the number of hypoxic cells should increase the possibility of cell kill by irradiation. Especially in the event that accessible brain distorting mass is present, surgical reduction in tumor burden is accomplished prior to implantation in recurrent tumors. This is undertaken to reduce further the tumor burden by protracted radiation of the remaining tumor cells. The implant procedure is initiated at the earliest time when wound factors and CT surgical artifact will permit the optimum localization of tumor target regions and percutaneous catheter placement (3–4 weeks).

The radiosensitivity of glioma cells in vitro is in the order of 143 cGy with an extrapolation number of approximately 1.4. The cell cycle time is estimated to be in the range of 75.6 + 45 hr. The growth fraction is estimated to be from 0.14 to 0.44. By protracting irradiation in the postoperative period, greater cell kill may be accomplished by arresting mitosis and preventing cell birth from preceding the cell kill in a manner similar to that achieved by superfractionation or multiple daily fractions delivered by teletherapy. However, local interstitial therapy will more reliably reduce the dose to "normal" tissues.

A peripheral tumor dose of 45 to 62 Gy has been delivered over a 4 to 5-day period.

Previously untreated individuals harboring neoplasms *without mass* are initially accessed by imaging-directed stereotactic biopsy. If a malignant and radiosensitive tumor is disclosed, regional teletherapy is initially delivered, imaging performed 2 to 4 weeks after completion of the course, and the residual mass is then treated with radiobrachytherapy technique.

Of importance is the cooperation and comprehension of basic issues and factors related to therapy by individuals concerned with the problems and disciplines of neurosurgery, radiation therapy, and radiation physics. Adjustment in combinations of catheter placement, isotope geometry, and dose rates are made according to lesion size, locale, and risk factors.

Surgical Technique.—Within the University of Southern California Medical Center Hospitals, multiple point source interstitial brachytherapy is undertaken with the assistance of a BRW stereotactic guidance system completely under local anesthesia.

Patients undergo application of the system's base ring in an operating room area and then are moved to the scanner unit where multiple-slice, or three-plane, tomography is undertaken with reference to a previously derived data base of three-dimensional CT, MRI, and digital subtraction venous angiographic imaging. Previously determined targets for transcutaneous catheter placement are verified at the scanner console by representatives of neurosurgical, radiation therapy, and radiation physics facilities, and the patient is transferred to the operating room for the remainder of the procedure (Fig. 4.34).

Employing x- and y-plane pixel coordinates of intralesional target points, as well as entry coordinates, three-dimensional trajectory transits are derived for placement of a *parallel catheter array* on an Epson HX-20 microcomputer.

Appropriate settings are entered into the stereotactic system's *arc,* and each trajectory

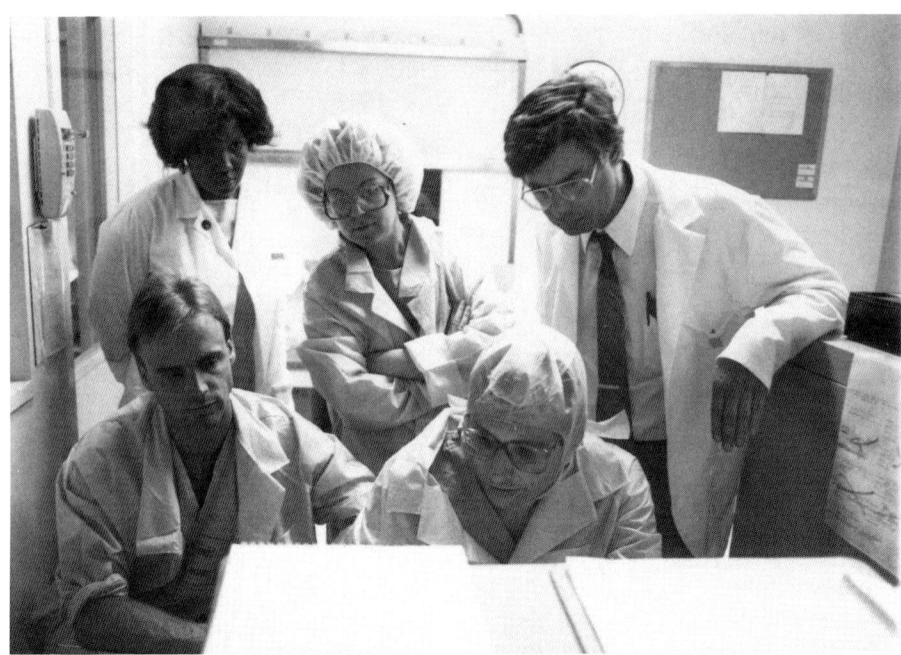

Figure 4.34. Members of neurosurgery, radiation oncology, and radiation physics services participate in finalization of multiple targeting at scanner console during operative procedure.

and target is individually checked extracranially on the *phantom base* unit.

Silastic catheters specially designed for afterloading with ^{192}Ir sources are transcutaneously introduced through 1/4-inch twist drill perforations made along trajectory lines in the arc system's rigid bushing holder (Figs. 4.35–45). Depending on the requirements of the procedure, 2 to 11 catheters have been introduced under local standby anesthesia, with the patient's full cooperation and response.

Following placement of the multiple catheter array, afterloading is completed in

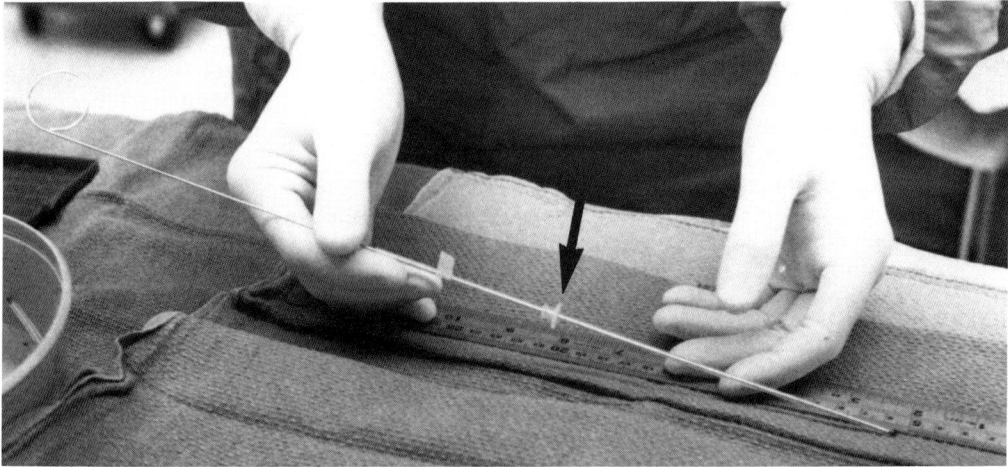

Figure 4.35. A 22-cm Silastic catheter is measured for depth of placement prior to stereotactic placement. This catheter is designed specifically for transcutaneous cerebral placement and afterloading with ^{192}Ir. *Arrow* indicates an adjustable Silastic cuff that is used to fix the catheter and source complex at the scalp surface.

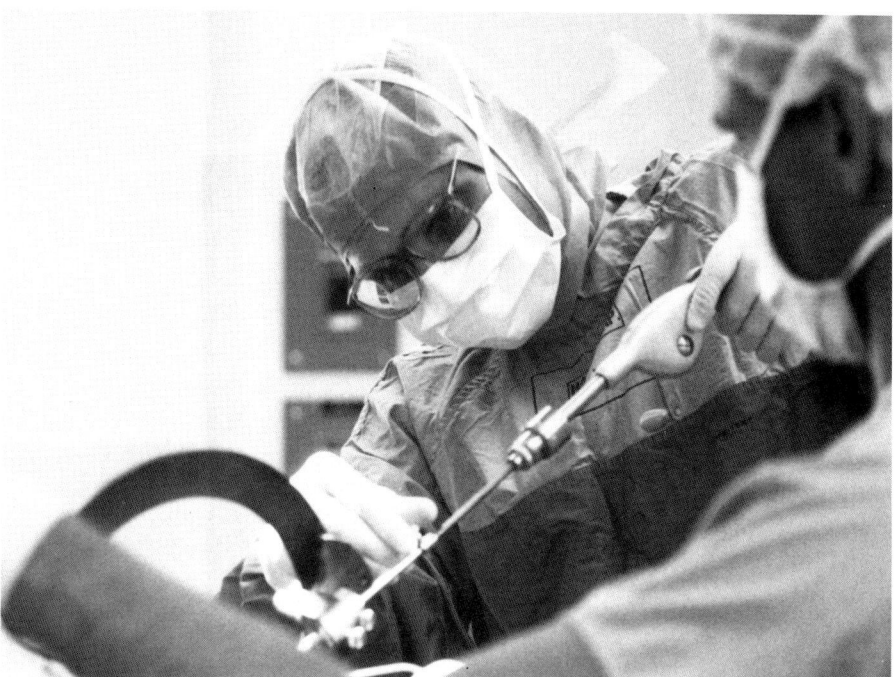

Figure 4.36. Following individual 6-mm incisions, multiple parallel catheters are introduced in an array through twist drill openings in the calvarium.

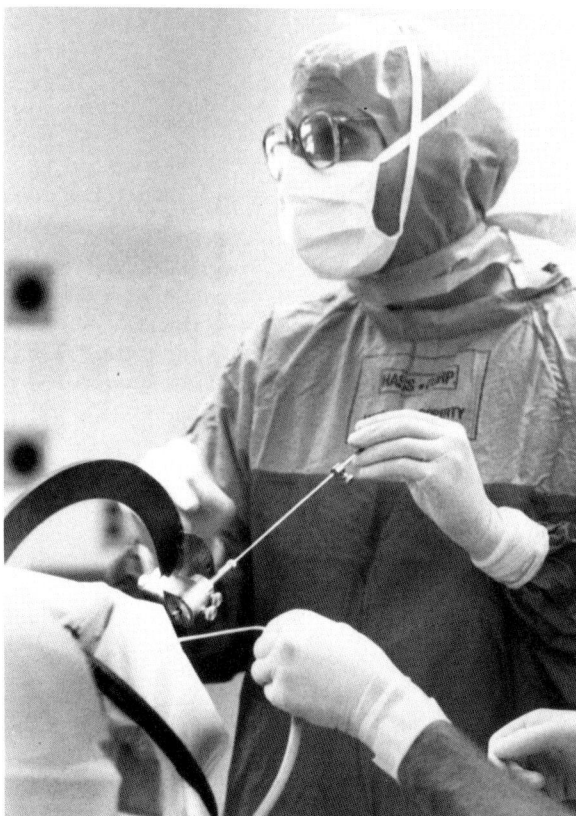

Figure 4.37. Surgeon alerts anesthesiologist prior to passage of a 14-gauge cannula through proposed track of catheter transit.

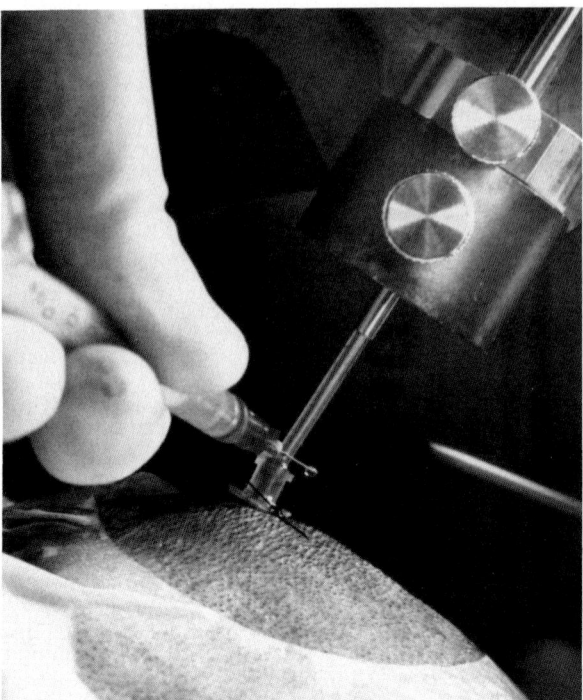

Figure 4.38. After Silastic cuff is sutured to scalp, catheter conduit is introduced to target site and temporarily fastened to cuff with AronAlpha Acrylic.

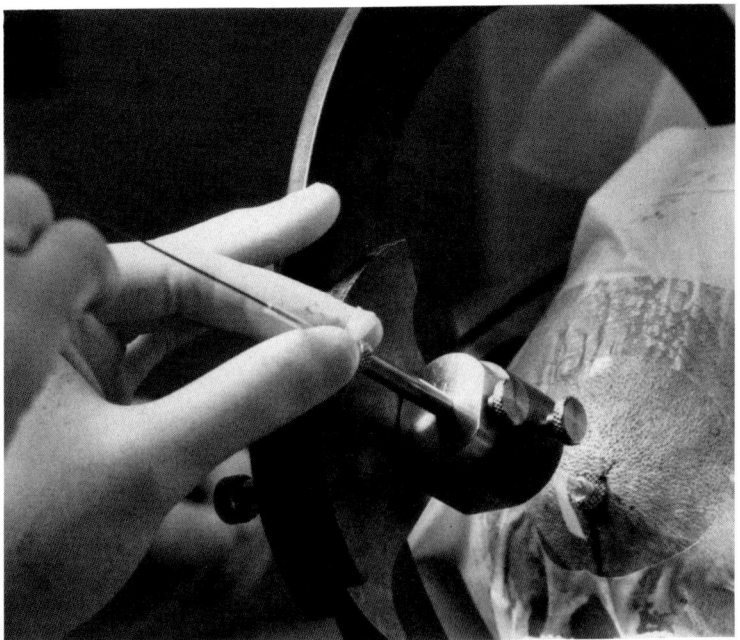

Figure 4.39. Steristrip is applied as a marker, stylet is removed from catheter, and catheter is trimmed.

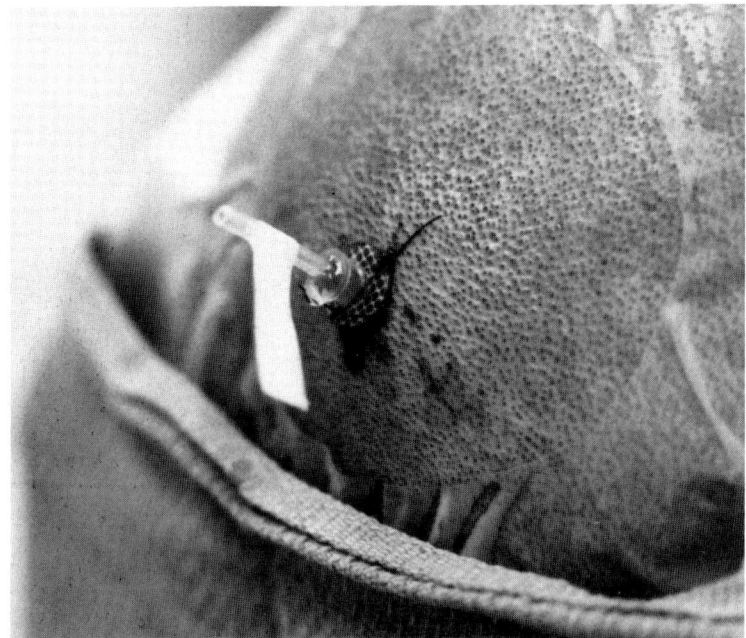

Figure 4.40. First catheter-cuff complex is completed in a proposed five-catheter array.

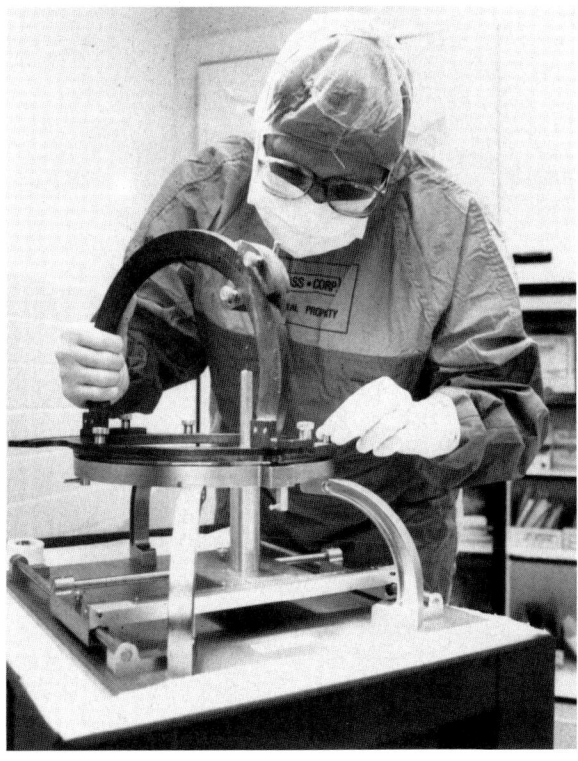

Figure 4.41. Surgeon makes appropriate settings in arc system for each catheter passage.

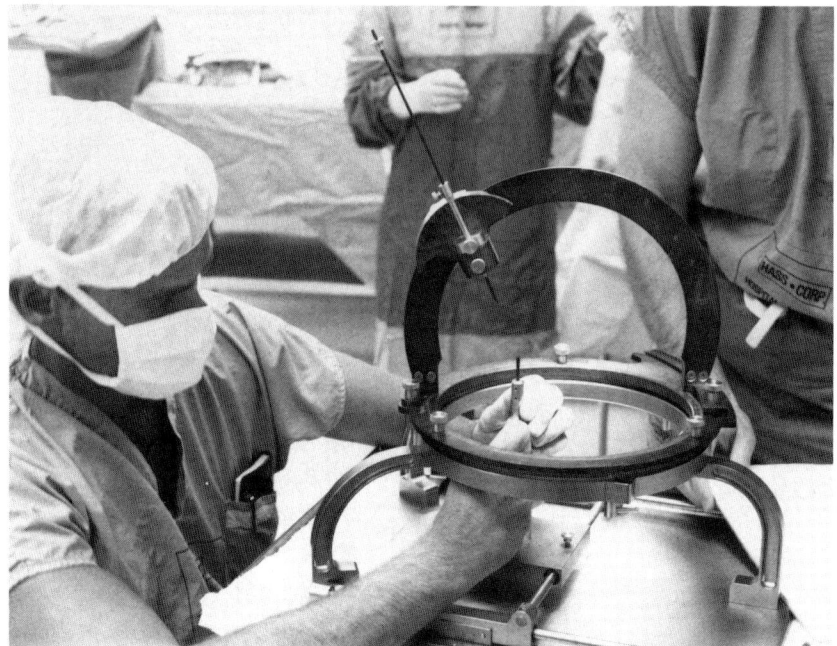

Figure 4.42. Individual targetings on phantom base are made to assure proper placement.

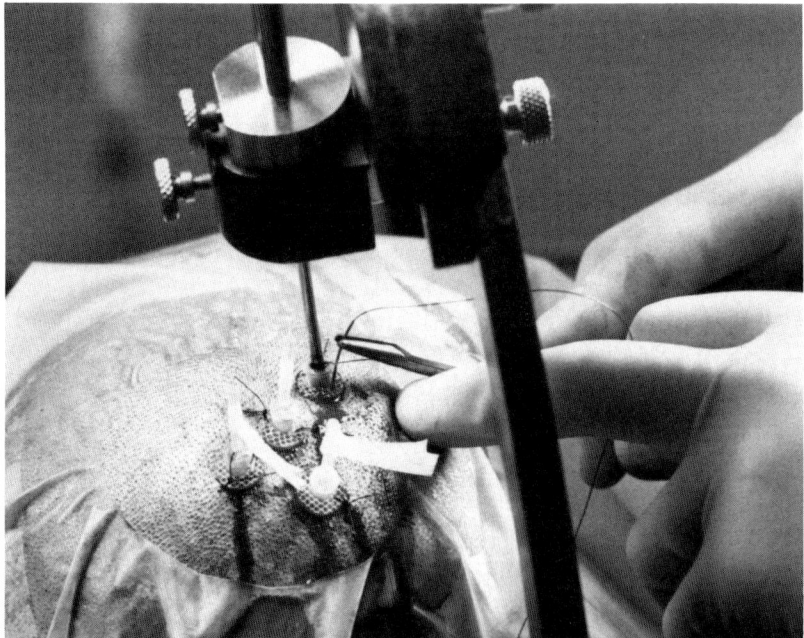

Figure 4.43. In process of placement of fourth catheter in a five-catheter array, method of fixation of cuff to scalp is noted. The 14-gauge cannula is passed through cuff to target site, and two monofilament sutures are employed to anchor cuff.

IMAGE-DIRECTED STEREOTACTIC SURGERY FOR INTRACRANIAL NEOPLASMS

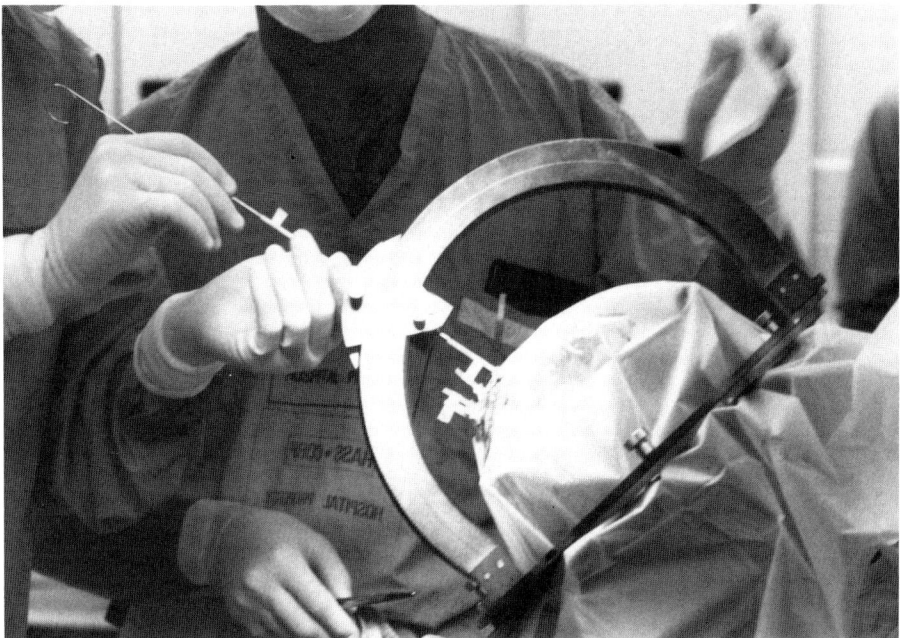

Figure 4.44. Catheter is introduced through cuff to target site.

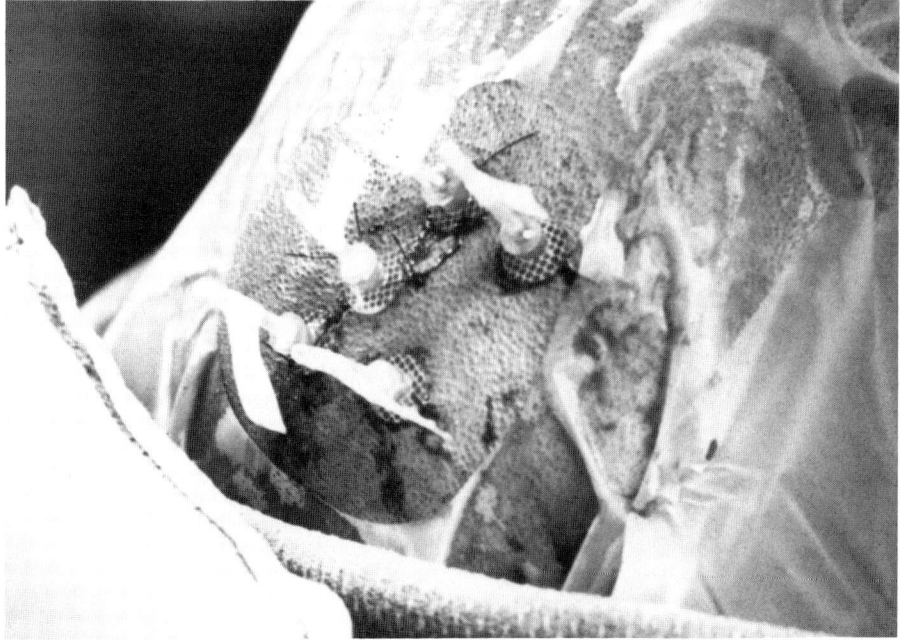

Figure 4.45. Five-catheter array is completed; irregularity is present because of irregular contours of tumor being treated.

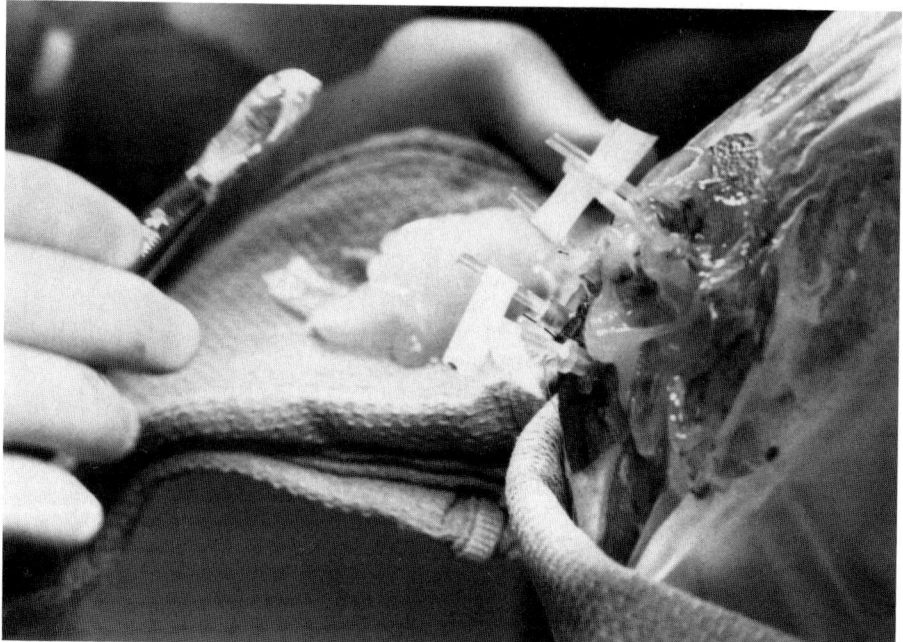

Figure 4.46. Antibiotic ointment is applied to base of complex.

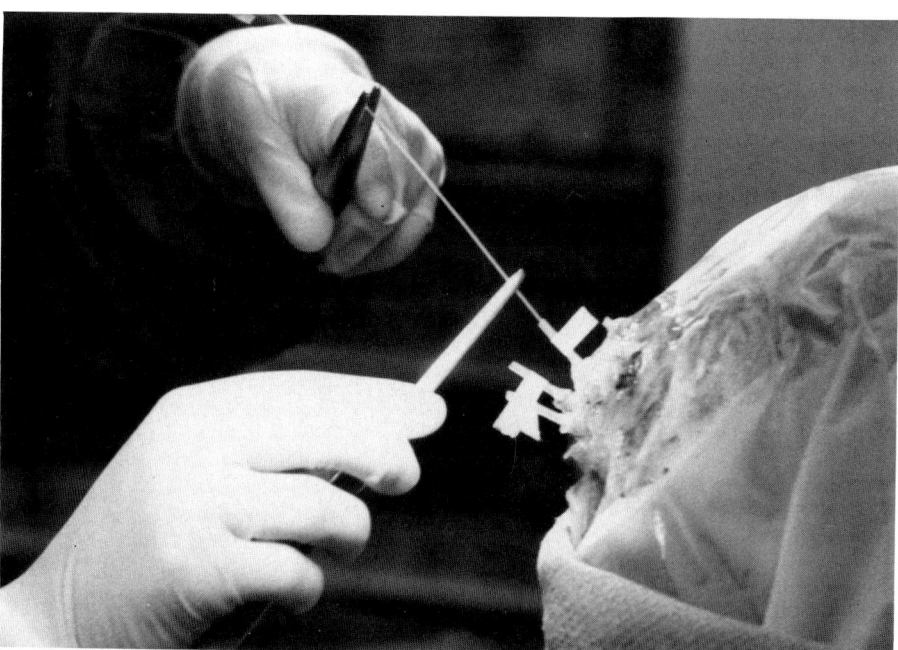

Figure 4.47. Catheters are individually afterloaded with seeds and length of sources varying in predetermined patterns.

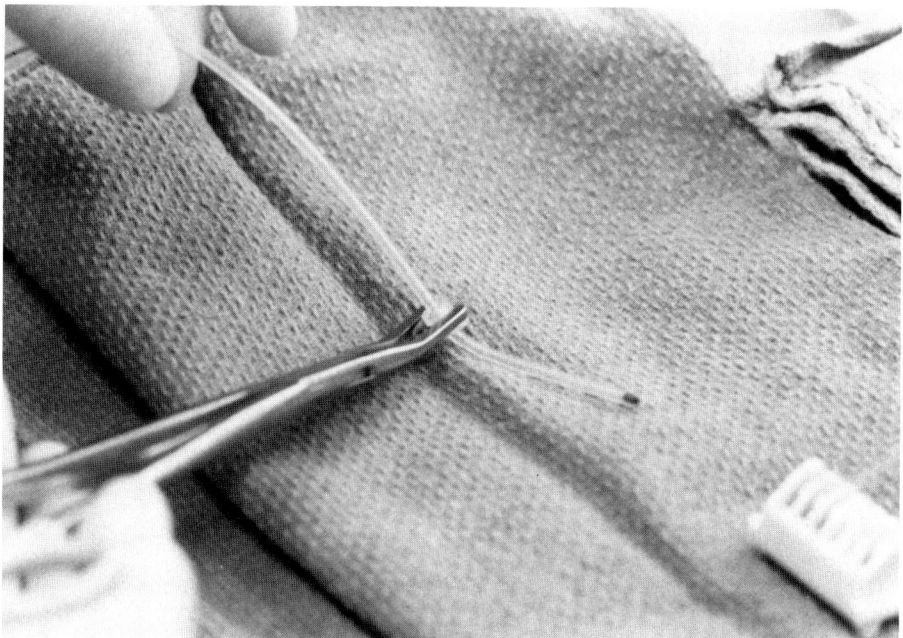

Figure 4.48. Demonstration of application of a Hemoclip to cuff-catheter complex.

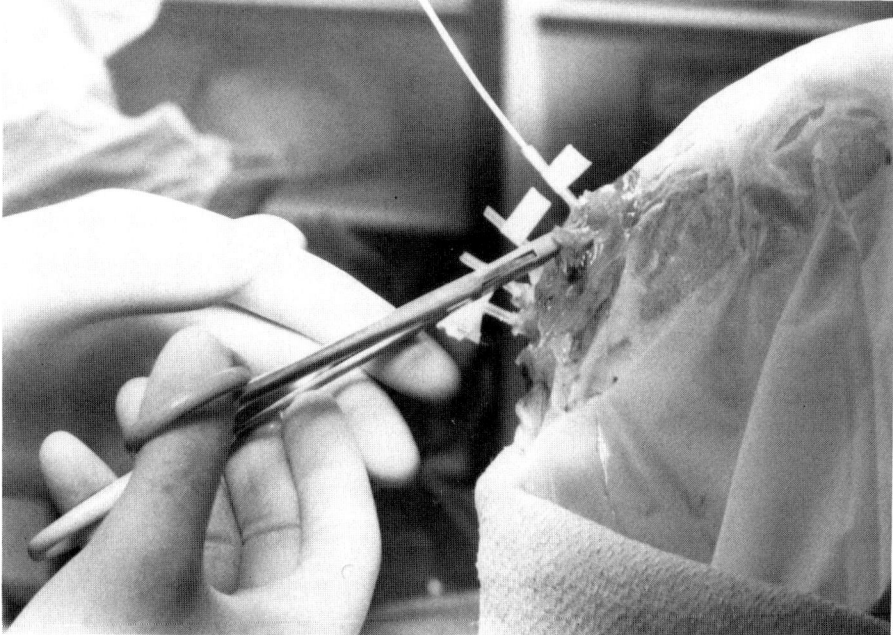

Figure 4.49. Following introduction of source ribbon, a Hemoclip is applied to cuff and catheter is fixing cuff-catheter-source complex at scalp level.

STEREOTACTIC NEUROSURGERY

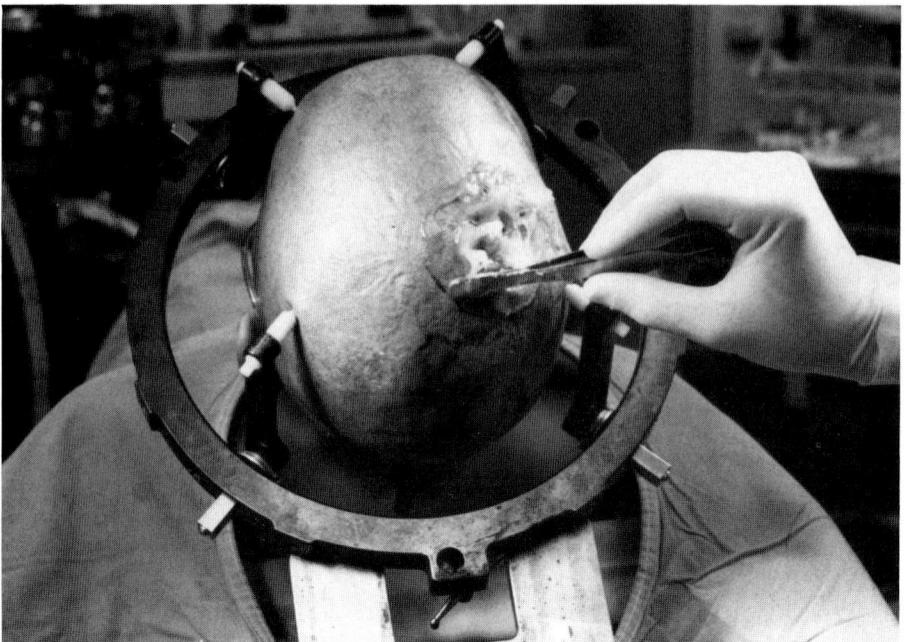

Figure 4.50. Catheters are trimmed to base of cuff and antibiotic ointment is applied.

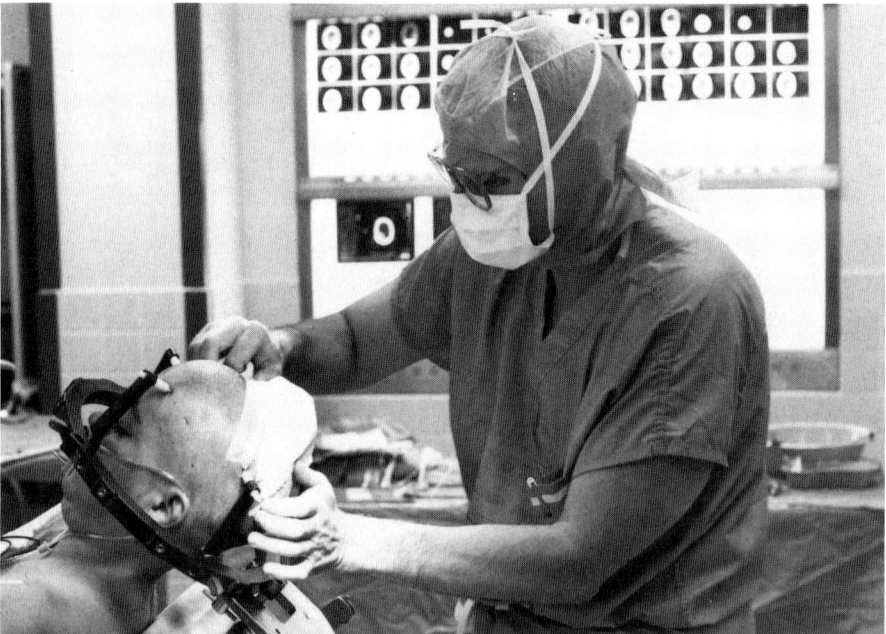

Figure 4.51. Fluff dressing is applied, which will remain intact over period of treatment. Following completion of this stage, the patient is taken to CT scanning suite for check films of actual catheter placement and nursed in an individual room until bedside catheter removal at completion of treatment period.

the operating room and the catheter-source ribbon complex is secured with a vascular clip prior to dressing application and radiographical assessment of the source placement (Figs. 4.46–51).

At dose schedules of 45 to 55 cGy/hr, patients are required to be hospitalized 4 to 6 days for completion of the individual therapeutic regimen. Catheters and sources are removed at the bedside with single sutures placed at each scalp incision site.

General Methodology and Results.—The patients are jointly evaluated for interstitial radiotherapy by a team consisting of a neurosurgeon, radiation oncologist(s), physicist, and nurse. All patients with recurrent and/or persistent invasive cerebral neoplasms are considered for therapy. For those patients seen at USC from the beginning of their treatment, the total dose of external beam radiotherapy of 45 Gy is given in five fractions per week at a daily dose of 18 Gy with 4-mV x-ray beam. As noted, the volume of interest in the treatment of malignant gliomas prior to 1984 was the whole brain. Due to a general lack of tumor recurrence outside of the primary site, and concern for neural injury in long-surviving patients, more conservative treatment fields are now used.

In all cases of solid lesion therapy, removable implants of ^{192}Ir have been used. Intensity of individual seeds has not exceeded 1 miCu. Geometrical arrangement of multiple sources, and varying intensity of sources in individual regions of the volume, fashions the desired isodose envelopes. *Personnel protection is not a problem* when employing this radionuclide provided education and vigilance is maintained at standards appropriate for any tertiary care facility. Total doses given depended on previous radiation received, site of the implant, and the radiation tolerance of surrounding structures. Brachytherapy doses did not exceed 55 cGy target volume to the periphery. No attempt was made to treat suspected tumor extensions not demonstrable on imaging studies. The dose rate was 40 to 55 cGy/hr. The reason for this low dose rate was an attempt to minimize the toxicity of radiotherapy. There is a strong laboratory evidence that high-dose radiotherapy may result in a greater incidence of serious late complications when compared with a lower dose rate radiotherapy. The clinical experience seems to support the laboratory data. In view of the available data on radiation toxicity, one is required to use meticulous technique both in brachytherapy and teletherapy to *limit the volume of tissue treated.* In teletherapy, a daily dose of 180 cGy is preferable, and in no clinical situation should it be substantially exceeded unless a long-term survival is not expected. Similarly, these authors have tried not to exceed interstitial brachytherapy at a dose rate of 55 cGy/hr. In order to promote dose homogeneity through the treated volume, at least two catheters are used, even for small lesions. In larger tumors, five or more catheters may be required. Due to the irregular shape of many lesions, five or less catheters may not give a totally satisfactory dose distribution (Fig. 4.52A–C).

In recent years, the authors have seen larger recurrent or persistent malignant gliomas. It is felt that an increase in the dose of radiation is not the answer. The incidence of complications related to large volume treatment would not be acceptable. We have elected to study interstitial microwave hyperthermia in combination with ^{192}Ir radiation. It is hoped that the *hyperthermia* and radiotherapy combination can address the problem of control of larger tumors, improving upon the interstitial radiotherapy modality. There is strong clinical and laboratory evidence that this can be accomplished and, therefore, a phase I and II clinical pilot study is in a preparatory stage.

Although available data does not permit a statistically valid (with multiple stratification) statement regarding the impact of this form of therapy on malignant gliomas, the current overall experience indicates a response rate (arrest in progression or reduction in volume of scan abnormality) of approximately 70% in *malignant astrocytomas* and 30% in *glioblastoma multiforme.* In responders, time to resumption of progression has had a mean of 10 months. Acute complications are rare (2%). Late complications, such as symptomatic radionecrosis, are also rare (3%). No case has required reexplora-

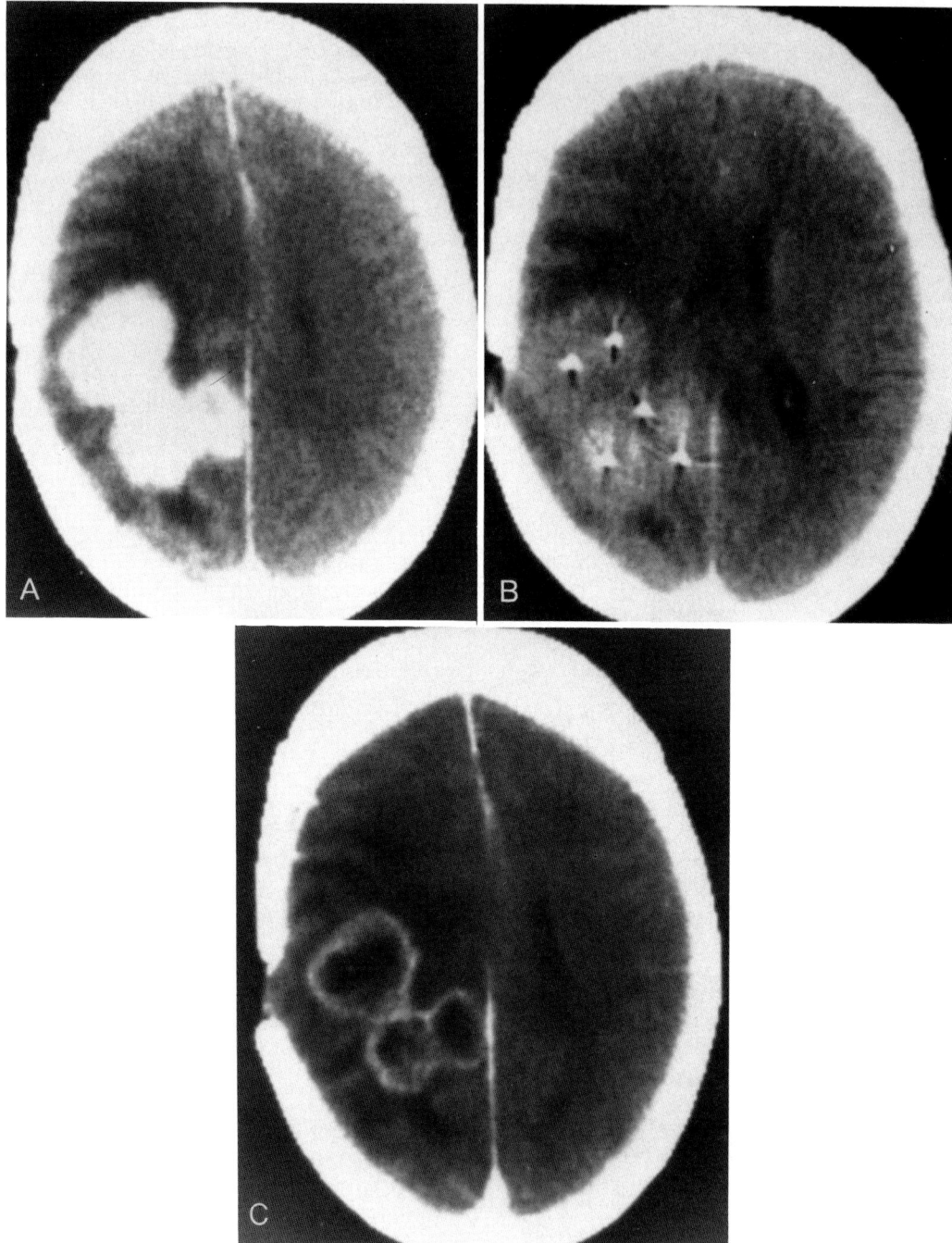

Figure 4.52. *A*) Irregular contour of anaplastic astrocytoma in right mid- and posterior hemisphere. *B*) Five-catheter placement within irregular target area. It should be noted that source intensity and number will vary according to requirements of catheter spacing. *C*) Same patient 3 months following catheter placement with alteration of scan picture indicating necrosis within target areas.

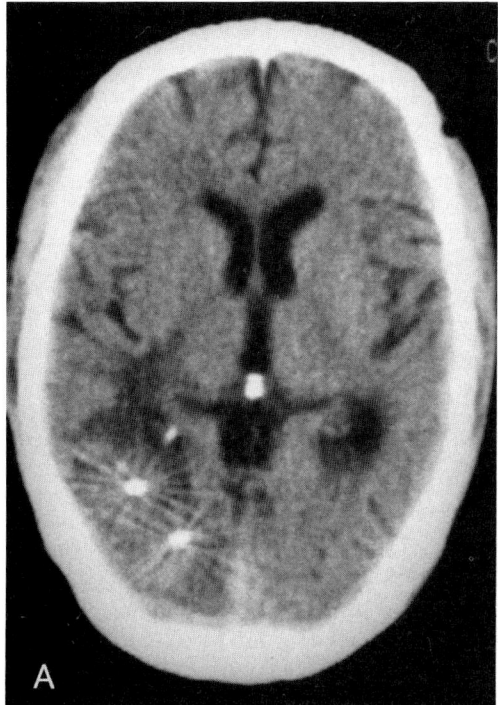 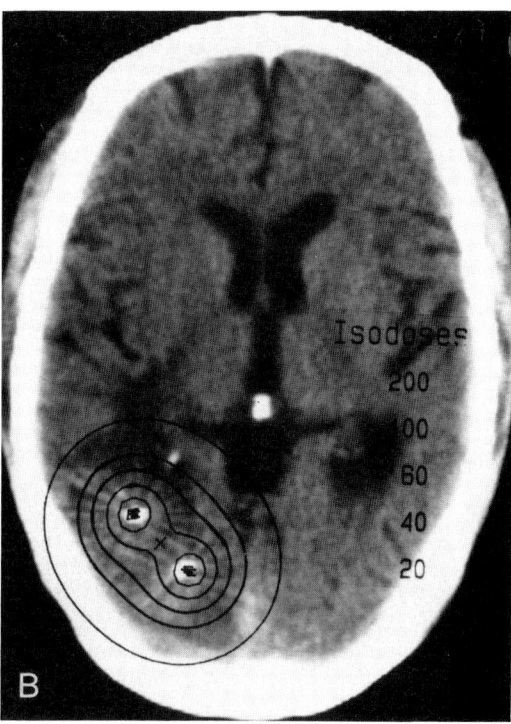

Figure 4.53. *A*) Two-catheter treatment of individual with primary cerebral lymphoma (without immunosuppressive disorder). *B*) Isodose curves in same case. Patient is now nearly 36 months after treatment without recurrence.

tion for a mass related to radionecrotic response. *Pineal region* and *primary cerebral lymphomas* (Fig. 4.53) have demonstrated persistent remission (12 to 48 months follow-up). No pattern of response has been observed in *metastatic lesions.*

The data suggest that the technique should be considered in individuals who have the following characteristics: (*a*) Histology, anaplastic astrocytoma or malignant mixed glioma, recurrent lymphoma, primary pineal, or germinoma tumor, or highly selected patients with solitary metastatic disease; (*b*) Age, less than 55 years; (*c*) Lesion size, less than 5 cm, maximal linear dimension (MR); (*d*) Lesion, CT or MRI definable; (*e*) No midline (MRI or CT) involvement; and (*f*) Initial performance status greater than 70 on the Karnofsky scale.

In our view, no data base is currently available to predict or define the value of optimal technique in applying this methodology in malignant invasive central nervous system tumors. Until such data are available the applications of the technique should be confined to major medical centers. Such centers are expected to have appropriate expertise to allow application of this complex technique in a multidisciplinary fashion for orderly and meaningful data accrual.

New Directions and Modifications.—Previous mention has been made of the concept of a *stereotactic work station* whose objective would be to develop a microcomputer environment to enhance the flexibility and data base for the standard available stereotactic guidance systems. Hardware systems, such as the Digital Equipment Corporation (DEC) Microvax II, could potentially be used to perform all standard software computations related to a stereotactic system for localization and targeting. Stereotactic volumetric computations and references could be translated into a computer graphic display based on a multiple composite-imaging data base.

Such a system would require and achieve:

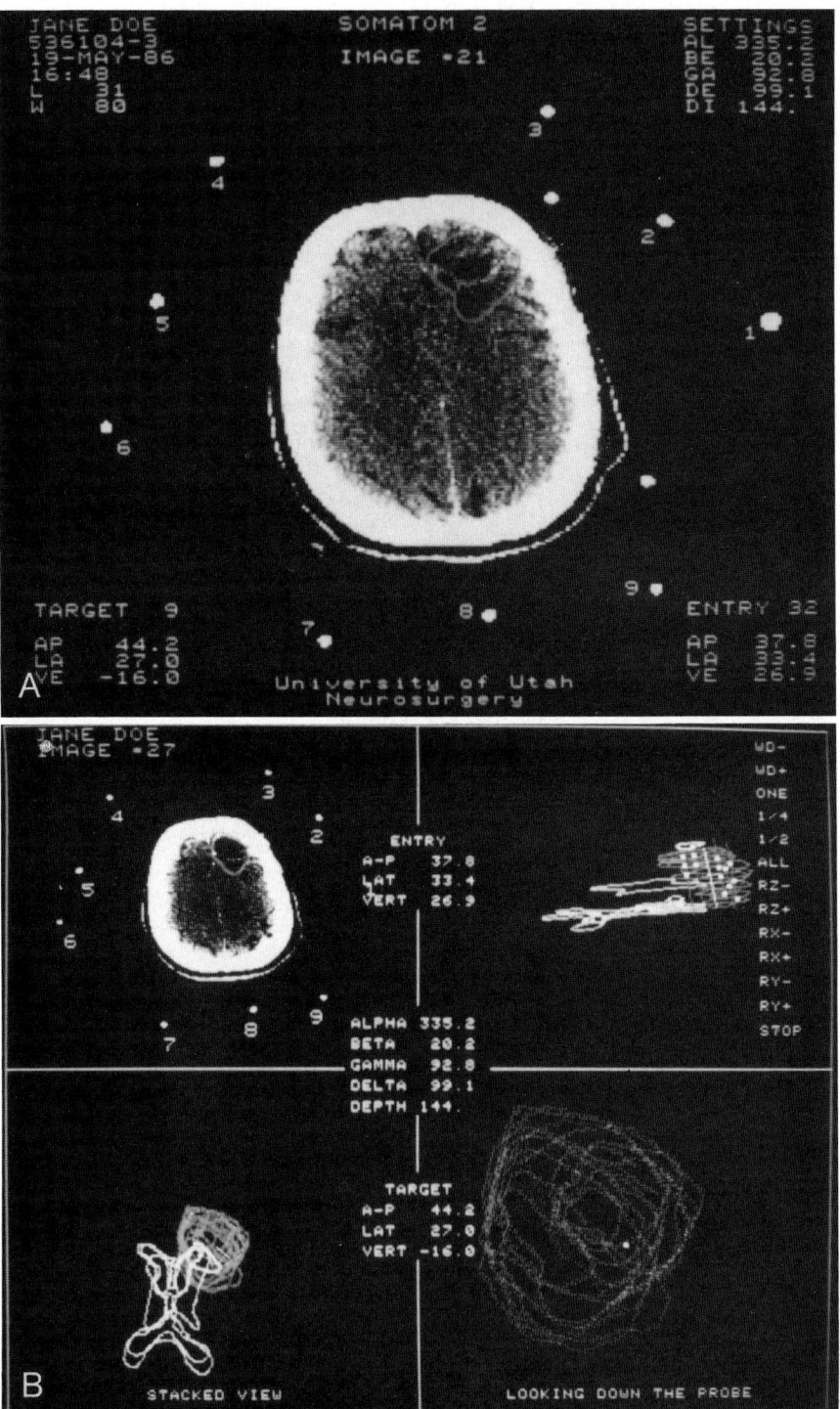

Figure 4.54. Stereotactic workstation (OR). Monitor data and graphic presentations in multicolor on screen (University of Utah). *A) BRW data processing* performed in workstation software package and presented on monitor screen. Note arc settings (upper right), entry coordinates (lower right), target coordinate (lower left). *B)* Development wireframe volumes from mouse tracing of structures from individual slices. Utilization of data for probe-tract relation to structure. *C)* Graphic depictions of radionuclide seeds with isodose curves available on each slice during course and planning for radiobrachytherapy procedure.

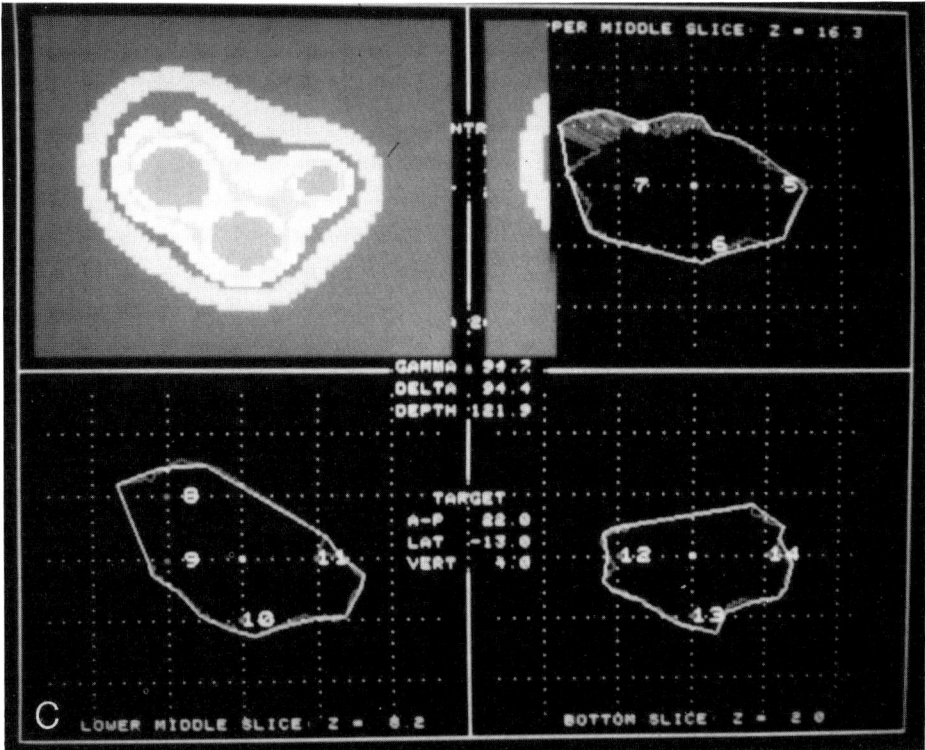

1. Access to imaging data from tape reserves and imaging devices either through a direct data link to such devices or through stored data formats of magnetic tape or magnetic floppy discs. Appropriate hardware and software would allow for all imaging data, including reconstructions to be viewed within an operating room area so that stereotactic computations and target localizations could be performed within the system remote from the scanner;
2. Previous analysis of imaging data which would permit that major intracranial structures such as tumor, brain, and vascular elements could be traced by a mouse-controlled cursor. These tracings could be converted from two-dimensional coordinates to three-dimensional stereotactic coordinates, which could be then preserved as a new data file. They could then be displayed as wireframe models of the anatomical structure with potential probe tracts to the target. These tracings could then be rotated and translated to provide multiple perspectives so that the specific structures at risk could be actively avoided; and
3. In conjunction with such a system, programs could be developed which would then reconfigure structures such as traced tumor borders perpendicular or orthogonal to an operator-selected probe track. These configurations would greatly simplify and increase the precision of planning for interstitial brachytherapy. The software data base could include isodose curves for specific points for brachytherapy which could then be superimposed on all of the graphic display information within the operating theatre, as the planning for probe pass and selective source placement could be developed in a more sophisticated fashion. There would thus be superimposition of a radionuclide source position to allow the tailoring of precision isodose curves with variability of parameters of intensity and spatial geometry. It is obvious that such abilities could be readily

expanded to include the biophysical aspects of phototherapy, including equations for light penetration in neural tissues and thermal gradients for hyperthermia probes (Fig. 4.54 *A-C*).

Stereotactic interstitial radiobrachytherapy delivers a controlled dose of radiation to a defined target region. The isodose envelope that is fashioned by the array of sources should strictly conform to the three-dimensional contour of the cellular neoplastic burden. The currently employed methodology is dependent on the volumetric contour as defined by images in stereotactic space.

The precise definition of the tumor contour and true *volume at risk* in relation to alteration of images may be accomplished by *multiple-tract biopsies* in relation to the imaging alterations and may serve as a predictor of response in relation to the extent of tumor involvement beyond an image-defined margin. This technique is complex and requires sophisticated support from neuropathologists and cytopathologists, but has the potential of offering a refinement in patient selection and modeling of radiation schema, thus improving results.

Initial studies have indicated that morphological contours and dispersions of tumor cells will vary in spite of uniformity of the histopathological type with cellular conglomerates ranging from compact to diffuse with poor localization on imaging studies.

Modification of dose delivery and parallel utilization of *hyperthermia* is an important area of current investigation.

Biochemical *protectors* of "normal" brain may effectively allow increased peripheral dose schedules and will impact upon the recurrence rate and survival.

Stereotactic radiosurgery directed at volumes at risk with appropriate peripheral gradients of isodose definition may prove to be an adjuvant methodology in malignant tumor management. Such techniques are readily available at major medical centers employing image-directed stereotactic systems and linear accelerator radiotherapy units. Their application in the management of malignant cerebral neoplasms is in an early stage of appraisal. However, the concept is proven in arteriovenous malformations and certain benign intracranial neoplastic processes. The relation and potential for this method of therapy to augment or obviate the need for interstitial brachytherapy is yet another important area for appraisal.

Hyperthermia

Historical Perspective

The idea of utilizing elevated temperatures to treat malignancies is an ancient concept. Hyperthermia, in the form of red-hot irons, was used by the early Greek physicians to treat small, superficial tumors. The first modern description of the therapeutic effects of hyperthermia on neoplasia cancer is that of Busch (1866), who reported the regression of a facial sarcoma after two febrile episodes in a patient with erysipelas (103). The first intentional use of hyperthermia in tumor treatment was by Coley (1896), who induced fevers of 39° to 40°C with bacterial toxins in an effort to reproduce the observations of Busch and others (103). The first application of local hyperthermia appears to be by Westermark (1898), who treated uterine cancer with a circulating-water system at 42° to 44°C for 48 hr (103). During the early part of this century, pioneering animal studies to define better the effects of hyperthermia were conducted by Stevenson (1918), Rohdenburg and Prime (1921), and Westermark (1927) (103). Over the past 25 years, the literature on hyperthermia in cancer treatment has grown dramatically, spurred primarily by the technological advances that have allowed for more precise heating within biological systems. In 1971, Sutton (103) introduced hyperthermia as a treatment modality for CNS neoplasms when he described a small group of patients treated with a combination of chemotherapy and invasive resistive heating. The following sections briefly summarize the biological considerations, methods of heat delivery, and current status of clinical trials in the field of hyperthermia as it applies to CNS malignancies.

Biological Considerations

The antineoplastic effects of heat are related to its ability to produce irreversible cell damage and, in addition, to its ability to potentiate the effects of ionizing radiation and chemotherapy. Cell killing from heat alone will be considered first.

In a number of neoplastic cell lines, temperature elevations above 42°C result in cell death. Furthermore, small changes in temperature result in relatively large changes in the necessary exposure time, as evidenced by the fact that above 42°C, a 1°C elevation requires halving the exposure time to achieve a similar survival curve in vitro (30). While this direct killing effect is potentially useful, the documented metabolic damage to neurons at temperatures greater than 43°C would appear to provide for a very narrow therapeutic index. Several factors, however, act to make hyperthermia more selective than these numbers would suggest. One factor is *thermal tolerance*. This is the ability of cells to survive otherwise lethal temperatures after previous exposure to sublethal temperature elevations. In vitro studies demonstrate that normal cells develop thermal tolerance more quickly than neoplastic cells. Furthermore, the phenomenon appears to be transient, lasting hours to days, with neoplastic cells losing thermal tolerance more rapidly than normal cells. This has led some investigators to suggest that loss of thermal tolerance is related to cell division (and subsequent dilution of "heat shock" proteins), a fact that may be particularly relevant in the brain where most normal cells are not dividing. A second factor that promotes the selectivity of hyperthermia is the fact that poorly vascularized tissues can be selectively heated to higher temperatures than surrounding normal tissue. This advantageous situation is further enhanced by the finding that heat frequently decreases blood flow even further in tumors, while having little effect or even increasing blood flow in normal tissues.

The exact mechanism of hyperthermic killing is not completely understood, although at least two targets appear to be involved—one being cell membranes (particularly the membranes of intracellular organelles) and the other being chromatin. Whether tumor cells are inherently more sensitive than normal cells to hyperthermia has never been conclusively demonstrated.

The observed differences in sensitivity may be attributable to physiological differences related to pH and nutrient levels (30).

Heat enhances the ability of ionizing radiation to kill mammalian cells. The mechanism of this action appears to involve interference with repair mechanisms in cells exposed to sublethal levels of radiation. While this effect can be realized with hyperthermia delivered either before or after irradiation, the greatest effect in vivo is achieved with concurrent administration of the two therapeutic modalities. In vitro results could conceivably differ from in vivo results due to physiological changes in the tumor induced by hyperthermia. It is of considerable importance to note that the effects of hyperthermia appear to be enhanced in hypoxic cells in the DNA-synthesis stage (S-phase) of the cell cycle, precisely those conditions that render cells relatively resistant to radiation therapy.

The potentiation of *chemotherapy* by hyperthermia may also be related to inhibition of cell repair, although increased uptake of the chemotherapeutic agent may also play a role. The potentiating effect of hyperthermia appears to be greatest for the nitrosoureas and cis-platinum.

In reviewing the biological effects of hyperthermia, one must consider the role of *immune responses*. Some investigators have suggested that hyperthermia stimulates an immune response that potentiates the direct effect of the heat. This concept stems mainly from experiments in which in vivo cure rates of 100% are obtained with hyperthermia at levels that produce no more than a log kill in vitro. Indeed, some authors have suggested that Coley's original work where hyperthermia was induced with bacterial toxins was purely an immunological phenomenon. However, in reviewing the role of the immune response in hyperthermia, Hahn (1982) concluded that no firm data existed to prove any correlation (39).

Methods of Heat Delivery

In discussing heat delivery systems it is convenient to divide the various systems into three categories: whole body systems, regional systems, and local systems. *Whole body systems* have been employed in the treatment of central nervous system tumors, but are, for obvious theoretical reasons, not well suited for the hyperthermia of brain tumors. *Regional systems,* while allowing for more focused heating in a noninvasive manner, still lack the spatial specificity of local systems and may be likened to external beam radiation in their ability to focus energy. Regional systems include magnetic induction techniques, ultrasound transducers, and certain types of rf and microwave applicators. *Local systems,* of necessity, are invasive instruments that may be likened to interstitial radiation implants in their ability to achieve spatial specificity. The most basic way to provide local heating is with resistive heating elements. Current interstitial techniques, however, generally utilize rf needle electrodes, ferromagnetic seeds that are magnetically induced or, most commonly, microwave antennas.

Microwave antennas, operating at higher frequencies than radiowaves, have the theoretical advantage of not heating fat preferentially (11). Operating at the allowable frequencies of 915 and 2450 MHz, interstitial microwave systems utilize an array of antennas inserted in parallel to achieve the desired geometry and treatment envelope. These elements are best placed stereotactically in a manner similar to placement of brachytherapy catheters.

The most significant problem in providing localized heating is to predict, with some degree of accuracy, the distribution of temperatures in a system where the dominant heat transfer mechanism is convection based on highly variable blood perfusion. This, coupled with the problem of obtaining accurate in vivo measurements (it must be remembered that metal temperature probes will, themselves, interact with the electromagnetic field and give falsely elevated readings), make the technical aspects of hyperthermia quite challenging.

Current Status of Clinical Trials

To date, only a few centers have utilized hyperthermia to treat intracranial tumors in man. All were essentially phase I studies. The results obtained from these centers are summarized below.

Salcman and Samaras (97) reported the use of single-microwave-antenna systems operating at 2450 MHz in six patients with malignant glial tumors. The patients received two 60-min sessions at 45°C separated by 48 hr. No permanent sequelae attributable to the hyperthermia sessions were reported.

Silberman *et al.* (99) reported the use of noninvasive regional heating by a magnetic-loop induction system in 10 patients with brain tumors (three primary and seven metastatic tumors). Normal brain temperatures ranged from 38.6 to 43.4°C with a median temperature of 41.1°C and an average of 40.9°C. Tumor temperatures ranged from 38.8 to 46.3°C with median and average temperatures of 42.5°C and 42.6°C, respectively. All patients but one received BCNU concurrently. These authors reported no mortality and minimal morbidity.

Winter *et al.* (114) reported on 12 patients with primary brain tumors treated with microwave antenna systems operating at 2450 MHz. Estimated peak tumor temperatures were 42.5°C for 1 hr. Several treatments spaced over a few days were employed. The authors reported no adverse effects due to the hyperthermia and favorable clinical responses in 75% of the patients.

Roberts *et al.* (93) reported a trial in six patients with malignant gliomas treated with interstitial hyperthermia and ^{192}Ir brachytherapy. Hyperthermia was delivered via a microwave antenna array operating at 915 MHz. Each patient received 60 min of hyperthermia with the objective of maintaining the tumor periphery at 42 to 43°C. After the hyperthermia treatment, the antennas and thermometry probes were removed and ^{192}Ir seeds were inserted into the same catheters. Twenty Gray were delivered over 3 to 9 days. One week later, the patients returned for conventional external-beam irradiation carried to 60GY over 6 weeks. The authors reported technical feasibility and reasonable patient tolerance. Intracranial pressures were transiently elevated in one patient.

Future Work

While hyperthermia appears to be a promising adjuvant therapy in the treatment of intracranial malignancies, many questions remain. First, technical problems relating to precise geometric localization must be overcome. Second, phase II trials are needed to determine optimum heat intensities, exposure times, and treatment sequences. Additional phase II trials are needed to determine the optimum timing of concomitant radiation or chemotherapy. Finally, phase III trials to determine the ultimate role of hyperthermia will be needed.

Immunotherapy

As imaging-directed stereotactic neurosurgery allows for precision access to points in a stereotactic volume within intracranial space, software programs that permit placement of multiple parallel catheters within a defined target envelope are ideal for the consideration of immunotherapy within a tumor volume. Although a number of potential techniques for immunotherapy by interstitial means are feasible, *adoptive* measures seem to hold intense interest. Currently, it has been demonstrated that incubation of peripheral blood lymphocytes in interleukin-2 (IL-2) for 3 to 4 days can generate cells highly lytic for a variety of human tumors including those of the brain (36, 51, 76, 77, 79, 94). These lymphokine-activated killer (LAK) cells are capable of mediating potent antitumor effects in vivo in animal models of tumor, especially when given concomitantly with IL-2, the latter being required for the continued proliferation and activity of LAK cells in vivo. Recently, IL-2 given alone has also been shown to have efficacy in vivo. The combination of LAK cells and IL-2 and also IL-2 alone have recently been shown to have a promising role in the therapy of patients with a variety of cancers refractory to conventional modes of treatment.

A regional approach using these modalities has been attempted in brain tumors with no signs of systemic or neural toxicity even after administration intraoperatively of up to 10^{10} LAK cells and 10^6 units of IL-2. However, these protocols employing LAK cells and IL-2 have not used the combination of IL-2 alone in a large enough number of patients and have used this therapy primarily during an open craniotomy when patients are intrinsically immunosuppressed and also usually receiving high-dose steroid drugs. Employment of stereotactic techniques with imaging guidance enables specific delivery of such components into the tumor and is required for optimum assessment of the employment of such a method of adoptive immunotherapy in the management of glial tumors.

Phototherapy

The concept of inactivation of biomolecules and biologial systems following exposure to certain dyes, visible light, and oxygen has been appraised for more than 80 years. More than 100 different dyes have been demonstrated to exert this photodynamic effect on systems ranging from isolated biomolecules to whole cells. This reaction is basically a photoinitiated oxidation involving energy transfer from the dye to oxygen to form singlet oxygen as a short-lived intermediate. Major emphasis has been placed on the photobiology of *porphyrins* in these schema, with molecular oxygen required for most porphyrin-sensitized reactions. These substances, especially hematoporphyrin (Hp), its acetic-sulphuric acid derivative (HpD) and, more recently, its chromatographic fractions, have demonstrated a preferential retention in neoplastic tissues as opposed to normal tissue. The long-lived photogenerator triplet state of the porphyrins reacts with oxygen by an energy transfer process to produce singlet oxygen which in turn damages the biological system. Electron transfer reactions are usually not important.

Only those wavelengths of light absorbed by the porphyrin molecule can lead to a photoreaction. From a physical standpoint, light is an electromagnetic radiation in the wavelength range from 10 nm to 20 µ. As discrete packets of energy or photons, light may be described by either wave principles or a quantum mechanics theory. To initiate a reaction, light must be absorbed by the molecule, and the probability for photon absorption is dependent upon factors of energy (wavelength) and the electron structure of the molecule. The porphyrins possess an absorption spectrum with peak absorption at 400 nm, the Soret band, and minor absorption bands of decreasing magnitude in the 500- to 640-nm regions. In particular, *blue* and *red light* actuate the porphyrin molecules.

Of singular importance in the consideration of this mechanism is the issue of *penetration* of *light* into tissue which is determined by the optical character of the tissue and the wavelength of light. The photon may be either absorbed, reflected, transmitted, or scattered. Light dosimetry related to either porphyrin activation or deterioration is a key issue, with the number of photons or the total number of photons delivered critical. Light penetration in the brain is limited, being on the order of 3 to 8 mm in an adult brain at 630 nm. There is extensive laboratory and clinical evidence that indicates the feasibility of pursuing the concept of photoactivation via an interstitial method in brain tumors. Multiple parallel catheter placement within a bridging-defined tumor burden may, in theory, serve as conduits for introduction of quartz fiber bundles for transmission of monochromatic *red light* that is generated via laser energy. Such a method could be applied to cystic lesions as well. The concept is currently experimental, but the body of knowledge related to phototherapy is growing and hopefully will permit clinical trials related to this concept during the course of the next decade (7, 31, 64).

Chemotherapy

Although extensive laboratory or clinical studies dealing with interstitial chemotherapy are not yet available, a number of reports have implied its potential feasibility and have recommended pursuit of further detailed investigations. The technical methodology related to imaging-directed stereotaxy no doubt will offer stimulation to those with expertise and interest in this topic (21, 60, 63, 108-111).

IMAGING-DIRECTED STEREOTACTIC RADIOSURGERY (LINEAR ACCELERATOR TECHNIQUE)

Background

Stereotactic radiosurgery is a method for treating intracranial lesions that are unsuitable for open surgical techniques. A high dose of radiation is delivered to a precisely defined volume of tissue with the normal tissues outside this volume receiving a low radiation dose, thus being minimally affected.

It is an attractive treatment modality because it may be applied and is effective in treating lesions in surgically "inaccessible" regions. Treatment complications reported to date are uncommon and hospitalization time is short.

The treatment combines the precision of stereotactic technique with radiobiologically more effective high doses of radiation.

In 1951, Leksell first introduced the term "radiation surgery" (63, 66, 67). He used very narrow beams of radiation (3, 5, 7 mm) stereotactically focused onto a cerebral brain target. As many as 179 beams were employed to achieve a very desirable steep dose gradient between the small treatment volume and the surrounding normal tissue (64, 65, 68). A single high dose of radiation sufficient to induce necrosis in the treatment volume was given. This is in contrast to the conventional method of giving radiation therapy in multiple fractions. A differential effect in cell kill is thereby achieved between tumor and normal tissue because normal tissues are better able to repair the damage from the much lower doses of radiation received.

In 1974, Leksell reported a modification of his radiosurgical method resulting in an increase in treatment volumes of lesions up to 14 mm in diameter. A significant limitation of this technique was the restricted range of volumes that could be treated. However, this method allowed diverse applications and has been used for treatment of benign conditions such as chronic pain, psychiatric disorders, Parkinson's disease, aneurysms, arteriovenous fistulas, acoustic neuromas, craniopharyngiomas, and pituitary adenomas. Treatment results were encouraging with few side effects being reported.

Radiosurgical techniques were expanded to include the "Bragg Peak" region (59-61) of a proton beam (Uppsala, Sweden and Boston, MA) and helium ions from synchrocyclotrons (Berkeley, CA). These radiation beams produced a dense region of ionization within the treatment volume while sparing normal tissues. Unfortunately, there have been very few facilities in the world capable of delivering such a treatment.

In 1985, Hartmann et al. (44) (Heidelberg, FRG) reported a method of modifying a conventional linear accelerator to achieve the same result by stereotactically localizing the center of the target volume, placing it at the isocenter of the treatment machine, and using a multiple arc technique. They stressed the importance of using less than six arcs and a narrow beam geometry achieved by employing additional collimators. These additional collimators allowed for more sharply defined x-ray beams. Such collimated-field diameters ranged from 9 to 29 mm. The use of multiple arcs resulted in a steep gradient between tumor and normal tissue of 7 to 15% change of relative dose/1 mm. Similar techniques and dosimetry studies were developed by Colombo et al. (Padua, Italy) using a 4-mV linear accelerator (23-25). Also, Barcia-Salario et al. (Valencia, Spain) (17) and Betti and Derechinsky (Buenos Aires, Argentina) (16) have described similar techniques using equipment available in most radiation therapy facilities.

In the United States, similar radiosurgical techniques were conceptualized (46) and practically implemented using a modified linear accelerator at the Joint Center in Boston (73). This method employs the BRW CT-guided stereotactic system and a 6-mV linear accelerator equipped with special collimators from 12.5 to 30 mm in diameter. The Boston group utilizes target localization via planar angiography (vascular lesions). Performance tests showed good accuracy in positioning the target point at the isocenter of the treatment machine.

The majority of studies have reported on the treatment of benign lesions. Few reports have discussed the treatment of small primary or metastatic brain tumors. Such studies are currently underway at the Norris Cancer Hospital and Research Institute (USC).

Current Experience, Concepts and Rationale for Radiosurgery

Radiation delivered in short interval (e.g., part of 1 day) requires a significantly lower dose to produce a stated effect than that required to produce the same effect over a long interval. Strandquist (70) studied radiation dose effect on skin tumors and constructed isoeffect curves for skin necrosis, cure of skin cancer, moist desquamation, etc. Lindgren (70) applied these principles to study the risk of producing brain necrosis and constructed isoeffect curves for brain tolerance and high risk of cerebral necrosis. He concluded that the threshold for radiation-induced brain necrosis was 45 Gy given over 30 days (or equivalent). In his opinion, by shortening the treatment interval to 1 day, cases of brain necrosis would start to occur at doses of 12 Gy and above. Lindgren's conclusions are often criticized because of a limited number of distribution points and for the assumption that the slope of the curves is the same as that of Strandquist.

The Berkeley Group observed in their study of injury following αparticle irradiation of the brain that higher doses will induce damage earlier.

Kjellberg (studying proton beam effects) performed a similar analysis on the threshold of brain necrosis in the monkey (59). He extrapolated the line out to 70 years in order to advance an hypothesis that would avoid long-term risks in patients being treated for benign conditions with a normal life expectancy. Kjellberg used his own animal and human data plus data from Zeman, Lungren, and Boden to relate the dose of radiation required to produce necrosis to volume being radiated. He showed that small volumes required greater radiation doses to produce the same effect. He felt that the Ellis Formula (used in radiobiology to compare different time, dose, or fraction size of radiation) has little use in radiosurgical procedures, which are usually carried out in one or two sessions. He considered *volume* radiated to be the crucially *important variable*. He observed that the lower limit of dose for brain necrosis of a 7-mm beam is about 5 times greater than for a 50-mm beam. He also observed the importance of the location of treatment site. Those in *corticospinal pathways, optic pathways,* and the *brainstem* were *more sensitive* than the "silent areas." He devised a lower dose schedule for arteriovenous malformations (AVMs) in those sensitive areas—a dose range in which no complications were witnessed by this group.

In conclusion, the rationale for radiosurgery is to deliver a dose to the central portion of the lesion that will produce necrosis, while at the same time ensuring that the dose to the adjacent normal tissue is below that which carries a significant risk of radiation necrosis.

Clinical Studies

Although the majority of clinical data deal with benign lesions, review of past experience permits estimations of guidelines for treatment volume, dosage, and expected complications related to a larger spectrum of neoplasia.

At the Karolinska Institute, where the concept of radiosurgery originated, its technique has been employed in the following areas (14, 67, 68, 90, 101, 102): (*a*) functional neurosurgery for chronic pain, psychiatric disorders, and Parkinson's disease; (*b*) vascular neurosurgery for aneurysms, AVMs, and carotid-cavernous fistulas; and (*c*) oncological neurosurgery for acoustic neuromas, craniopharyngiomas, and pituitary adenomas.

Data indicated good results with few serious side effects with their technique. The diameter of the treatment volume was limited to 2.5 cm because of technical limitations. Currently, single treatments of 50 Gy are being given there for AVMs. In a series of 135 patients with AVMs, 95% whose AVMs were completely encompassed by the treatment volume achieved complete or partial cure.

Barcia-Solario *et al.* (17) have treated acoustic neuromas and AVMs by inducing focal lesions since 1977. They report lesions up to 30 mm in diameter. For acoustic neuroma, 40 Gy were delivered to the center and 25 Gy to the surface (50% isodose line). For AVMs, 45 Gy were delivered to the center and 30 Gy to the surface. They have noted the appearance of an area of central necrosis at 6 months and regression of treated lesions over 1 year.

Initial studies on the feasibility of using the proton beam in radiosurgical techniques were carried out by Larsson using the 183-MeV cyclotron at the Gustav Werner Institute in Uppsala, Sweden. Kjellberg introduced stereotactic proton beam Bragg Peak radiosurgery with 165-MeV cyclotron in Boston.

By 1979, Kjellberg had treated 1215 patients (60, 61). These included pituitary adenoma (812 cases), other sellar tumors (eight cases), normal pituitary suppression (220 cases), benign tumors (23 cases), malignant tumors (33 cases), AVMs (114 cases), and other (five cases). He employed dose ranges from 9 to 50 Gy for AVMs depending on treatment volume and location in sensitive sites. In 1983, results of the first 75 patients treated for AVMs (follow-up 2–16 years) indicated that in 66 of 75 patients there were no complications. Four of the first 27 patients treated had complications felt to be dose related. The treatment volumes were in the upper range (2–5 cm), and associated with corticospinal pathways. Subsequent protocol changes were instituted. Four other patients had what were considered to be nontreatment-related complications, i.e., hemorrhages within 18 months of treatment. He concluded that none of the group had died of procedure-related causes. Data were interpreted to indicate no infections, procedure-related hemorrhages, or thromboembolic events.

In 1984, the Berkeley California Group published their first clinical report (55 patients) of the use of stereotactically directed narrow beams of helium ions from an 184-inch synchrocyclotron. Their series included deep-seated and life-threatening AVMs and carotid-cavernous fistulas. The physical properties of their treatment modality are similar to those of the proton beam. They gave 4500 rads to the center of a volume up to 3 x 3 x 3 cm with rapid fall-off at the edges (surface dose not specified). They had no early complications at 3 years, and have not observed any early demyelinative changes that might be a predictor of late complications. The majority of cases of brain necrosis occur within 3 years of treatment. Infrequent late cases may occur up to 30 years after treatment. Hartmann *et al.* (44) have treated 17 patients with AVMs or isolated brain metastases. Treatment consisted of a single dose in the range of 20 to 38 Gy using a 15-mV x-ray beam from a linear accelerator.

In Italy, Colombo *et al.* (23) recently reported on six cases of malignant brain lesions up to 4 cm in diameter. He utilized two fractions of treatment 2 weeks apart with doses varying from 10 to 25 Gy/fraction. Data cannot be evaluated since some cases also had external beam therapy, or because the follow-up time was limited. They stated that only one lesion failed to respond and there were no acute complications. It is too soon to evaluate late complications. Some of the lesions they treated were 4 to 5 cm in diameter.

General Methodology (BRW System)

The stereotactically guided small volume irradiation procedure uses CT (or MRI) information obtained from patient scans carried out with the base ring in place to calculate the coordinates of the chosen target point relative to the base ring. The base ring assembly, still fixed to the patient, is later supported by the BRW floor stand, built to attach to the base ring with precise reproducibility. The patient is supported by the radiotherapy treatment couch while the head ring is attached to the floor stand. Initially, however, the floor stand is fitted with an identical base ring that is not attached to the patient. This simulation base ring is fitted with a machined target assembly that has in turn been adjusted on a phantom base so as to locate the target point relative to the base ring (Fig. 4.55). (The adjustment on the phantom base follows the standard BRW procedure for locating the target using the coordinates calculated from the digital CT or MRI data.) The result of this stage of the procedure is the precise placement of a target attached to the BRW floor stand. The target represents the location of the chosen cranial target point relative to an identical base ring attached to the patient.

The floor stand, which has three orthogonal drives, is now adjusted so that the target is located at the *isocenter* of the radiotherapy accelerator. The isocenter is defined as the common point of intersection of the beam central ray, the horizontal axis of rotation of

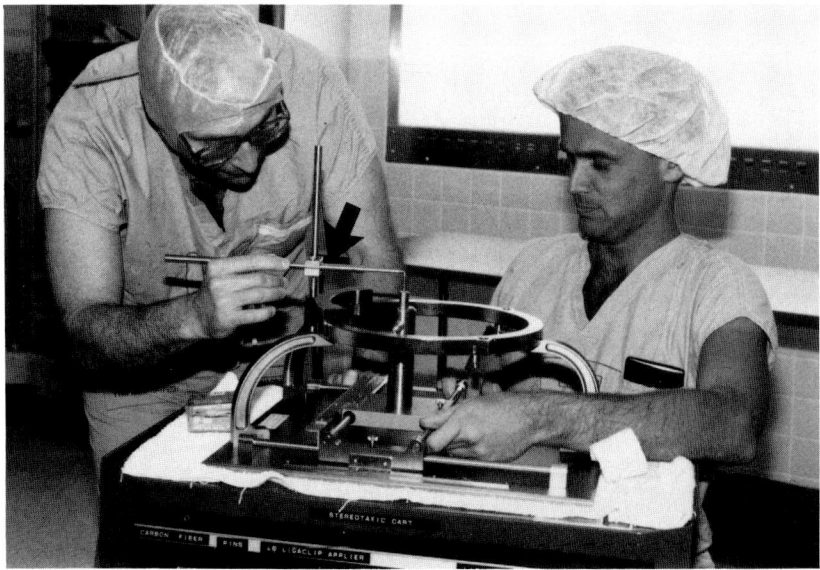

Figure 4.55. Translation of imaging data with center of target volume determined on phantom base with treatment volume isocenter transferred to isocenter of linear accelerator unit by targeting assembly (phantom pointer).

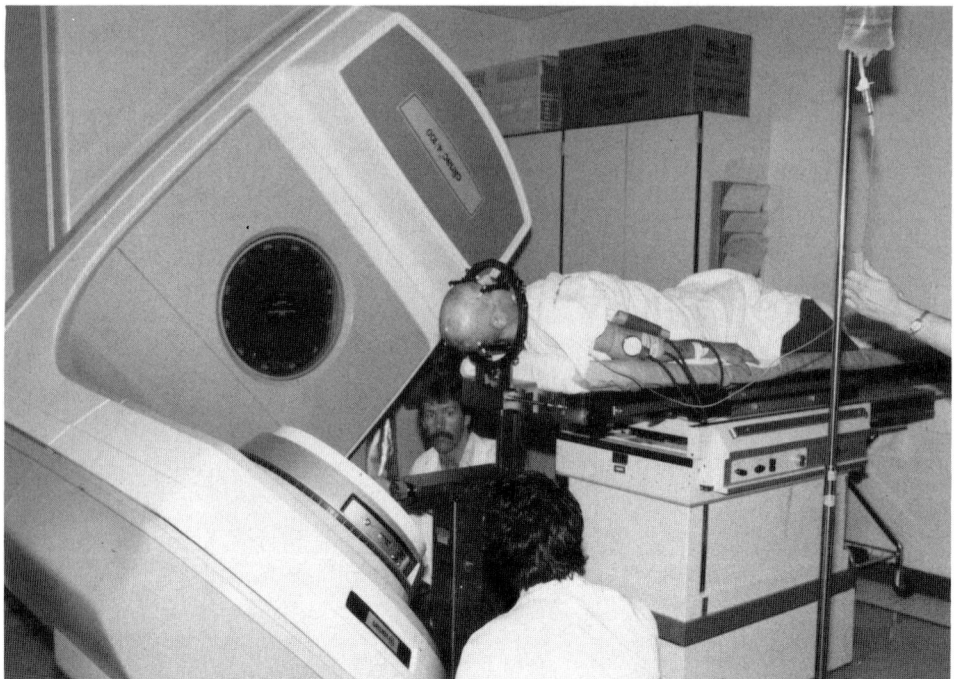

Figure 4.56. Treatment arcs are checked with center of the tumor volume fixed at isocenter of rotation of linear accelerator unit.

the gantry, and the vertical axis of rotation of the treatment couch. Gantry rotation through 360° of arc is specified to result in the beam central axis always passing through a 1-mm radius spherical volume that defines the isocenter. Couch rotation is also specified in such a way that turntable rotation over the complete 180° of rotation possible would retain within a 1-mm radius sphere, a pointer at isocenter that is attached to the couch. Attachment to the turntable is more direct, being subject to fewer mechanical tolerances.

The floor stand is adjusted so that the target is located at isocenter. Its location may be observed with the aid of room lasers and adjusted to project light beams to isocenter. An adjustable supplemental collimator assembly attached to the treatment head of the accelerator may be adjusted so that it is centered on the target. This adjustment employs the accelerator's optical projection field, which is coincident with the x-ray field. Turntable and couch rotations are then used to test the correctness of target placement relative to the isocenter and the adjustment of the supplemental collimator. The simulation base ring and its associated target are now removed and, without moving the floor stand, the patient and attached base ring are placed on the treatment couch and the base ring holder of the floor stand. The number of arcs and total dose to be used for the treatment having been decided beforehand, the dose to the isocenter for each arc is known. Each arc is then simulated on the patient with the light field from the treatment head (Fig. 4.56). The limits of each arc are determined from the constraints that the x-ray beam not pass through the eyes and that the gantry not collide with the floor stand or the adapter to the turntable. This will generally permit an arc of 100° or more to be used for each orientation of the treatment table.

This method, elegant in its simplicity, promises to expand the treatment option of stereotactic radiosurgery to a greater population of patients. Again, it is apparent that carefully controlled studies are in order prior to general employment of this technique.

REFERENCES

1. Adams JH, Graham D, Doyle D: *Brain Biopsy: The Smear Technique for Neurosurgical Biopsies.* Philadelphia, JB Lippincott, 1981.
2. Allen JC, Nisselbaum J, Epstein F, et al: Alpha-fetoprotein and human chorinic gonadotropin determination in cerebrospinal fluid. *J Neurosurg* 51: 368-374, 1979.
3. Apuzzo MLJ: CT guidance stereotaxis in the management of 94 lesions of the third ventricular region. In: *Surgery in and Around the Brain Stem and the Third Ventricle,* Berlin-Heidelburg, Springer-Verlag, 1986.
4. Apuzzo MLJ, Chandrasoma PT, Zelman V, Giannotta SL, Weiss MH: Computed tomographic guidance stereotaxis in the management of lesions of the third ventricular region. *Neurosurgery* 15: 502-508, 1984.
5. Apuzzo MLJ, Sabshin JK: Computed tomographic guidance stereotaxis in the management of intracranial mass lesions. *Neurosurgery* 12: 277-285, 1983.
6. Apuzzo MLJ, Heifetz MD, Weiss MH, Kurze T: Neurosurgical endoscopy using the side-viewing telescope: Technical note. *J Neurosurg* 46: 398-400, 1977.
7. Apuzzo MLJ, Jepson JH, Luxton G, Little FM: Ionizing and nonionizing radiation treatment of malignant cerebral gliomas: Specialized approaches. *Clin Neurosurg* 31: 470-496, 1984.
8. Apuzzo MLJ, Chandrasoma PT, Zelman V, von Hanwehr RI, Fredericks CA: Applications of computerized tomographic guidance stereotaxis. In Apuzzo, MLJ (ed): *Surgery of the Third Ventricle.* Baltimore, Williams & Wilkins, pp 751-792, 1987.
9. Apuzzo MLJ, Chandrasoma PT, Cohen D, Zee CS, Zelman V: Computed imaging stereotaxy: Experience and perspective related to 500 procedures applied to brain masses. *Neurosurgery* 20: 930-937, 1987.
10. Arita N, Bitoh S, Ushio Y, et al: Primary pineal endodermal sinus tumor with elevated serum and CSF alphafetoprotein levels. *J Neurosurg* 53: 244-248, 1980.
11. Atkins ER: Hyperthermia techniques and instrumentation. In Storm FK (ed): *Hyperthermia in Cancer Therapy.* Boston, MA, G.K. Hall Medical Publishers, pp 233-256, 1983.
12. Backlund EO: Role of stereotaxis in the management of midline cerebral lesions. In Apuzzo MLJ (ed): *Surgery of the Third Ventricle.* Baltimore, Williams & Wilkins, pp 802-805, 1987.
13. Backlund EO: Studies on craniopharyngiomas: III. Stereotaxic treatment with intracystic yttrium-90. *Acta Chir Scand* 139: 237-247, 1973.
14. Backlund EO: Studies on craniopharyngiomas. Stereotaxic treatment with radiosurgery. *Acta Chir Scand* 139: 344-351, 1973.
15. Backlund EO: Stereotactic treatment of craniopharyngiomas. *Acta Neurochir* (Suppl) 21: 177-183, 1974.
16. Betti O, Derechinsky V: Irradiation stereotaxique multifaisceaux. *Neurochirurgie* 29: 295-298, 1983.
17. Barcia-Solario JL, Hernandez G, Ciudad J, Bordes V: Stereotactic radiosurgery in acoustic neuromas. *Acta Neurochir* (Suppl 33): 1984.
18. Bernstein M, Gutin PH: Interstitial irradiation of brain tumors: A review. *Neurosurgery* 741-750, 1981.
19. Borit A: Embryonal carcinoma of the pineal region. *J Pathol* 97: 165-168, 1969.
20. Bosch DA: Indications for stereotactic biopsy in brain tumours. *Acta Neurochir* (Wien) 54: 167-179, 1980.
21. Bouvier G, Penn RD, Kroin JS, Beique R, Guerard MJ: Direct delivery of medication into a brain tumor through multiple chronically implanted catheters. *Neurosurgery* 20: 286-291, 1987.
22. Brezovich IA, Atkinson WJ, Lilly MB: Local hyperthermia with interstitial techniques. *Cancer Res* 44: 4752-4756, 1984.
23. Colombo F, Angrilli F, Zanardo A, Pinna V, Alexandre A, Benedetti A: A new method for utilizing CT data in stereotactic surgery: Measurement and transformation technique. *Acta Neurochir* (Wien) 57: 197-203, 1981.
24. Colombo F, Benedetti A, Pozza F, Avanzo RC, Marchetti C, Chierego G, Zanardo A: External stereotactic irradiation by linear accelerator. *Neurosurgery* 16: 154-160, 1985.
25. Coughlin JCT, Douple EB, Strohbehn JW, Eaton WL, Trembly BS, Wong TL: Interstitial hyperthermia in conjunction with brachytherapy. *Radiology* 148: 285-288, 1983.
26. Crain BJ, Bigner SH, Johnston WW: Fine needle aspiration biopsy of deep cerebrum. A comparison of normal and neoplastic morphology. *Acta Cytoligica* (Balt) 26: 772-778, 1983.
27. Daumas-Duport C, Blond S, Vedrenne CL, Szikla G: Radiolesion versus recurrence: Bioptic data in 39 gliomas after interstitial, or combined interstitial and external radiation treatment. *Acta Neurochirurgica* (Suppl), 33: 291-299, 1984.
28. Daumas-Duport C, Monsaingeon V, Szenthe L, and Szikla G: Serial stereotactic biopsies: A double histological code of gliomas according to malignancy and 3-D configuration, as an aid to therapeutic decision and assessment of results. *Appl Neurophysiol* 45: 431-437, 1982.
29. Dayan AD, Marshall AHE, Miller AA, et al: Atypical teratomas of the pineal and hypothalamus. *J Pathol Bacteriol* 92: 1-28, 1966.
30. Dewey WC, Holahan EV: Hyperthermia—basic biology. Prog. exp. *Tumor Res* 28: 198-219, 1984.
31. Dougherty TJ, Thomas RE, Goyle DG, Weishaupt KR: Interstitial photoradiation therapy for primary solid tumors in pet cats and dogs. *Cancer Res* 41: 401-404, 1981.
32. Eisenhardt I, Cushing H: Diagnosis of intracranial tumors by supravital technique. *Am J Pathol* 6: 541-552, 1930.
33. Emami B, Mittal BM, Sapareto S: Sequencing of

the total course of hyperthermia and irradiation. *Cancer Res* 44: 4731–4732.
34. Fulling KH, Nelson JS: Cerebral astrocytic neoplasms in the adult. Contribution of histologic examination to the assessment of prognosis. *Seminars in Diagnostic Pathology* 1: 152–163, 1984.
35. Giovanella BC: Thermosensitivity of neoplastic cell in vitro. In F Kristian Storm (ed): *Hyperthermia in Cancer Therapy.* Boston, MA, G.K. Hall Medical Publishers, pp 55–62, 1983.
36. Grimm EA, Mazumder A, et al: The human lymphokine activated killer cell phenomenon. *J Exp Med* 155: 1823, 1982.
37. Gutin PH, Phillips TL, Hosobuchi Y, et al: Permanent and removable implants for the brachytherapy of brain tumors. *Int J Radiat Oncol Biol Physio* 7: 1371–1381, 1981.
38. Gutin PH, Phillips TL, Wara WM, et al: Brachytherapy of recurrent malignant brain tumors with removable high activity iodine-125 sources. *J Neurosurg* 60: 61–68, 1984.
39. Hahn GM: *Hyperthermia and Cancer.* New York, Plenum Press, 1982.
40. Hall EJ: *Radiobiology for the Radiologists.* Second Edit. New York, Harper & Row, 1978.
41. Hall EJ (ed): The oxygen effect. In *Radiobiology for the Radiologist, ed 2.* New York, Harper & Row, 1978.
42. Hall EJ (ed): Radiosensitivity and cell age in the mitotic cycle. In *Radiobiology for the Radiologist, ed. 2.* New York, Harper & Row, 1978.
43. Hall EJ, Roizin-Towle L: Biological effects of heat. *Cancer Res* 44: 4708–4713, 1984.
44. Hartmann B, Schlegel W, Sturm V, Kober B, Pastyr O, Lorenz W: Cerebral radiation surgery using moving field irradiation at a linear accelerator facility. *Int J Radiat Oncol Biol Physl* 11: 1185–1192, 1985.
45. Hasse J, Neilsen K: Value of tumor markers in the treatment of endodermal sinus tumors and choriocarcinomas in the pineal region. *Neurosurgery* 5: 485–488, 1979.
46. Heifetz MD, Wexler M, Thompson R: Single-beam radiotherapy knife: A practical theoretical model. *J Neurosurg* 60: 814–818, 1984.
47. Heilbrun MP: Computed tomography-guided stereotactic systems. *Clin Neurosurg* 31: 564–581, 1983.
48. Heilbrun MP, Roberts TS, Apuzzo MLJ, Wells TH, Sabshin JK: Preliminary experience with Brown-Roberts-Wells computerized tomography stereotaxic guidance system. *J Neurosurg* 59: 217–222, 1983.
49. Hochberg FH, Pruitt A: Assumptions in the radiotherapy of glioblastoma. *Neurology* 30: 907–911, 1980.
50. Iizuka J: Development of a stereotaxic endoscopy of the ventricular sys. *Confin Neurol* 37: 141–149, 1975.
51. Jacobs SK, Wilson DJ, et al: Interleukin-2 and autologous lymphokine activated cells in the treatment of malignant glioma. *J Neurosurg* 64: 743, 1986.
52. Jane JA, Bertrand G: A cytological method for the diagnosis of tumors affecting the central nervous system. *J Neuropath & Exp Neurol* 21: 400–409, 1962.
53. Kelly PJ: Computer-assisted stereotaxis: New Approaches for the management of intracranial intra-axial tumors. *Neurology* 36: 535–541, 1986.
54. Kelly PJ: Computer-assisted stereotaxic laser microsurgery. In Apuzzo MLJ (ed): *Surgery of the Third Ventricle.* Baltimore, Williams & Wilkins, pp 811–828, 1987.
55. Kelly PJ, Kall BA, Goerss S: Transposition of volumetric information derived from computed tomography scanning into stereotactic space. *Surg Neurol* 21: 465–471, 1984.
56. Kelly PJ, Kall BA, Goerss S: Computer simulation for the stereotactic placement of interstitial radionuclide sources into computed tomography-defined tumor volumes. *Neurosurgery* 14: 442–448, 1984.
57. Kelly PJ, Kall BA, Goerss S, Earnest F. IV: Computer-assisted stereotaxis laser resection of intra-axial brain neoplasms. *J Neurosurg* 64: 427–439, 1986.
58. Kirshner JJ, Ginsberg SJ, Fitzpatrick AV, Comis RL: Treatment of a primary intracranial germ cell tumor with a systemic chemotherapy. *Med Pediatr Oncol* 9: 361–365, 1981.
59. Kjellberg RN: Isoeffective dose parameters for brain necrosis in relation to proton radiosurgical dosimetry. Stereotactic cerebral irradiation. INSERM Symposium No. 12, 1979.
60. Kjellberg RN: Stereotactic bragg peak proton radiosurgery results. Stereotactic cerebral irradiation, INSERM Symposium No. 12, 1979.
61. Kjellberg RN, Hanahamura T, Davis KR, Lyons SL, Adams RD: Bragg-peak proton-beam therapy for arteriovenous malformations of the brain. *New Eng J Med* 309: 269–274, 1983.
62. Kobayashi T, Kageyama N, Ohara K: Internal irradiation for cystic craniopharyngioma. *J Neurosurg* 55: 896–903, 1981.
63. Kroin JS, Penn RD: Intracerebral chemotherapy: Chronic microinfusion of cis-platinum. *Neurosurgery* 10: 349–354, 1982.
64. Laws ER Jr, Cortese DA, Kinsey JH, et al: Photoradiation therapy in the treatment of malignant brain tumors. A phase I (feasibility) study. *Neurosurgery* 9: 672–678, 1981.
65. Leibel SA, Gutin PH, Phillips TL: Interstitial implantation of high-activity iodine-125 sources for treatment of recurrent malignant brain tumors. *Int J Radiat Oncol* 10: 144, 1984.
66. Leksell L: The stereotaxic method and radiosurgery of the brain. *Acta Chir Scand* 102: 316–319, 1951.
67. Leksell L: *Stereotaxis and Radiosurgery: An Operative System.* Springfield, IL, Charles C Thomas, 1971.
68. Leksell L, Backlund O: Stereotactic gammacapsulotomy. In Hitchcock ER, Ballantine HT, Meyerson B (eds): *Modern Concepts in Psychiatric Surgery.* Amsterdam, Elsevier, pp 213–216, 1979.
69. Leksell L, Leksell D, Schwebel J: Stereotaxis and

nuclear magnetic resonance. *J Neurol, Neurosurg and Psychiatry* 48: 14–18, 1985.
70. Lindgren M: On tolerance of brain tissue and sensitivity of brain tumors to irradiation. *Acta Radiol* 170: 1–73 (Suppl.), 1958.
71. Liwnicz BH, Henderson KS, Masukawa T, Smith RD: Needle aspiration cytology of intracranial lesions. A review of 84 cases. *Acta Cytologica* 26: 779–786, Baltimore, 1982.
72. Lunsford LD, Martinex AJ, Latchaw RE: Stereotaxic surgery with a magnetic resonance- and comuterized tomography-compatible system. *J Neurosurg* 64: 872–878, 1986.
73. Lutz W, Winston KR, Maleki N: A system for stereotactic radiosurgery with a linear accelerator. Joint Center for Radiotherapy, Department of Neurosurgery, Harvard Medical School, *Neurosurgery*, (in press).
74. Lyons BE, Britt RH, Strohbehn JW: Localized hyperthermia in the treatment of malignant brain tumors using an interstitial microwave antenna array. *IEEE Trans Biomed Engin* 31: 53–62, 1984.
75. Lyons BE, Strohbehn JW, Roberts DW, Wong TZ, Britt RH: Interstitial microwave hyperthermia for the treatment of brain tumors. In Leopold J, Anghileri CT, Robert J (eds): *Hyperthermia in Cancer Treatment.* Boca Raton, Florida, CRC Press, pp 25–45, 1986, vol 3.
76. Mazumder A, Eberlein TJ, *et al:* Phase I study of adoptive immunotherapy of cancer with activated autologous mononuclear cells. Cancer 53: 896, 1984.
77. Mazumder A, Rosenberg SA: Successful immunotherapy of NK-resistant established pulmonary metastases by syngeneic lymphocytes activated by interleukin-2. *J Exp Med* 159: 495, 1984.
78. Morris AA: The use of the smear technique in the rapid histological diagnosis of tumors of the central nervous system: Description of a new staining method. *J Neurosurg* 4: 497–504, 1947.
79. Mule JJ, Shu S, *et al:* Adoptive immunotherapy of established pulmonary metastases with LAK cells and recombinant interleukin-2. *Science* 225: 1487, 1984.
80. Mundinger F: The treatment of brain tumors with radioisotopes. *Progr Neurol Surg* 1: 202–257, 1966.
81. Mundinger F, Hoefer T: Protracted long-term irradiation of inoperable midbrain tumors by stereotactic Curie-therapy using Iridium-192. *Acta Neurochir* 21: 93–100, 1974.
82. Mundinger F: Implantation of radioisotopes (Curie-therapy). In Schaltenbrand G, Walker AE (eds): *Stereotaxy of the Human Brain.* New York, Thieme-Stratton, 1982.
83. Mundinger F: Rationale and methods of interstitial Ir-192 brachytherapy and Ir-192 and I-125 protracted long-term irradiations. In Szikla G, (ed): *Cerebral Irradiations.* Amsterdam, Elsevier, pp 101–117, 1979.
84. Mundinger F, Weigel K: Long-term results of stereotactic interstitial curietherapy. *Acta Neurochirurgica Suppl* 33: 367–371, 1984.
85. Ostertag CB: Biopsy and interstitial radiation therapy of cerebral gliomas. *Ital J Neurol Sci* (Suppl.) 2: 121–128, 1983.
86. Ostertag CB, Groothuis D, Kleihues P: I. Effects of tumour and brain. Experimental data on early and late morphologic effects of permanently implanted gamma and beta sources (iridium-192, iodine-125 and yttrium-90) in the brain. *Acta Neurochir* (Suppl) 33: 271–280, 1984.
87. Ostertag CB, Weigel K, Birg W: CT-changes after long-term interstitial iridium-192 irradiation of cerebral gliomas. In Szikla G (ed): *Stereotactic Cerebral Irradiation.* Amsterdam, Elsevier, 1979, pp 149–155.
88. Petrovich Z, Apuzzo MLJ, Luxton G, Jepson JH, Cohen D: Interstitial radiobrachytherapy of malignant cerebral gliomas. In Walker M, Kornblith P (eds): *Contemporary Concepts in Neurooncology.* Futura Publishers, 1987.
89. Powell MP, Torrens MJ, Thomas JLG, *et al:* Isodense colloid cysts of the third ventricle: A diagnostic and therapeutic problem resolved by ventriculoscopy. *Neurosurgery* 13: 234–237, 1983.
90. Rahn T, Thorin M, Hall K, Backlund EO: Stereotactic radiosurgery in the treatment of MB Cushing. *Stereotactic Cerebral Irradiation,* INSERM Symposium No. 12, 1979.
91. Rao DV, Simpson JR, Marchosky JA: Afterloading interstitial irradiation for CNS tumors. *Int J Radiat Oncol* 10: 144, 1984.
92. Rivas JJ, Lobato RD: CT-assisted stereotaxic aspiration of colloid cysts of the third ventricle. *J Neurosurg* 62: 238–242, 1985.
93. Roberts DW, Coughlin CT, Wong TZ, Fratkin JD, Douple EB, Strohbehn JW: Interstitial hyperthermia and iridium brachytherapy in treatment of malignant glioma. *J Neurosurg* 64: 581–587, 1986.
94. Rosenberg SA, Lotze MT, *et al:* Observations on the systemic administration of autologous lymphokine-activated killer cells and recombinant interleukin-2. *New Eng J Med* 313: 1485, 1985.
95. Russell DS, Krayenbuhl H, Cairns H: The wet film technique in the histological diagnosis of intracranial tumors. A rapid method. *J Pathol* 45: 501–505, 1937.
96. Salcman M: Feasibility of microwave hyperthermia for brain tumor therapy. *Prog exp tumor Res* 28: 220–231, 1984.
97. Salcman M, Samaras GM: Hyperthermia for brain tumors: Biophysical rationale. *Neurosurgery* 9: 327–335, 1981.
98. Sheithauer BW: Neuropathology of pineal region tumors. *Clin Neurosurg* 32: 351–383, 1985.
99. Silberman AW, Rand RW, Storm FK, Drury B, Benz ML, Morton DL: Phase I Trial of thermochemotherapy for brain malignancy. *Cancer* 56: 48–56, 1985.
100. Silberman AW, Rand RW, Krag DN Storm FK, Benz ML, Drury B, Morton DL: Effect of localized magnetic induction hyperthermia on

the brain. *Cancer* 57: 1401-1404, 1986.
101. Steiner L: Treatment of arteriovenous malformations by radiosurgery. In Wilson CB, Bennet MS (eds): *Intracranial Arteriovenous Malformations.* Baltimore, Williams & Wilkins, 1984.
102. Steiner L, Leksell L, Forster DM, Greitz T, Backlund O: Stereotactic radiosurgery in intracranial arteriovenous malformations. *Act Neurochir (Suppl)* 21: 195-209, 1974.
103. Storm FK: Background, principles, and practice. In Storm FK (ed): *Hyperthermia in cancer therapy.* Boston, MA, G.K. Hall Medical Publishers, pp 1-8, 1983.
104. Szikla G, Peragut JC: Irradiation interstitielle des gliomes. *Neurochir* (Suppl 2) 21: 187-228, 1975.
105. Szikla G: Stereotactic cerebral irradiation. North Holland, Elsevier, 1979.
106. Szikla G, Schlienger M, Betti O, Talairach J, Cohadon F, Rougier A, Pigneux J, Benabid AL, Vrousos P, Chiroussel J, Sedan R, Peragut JC, Farnarier P, Pecker J, Scarabin JM, Vallee B, Gilbert P: Combined interstitial and external irradiation of gliomas. A progress report. In Szikla G (ed): *Stereotactic Cerebral Irradiation.* New York, Elsevier, pp 329-338, 1979.
107. Szikla G, Schlienger M, Blind S, Daumas-Duport C, Missir O, Miyahara S, Musolino A, Schaub C: Insterstitial and combined interstitial and external irradiation of supratentorial gliomas. Results in 61 cases treated 1973-1981. *Acta Neurochir Suppl* 33: 355-362, 1984.
108. Tator CH: Intraneoplastic injection of CCNU for experimental brain tumor chemotherapy. *Surg Neurol* 7: 73-77, 1977.
109. Tator CH, Day A, Ng R, Liberman L: Chemotherapy of an experimental glioma with nitrosoureas. *Cancer Res* 37: 476-481, 1977.
110. Tator CH, Wassenar W: Intraneoplastic injection of methotrexate for experimental brain tumor chemotherapy. *J Neurosurg* 46: 165-174, 1977.
111. Tator CH, Wassenaar W, So WS: Therapy of an experimental glioma with systemic or intraneoplastic methotrexate or radiation. *J Neurosurg* 46: 175-184, 1977.
112. Weigel K, Ostertag CB, Mundinger F: Interstitial long-term irradiation of tumors in the pineal region. Stereotactic cerebral irradiation. INSERM. Symp. No. 12, 1979, pp 283-292.
113. Willems JS: Aspiration biopsy cytology of tumors of the central nervous system and base of the skull. In Linsk JA, Franzen S (eds): *Clinical Aspiration Cytology.* Philadelphia, JB Lippincott, 1983.
114. Winter A, Laing J, Paglione R, Sterzer F: Microwave hyperthermia for brain tumors. *Neurosurgery* 17: 387-399, 1985.

Chapter 5

Contemporary Stereotactic Ventralis Lateral Thalamotomy in the Treatment of Parkinsonian Tremor and Other Movement Disorders

PATRICK J. KELLY, M.D.

In the late 1950s and early 1960s, stereotactic surgery found its greatest application in the production of subcortical lesions for the treatment of parkinsonian tremor and other movement disorders. As clinical experience accumulated, surgical methods became more sophisticated, and postoperative results improved. However, the advent of L-dopa in 1968 brought about a precipitous decline in the number of stereotactic procedures being performed. Following 1968, stereotactic thalamotomy was done only in the rare patient with Parkinson's disease who was unable to take L-dopa, or who failed to derive significant benefit from L-dopa. Occasional procedures were still performed for the treatment of other types of movement disorders and chronic pain.

In the late 1970s, stereotactic technique underwent a renaissance. This was reflected to a significant degree by the development of CT-guided stereotactic methods; the major application for these procedures was in the biopsy and treatment of intraaxial neoplasms. However, these new techniques were also of benefit to patients undergoing thalamic neuroablative surgery. Incorporation of imaging technology and neurophysiological methods for localization of structures and optimal lesion sites have increased the precision of stereotactic neuroablative procedures that maximize the therapeutic benefits and reduce the surgical risk.

Because technology has resulted in improved postoperative results and lower risk, perhaps it is now time to reassess the role of stereotactic thalamotomy in the management of patients with Parkinson's disease as well as in those having other types of movement disorders. After almost 20 yr of experience with L-dopa and L-dopa/carbidopa in Parkinson's disease, it is clear that there are many individuals whose tremor is not well controlled medically. These patients can be helped by a stereotactic thalamotomy which will delay the onset of disability for many years before bradykinesia becomes a significant problem. The following will review the history for movement disorder surgery and describe contemporary techniques for stereotactic ventralis lateral (VL) thalamotomy.

HISTORICAL ASPECTS

Surgeons have placed lesions in various locations within the extrapyramidal system and have noted beneficial results on the treatment of tremor and rigidity associated with Parkinson's disease. Horsley (30) in 1909, and later Bucy (17) extirpated the motor cortex and noted ablation of resting tremor. Meyers lesioned the ansa lenticularis by means of craniotomy and transventricular approach in 1942 (42). He also noted cessation of tremor. He concluded that destruction of the pallidothalamic tracts was the key to the control of tremor and rigidity. Utilizing a less hazardous subfrontal route, Fenelon (22) in Paris in 1950 successfully produced lesions of the ansa lenticularis by inserting a coagulating electrode. This open procedure was adopted by others, notably Guiot and Briot (24) of Paris and Gillingham of Edinburgh. These workers then developed a stereotactic instrument for thermocoagulation of medial segment of the globus pallidus—the point of origin of the ansa lenticularis. About that time, stereotactic pallidoansotomy had also been developed by Spiegel and Wycis in the United States (47).

Human stereotactic instruments have been available since Spiegel and Wycis first introduced mechanical three-dimensional control of subcortical probe placement (46, 48). In addition, Spiegel and Wycis also proposed the use of ventricular system landmarks for the stereotactic localization of subcortical targets (47). Cooper and Poloukhine (19) and Guiot and Brion (24) placed stereotactic lesions in the internal segment of the globus pallidus in the late 1950s and reported beneficial results in the treatment of tremor and rigidity. Later Bravo and Cooper (14) and Hassler (27) found that lesions in the ventral lateral thalamus more effectively abolished tremor and rigidity with acceptable levels of morbidity. This target, ventralis lateral (VL), remains the most common contemporary lesion site for the control of many types of movement disorders.

SURGICAL INDICATIONS FOR VL THALAMOTOMY

Parkinson's Disease: Tremor and Rigidity

No therapy alters the relentless progression of Parkinson's disease. Therapy is symptomatic with a goal of palliating the symptoms causing the disability. Initially, tremor and rigidity are responsible for the disability. Later in the course of the disease, bradykinesia results in significant disability and debilitation. Surgery is of particular benefit in patients with unilateral tremor who do not develop "midline symptoms" (i.e., bradykinesia, mental deterioration, and speech and gait disturbances). However, in patients with bilateral tremor, bilateral VL thalamotomy staged at least 3 months apart can provide effective long-term palliation from tremor and rigidity (38–40). Surgery is of no benefit in patients having rigidity and bradykinesia without tremor and in those who have rapidly progressive parkinsonism.

Intention Tremor

Selected patients with multiple sclerosis disabled by intention tremor can be helped by VL thalamotomy (41). Unfortunately, because of the degenerative nature of the disease, the ultimate long-term results will not be gratifying. In addition, younger patients having intention tremor related to cerebellar injuries can have good palliation by VL thalamotomy.

Essential or Familial Tremor

These patients do not have a degenerative disease. They are excellent candidates for stereotactic thalamotomy when disabling tremor is refractory to medication such as anticholinergics and Inderal®.

Dystonia Musculorum Deformans

In some hands, good results can be obtained in patients with dystonia (9, 18). The results of VL thalamotomy are better if the patient's dystonia is confined distally to an extremity (10, 18). Patients having midline dystonic syndromes including torticollis and retrocollis do not usually derive lasting benefit from central stereotactic procedures, and require peripheral intervention as well (10).

Cerebral Palsy

Some authors have reported favorable results with tension athetosis involving the upper extremities (16). It must be recognized that the basic pathological process has resulted in considerable destruction of cortex and basal ganglia. Therapeutic subcortical lesions may result in significant gait, speech, or intellectual complications, even though the surgery may have a beneficial effect on the tension athetosis.

ANATOMICAL CONSIDERATIONS

To greatly oversimplify the pathophysiology, tremor and other movement disorders result from disinhibition of a facilitory neuronal loop extending from cortex to striatum to pallidum to VL thalamic nuclear mass and back to cortex. In Parkinson's disease, neuronal loss in the substantia nigra, reduction of striatal dopamine, and reduced inhibition by the nigral-striatal pathway results in tremor and rigidity early in the course of the disease. Lesions of the subthalamic area and nucleus result in disinhibition of the cortical-striatal-pallidal-thalamic-cortical loop at the pallidum and result in hemiballismus. Disruption of the inhibitory γ-aminobutyric acid-mediated (GABA-mediated) pathways of the brachium conjunctivum result in disinhibition of the loop in the thalamus and intention tremor results.

Lesions anywhere in this loop will abolish most movement disorders in general and parkinsonian tremor in particular. As stated above, the most common target is in VL.

The Hassler terminology, most frequently used in the description of stereotactic thalamic surgery divides the lateral thalamic nuclear mass into lateral polaris (LPO), ventralis oralis anterior (VOA) (LPO and VOA correspond to ventralis anterior in Anglo-American terminology), ventralis oralis posterior (VOP) and ventralis intermedius (VIM) (which corresponds to VL) and ventralis caudalis (VCE and VCI) (which correspond to ventralis posterior [VP], VL, and ventralis medialis [VM], respectively). VOA is the most commonly used target for rigidity, while VOP and VIM are the best targets for tremor.

RADIOGRAPHICAL ESTABLISHMENT OF INTRACRANIAL TARGETS

Several tools at the neurosurgeon's disposal facilitate subcortical target localization. These are positive-contrast ventriculography, stereotactic atlases, stereotactic CT scanning, and neurophysiological investigations. Contrast studies are done with the patient in the stereotactic frame in order to establish the approximate position of anatomical structures.

Ventriculography

Ventriculography determines the position of anatomical structures that lie close to the midline and adjacent to the ventricular system. However, inaccuracy increases in direct relationship to the distance that the target structure lies from the radiologically determined ventricular system landmark (15, 52). Even though landmarks within the third ventricle are accurate in establishing the position of midline thalamic nuclei, they are less accurate in predicting the position of substructures in the lateral nuclear group. Therefore, a part of the ventricular system lying as close as possible to the desired target is selected when determining stereotactic coordinates.

For stereotactic thalamotomy, a positive-contrast third ventriculogram is utilized. It must demonstrate: (*a*) the anterior and posterior commissures, (*b*) the foramen of Monro, (*c*) the floor of the lateral ventricle, (*d*) the pineal recess, and (*e*) the aqueduct of Sylvius. Important calculations are based on the ability to reliably identify and confirm these landmarks.

DELINEATION OF SUBCORTICAL STRUCTURES FROM VENTRICULOGRAPHY

Three planes are constructed: a horizontal plane from anterior and posterior commissures, a vertical plane oriented perpendicular to the anterior commissure-posterior commissure (AC-PC) plane midway between anterior commissure and posterior commissure, and the midline plane. These form the baseline for determination of height, anterior-posterior coordinates and laterality coordinates, respectively. The approximate position of mesencephalic or diencephalic targets may be defined in coordinates based on these baselines. The coordinates for the target structures may be derived empirically, by geometrical methods (see "Procedure for VL Thalamotomy") or by utilizing a stereotactic atlas.

Stereotactic Atlases

A stereotactic atlas consists of cadaver brain sections sliced in accurate relationship to coordinate axes defined by ventricular system landmarks.

Spiegel and Wycis Atlas

The first human stereotactic atlas based on ventricular system landmarks was that of Spiegel and Wycis in 1952 (46). Thirty brains were sectioned and a variability study performed. The atlas consisted of 12 frontal sections of the cerebrum, fourteen myelin-stained diencephalic sections, selected sections sliced at angles to the base line, and other sagittally and horizontally sectioned brain specimens. Each of the 71 plates in the atlas is surrounded by a frame calibrated in millimeters. The variability study shows an impressive range in the position of subcortical structures in individual brains with respect to the base line coordinate axes (the posterior commissure, Frankfort's line, and the intraaural plane).

Talairach Atlas

In 1957, Talairach stressed the importance of having two intraventricular reference points: the anterior and posterior commissures (49). Each target nucleus or tract is defined by a set of geometrical constructs based on a grillwork established by subdivisions of the anterior commissure-posterior commissure line and thalamic height.

Schaltenbrand and Bailey Atlas

This atlas (1959) (45) and the later version by Schaltenbrand and Wahren consist of horizontal, coronal, and sagittal brain sections parallel to the AC-PC plane, a plane perpendicular to the AC-PC line at its midpoint, and the midline, respectively. Macroscopic slices (2× magnification) show the entire brain section with the coordinate grid. Microscopic slices of diencephalic structures (4× magnification) are presented in sagittal, coronal, and horizontal planes with the coordinate axes. Transparent acetate overlays outline the anatomical limits of the various subnuclei labeled according to the Hassler terminology and may be superimposed on the microscopic sections.

Andrew and Watkins Atlas

This atlas (1960) is based on a study of 26 hemispheres (6). The coordinate axes are: the midline, a horizontal plane developed between the foramen of Monro and the posterior commissure, and a line perpendicular to the foramen of Monro and the posterior commissure line at its midpoint, which forms the zero plane in the anterior-posterior dimension. Each diencephalic structure has been carefully measured with respect to these reference planes. Frequency distribution charts are tabulated and graphically portrayed as quadrangles showing the medial location of the structure with respect to the coordinate axes and variability range.

Van Buren and Borke Atlas

The first part of this atlas (1973) depicts stained sections of the human thalamus in 10 sagittal, eight horizontal, and 10 frontal sections (51). The second section graphically displays serial sections in three planes for each of the 24 thalamic nuclear substructure with respect to axes based on the AC-PC line. Sections are at 5-mm intervals. Superimposed outlines from several brains demonstrate variability of up to 5 mm in most of the main thalamic nuclear divisions. A simpler labeling system for the thalamic nuclei than Hassler's is used in this atlas.

Use of Stereotactic Atlas

Landmarks used to define the coordinate axes on which the stereotactic atlases being used is based must be defined in the patient by positive-contrast ventriculography. The surgeon then refers to the atlas and finds the desired anatomical target on a coronal, sagittal, or horizontal section and reads the actual stereotactic coordinates from the coordinate axis scale. These coordinates are corrected for radiographical magnification and transferred to the ventriculogram radiographs. The actual mechanical adjustments on the stereotactic frame that will target the structure are then derived.

All stereotactic atlases are inaccurate to some degree. This is due to fixation artifact and spatial anatomical variability in the relationship between subcortical structures and radiographically determined landmarks between individual brains (15, 52). Spatial variability increases the further the target structure lies from the radiologically determined landmarks. Proportional grid systems described by Talairach may improve localization accuracy somewhat. However, the variability studies of Andrew and Watkins (6) or Van Buren and MacCubbin (52) should make surgeons cautious in the use of stereotactic atlases as the sole means of deriving target coordinates. Atlases are therefore used to determine *approximate* target coordinates in functional stereotactic neurosurgery. The precise locations of subcortical structures are established by neurophysiologic methods.

STEREOTACTIC CT SCANNING

The CT scan establishes the axial configuration of the third ventricle and of the thalamus and stereotactically demonstrates the laterality of the internal capsule in an individual patient. Measurements may be taken off diagnostic CT scan slices that are obtained parallel to the AC-PC line. Alternatively, the use of a CT-compatible stereotactic head frame for data acquisition provides a mechanism by which stereotactic coordinates of any point selected on CT images may be accurately calculated (32).

Neurophysiological Localization

In early functional stereotactic procedures, targets were localized radiologically and a lesion was progressively enlarged until the desired clinical effect was attained. Lesions therefore tended to be quite large in some patients in order to compensate for the inaccuracy of early stereotactic instrumentation and variations in individual spatial anatomy. Therapeutically effective but unnecessarily large lesions had undesirable side effects: resting tremor was not infrequently converted to intention tremor, dysphasic speech became aphasic or dysphonic, and bradykinetic gait was replaced by ataxic gait.

In addition, ventriculography cannot detect variations of the medial-lateral width of the thalamus between individual patients. This set the stage for more severe complications. In patients with narrow thalami, large lesions could damage the internal capsule, situated in these patients more medially than usual. On the other hand, medial spread of a large lesion in an unusually wide thalamus could disrupt the fibers of the mammilothalamic tract and produce recent memory loss following bilateral procedures. Other patients having short thalami in the anterior-posterior dimension occasionally complained of contralateral and sometimes painful sensory dysesthesia following lesions of VL due to spread of the lesion into the sensory relay nucleus (VP) (29). Extension of lesions inferiorly occasionally damaged the subthalamic nucleus, which traded hemiballismus for resting tremor (20).

Because of these side effects and complications, surgeons developed physiological controls to corroborate targets prior to production of lesions. The most commonly used methods are electrical stimulation and microelectrode recording.

Electrical Stimulation

Modern rf generators have an option for electrically stimulating the lesion-producing electrode tip. Important physiological localizing information can be derived from low- and high-frequency electrical stimulation of a radiologically determined target site prior to producing the lesion. (5, 7, 28). In patients undergoing VL thalamotomy for movement disorders, low-frequency electrical stimulation of a properly sited electrode frequently accentuates tremor; high-frequency stimulation may abolish it.

Electrical stimulation of electrodes sited too far lateral result in internal capsular responses—twitching in the contralateral musculature in synchrony with stimulation at low frequencies or tonic contractions when 60 to 100 Hz stimulation is employed. In addition, stimulation of electrodes located too far posteriorly produce sensory dysesthesia contralaterally due to stimulation of VP. Visual, vestibular, auditory, temperature alteration, oculomotor, or fear responses indicate that the electrode is in the subthalamus or midbrain.

Current spread may result in stimulation of structures far away from the electrode tip. It is, therefore, important that the surgeon evaluate the effects of stimulation at threshold levels only (4, 50). In practice, stimulation is begun at low current levels (0–1 mA) with low frequency (2–5 Hz) and the current progressively increased to 1 mA or until physiological effect is noted. Next the current is reduced to below threshold levels and frequency is slowly increased up to 300 Hz or until a response is obtained. Careful physiological mapping of the sensory relay nucleus with 1.1-mm diameter bipolar concentric electrodes can give precise information regarding the medial-lateral organization of an individual patient's thalamus (21, 44, 50). The somatotopy of VP reflects the topographic organization of the contralateral body in VL and ventralis anterior (VA).

Microelectrode Recording

The recording of single unit activity by microelectrode has been used to help some surgeons in locating cellular groups firing in synchrony with tremor (12, 13, 31). Ablation of these cellular groups has been shown effective in the control of tremor (33). Unfortunately, there are so much data generated by single unit activity that, in this author's opinion, it is not an expedient means for localization during human stereotactic procedures. Nevertheless, computerization of this information and the use of graphics may render this data more manageable in the future (8, 11, 50).

Semimicroelectrode Recording

Semimicroelectrode recording establishes the position of junction between grey masses and fiber pathways (e.g., thalamus, internal capsule) and defines nuclear subgroups (1–3, 23, 26, 43). The technique employs a bipolar concentric electrode with 10 to 50 μm tip- and 400 μm tip-to-ring measurement. A preamplifier head stage attaches the microelectrode to a DC amplifier and thence to an oscilloscope and audio monitor.

Cellular "noise" is encountered in the cortex and all subcortical nuclear groups. White matter fiber tracts are essentially silent (1, 2, 23). Characteristic amplitude and frequency patterns aid in the identification of individual nuclear subgroups. Ventralis posterior is identified by high amplitude- (150 μV) evoked responses obtained (without averaging) when a part of the contralateral body is tapped or brushed. These somatosensory responses are so specific that it is possible to establish the VP thalamic representation of body parts in the individual patient. This information can serve as a "navigational landmark" with which to define the orientation of the body in the other nuclei of the VL nuclear mass (36).

PROCEDURE FOR VL THALAMOTOMY

There is some variation in the target localization methodology for VL thalamotomy as performed in different centers. In general, the stereotactic neuroradiological investigation establishes the *approximate position* of the subcortical target structures in reference to the stereotactic frame. The precise position of the target of the target structure is established by microelectrode recording and/or subcortical stimulation.

We use a Todd-Wells stereotactic frame and a preoperative data base consisting of stereotactic CT scanning, a computer resident stereotactic atlas, positive-contrast ventriculography, and microelectrode exploration. Lesion sites are corroborated by stimulation and lesions are made with an rf system. Stereotactic neuroablative procedures are usually done under mild sedation and local anesthesia in order to carefully monitor the clinical effects of stimulation and lesion production. The operation is performed in two sessions: first, a data acquisition procedure and, second, a microelectrode recording and lesioning procedure.

Data Acquisition

A CT-compatible stereotactic head frame is applied to the patient under local anesthesia and mild sedation, as described in previous reports (32–35, 37, 39). This fixes to the skull by four carbon fiber pins inserted in holes drilled in the outer table of the skull into the diploe. The depth of the pins in relationship to the vertical support elements of the head frame is measured by micrometers.

The patient then undergoes stereotactic CT scanning on a General Electric 8800 or 9800 CT scanning unit. A CT localization system containing nine carbon fiber rods in the shape of the letter "N" on either side of the head and anteriorly, attaches to the stereotactic head holder (Fig. 5.1).

This produces nine reference marks on each CT slice which allow calculation of

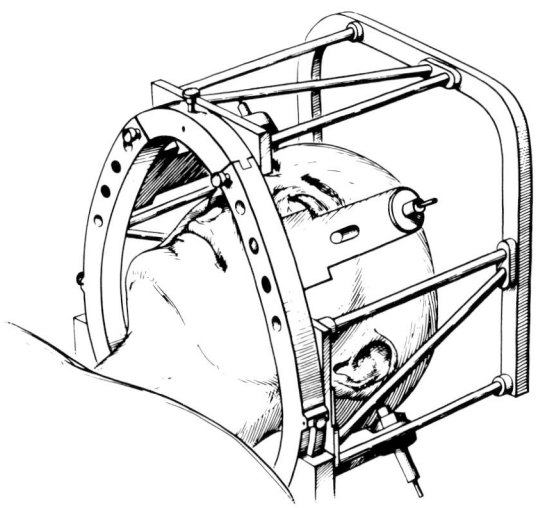
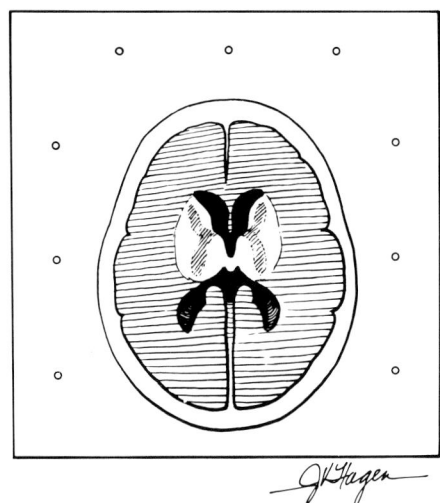

Figure 5.1. Stereotactic CT scanning. Patient's head is fixed in CT-compatible stereotactic headholder. Localization system attached to base of the head holder creates nine reference marks on each CT slice from which stereotactic coordinates of any selected point on slice may be calculated.

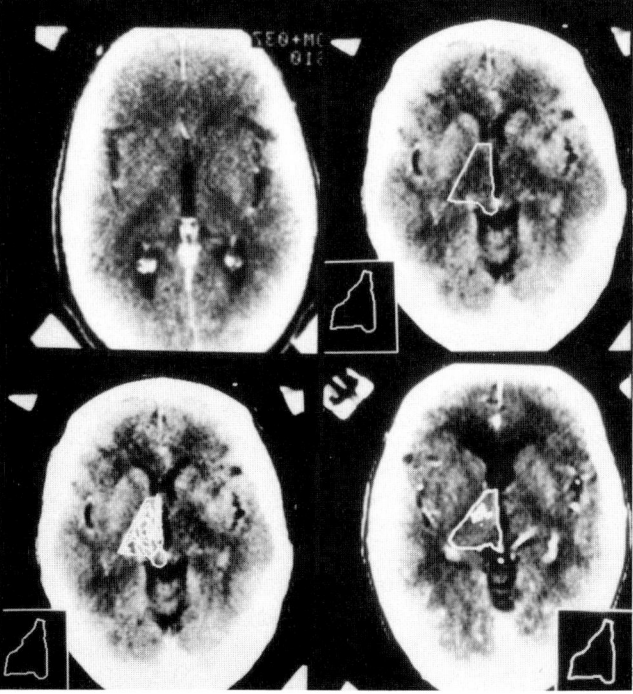

Figure 5.2. A computer resident stereotactic atlas is superimposed upon reformatted CT slice. *Top left,* Paraxial CT slice reconstruction is generated at required height and in plane parallel to desired horizontal atlas sections in relationship to anterior and posterior commissure, which have been identified on a sagittal reconstruction. *Top right,* Surgeon desinates bouondaries of thalamus on paraxial CT reconstruction. *Bottom left,* Computer scales and displays all of thalamic substructures to fit within designated boundary. *Bottom right,* Substructure of interest (in this case VIME) is selected and displayed. Surgeon then positions a cursor within this substructure and stereotactic coordinates of that selected point are calculated and displayed.

stereotactic coordinates of any selected point on the CT slice. Five-millimeter CT slices overlapping at 3-mm intervals are obtained through the region of the third ventricle. The CT data are then transferred to an operating room computer system. A computer resident digitized Shaltenbrand-Wahren stereotactic atlas is scaled by computer and superimposed on the CT slice within defined landmarks (the lateral wall of the third ventricle, pulvinar, and medial border of the internal capsule, Fig. 5.2). The computer-scaled outlines of individual thalamic nuclei are then drawn in over the CT slice by the computer. Any thalamic nucleus may be selected by cursor on the display console and stereotactic coordinates calculated as has been described previously (32).

STEREOTACTIC VENTRICULOGRAPHY

The lateral ventricle is tapped stereotactically through a burr hole made 12 cm posterior to the nasion, 2.5 cm from the midline and a contrast ventriculogram is done utilizing a 200 mg/100 ml concentration of metrazimide. The anterior and posterior commissures are identified (Fig. 5.3). The approximate location of the various thalamic subnuclei are determined utilizing a method developed by Guiot and described elsewhere (36). Following this procedure, the wound is closed and the patient removed from the stereotactic frame for that day.

Semi-Microelectrode Recording

The patient is returned to the operating room on the next operating day for reapplication of the frame. Reapplication in the same frame position is assured by the fact that the head holder fixes to the patient's skull by pins inserted into holes drilled in the outer table of the patient's skull which were made during the first application of the head holder. The head holder's position is checked by micrometer settings which measure the depth of the fixation pins relative to the vertical supports of the head holder.

Under sedation and local infiltration anesthesia the patient is replaced in the stereotactic frame and the coronal wound opened. A bipolar concentric microelectrode with a 10- to 50-µm active recording tip and a 400-µm tip-to-ring distance is directed from the coronal burr hole to an intracranial target point, 1 mm anterior to the posterior commissure on the AC-PC line and 11.5 to 13 mm lateral to the lateral wall of the third ventricle. The electrode is connected to a head stage preamplifier and DC amplifier (DAM 5A). The recorded electrical activity is presented aurally and visually by audio monitor and oscilloscope, respectively. Distinctive cellular activity is encountered at the cortex, the caudate nucleus, and dorsal thalamus (Fig. 5.4). Background amplitude of the cellular activity increases as the electrode enters VP. At this point, the contralateral side of the patient's body is tapped or brushed. High-amplitude (150 mV) responses are obtained when touching the part of the face, trunk, arm, leg, or digits represented by the part of the thalamus in which the electrode lies. Using this method, it is possible to establish the VP representation of specific body parts within an individual patient's thalamus. Somatosensory-evoked responses recorded in VP are used to define the neurophysiological lateral position of the proposed lesion site (33, 36).

Averaged median and tibial nerve somatosensory-evoked responses are used to determine the electrophysiological "floor" (inferior boundary) of the sensory thalamus. Here, reversal of polarity of the N_{14} wave is noted as the electrode passes from the sensory thalamus into the fibers of the medial lemniscus (Fig. 5.5). Responses to nerve stimulation are quite focal and specific within VP. As the electrode enters the medial lemniscus, responses become more generalized with evoked potentials recorded at one site with stimulation of different nerves on different limbs (Fig. 5.6). The inferior aspect of the thalamus frequently but not always corresponds to the AC-PC line. AP and lateral radiographs that demonstrate the position of the tip of the microelectrode are obtained. These are compared to the ventriculogram. This information is useful in determining the final height coor-

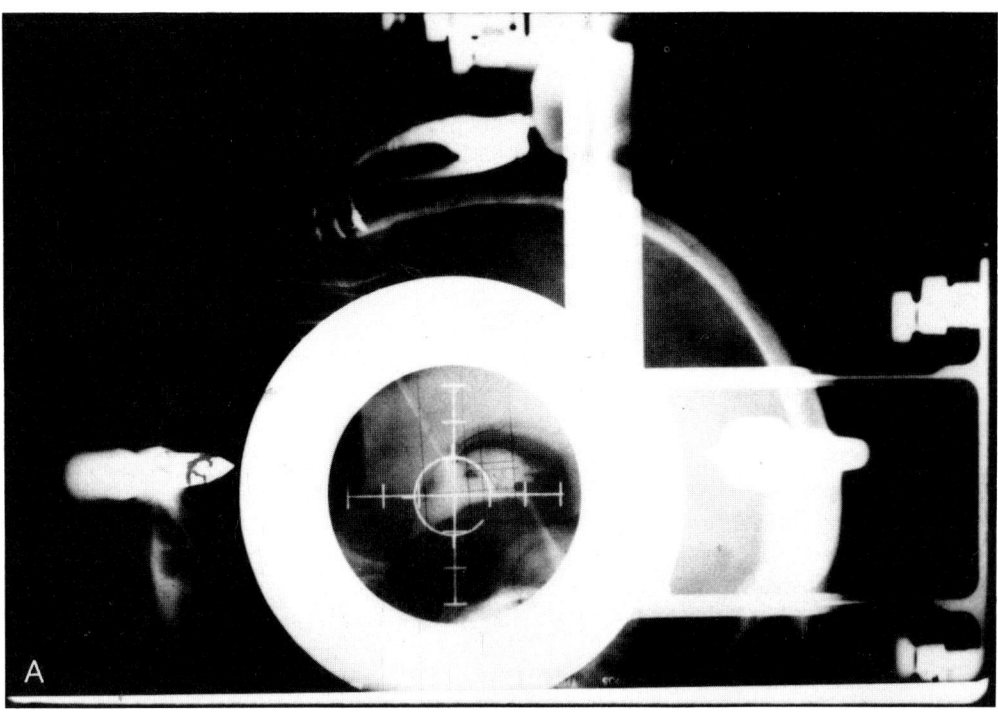

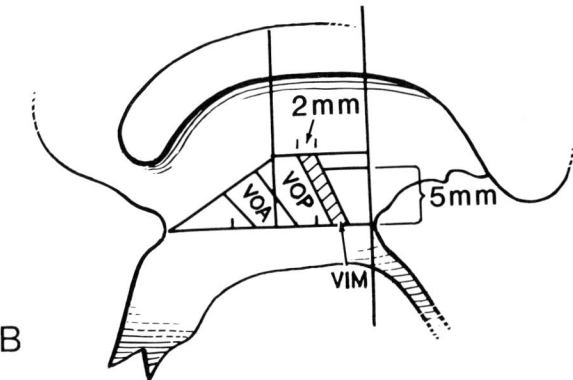

Figure 5.3. *A*) Positive-contrast ventriculogram which demonstrates anterior (AC) and posterior commissures (PC). *B*) Derivation of ventrolateral nuclear subgroups based on AC-PC line and thalamic height.

dinate for the lesion site in relationship to the physiological inferior thalamic boundary.

Lesioning Procedure

The target point for the lesion site is 2.5 mm above the inferior boundary of the thalamus, 3 mm posterior to the midpoint of the AC-PC line, and at a lateral position determined from the microelectrode recording.

For the treatment of upper extremity tremor, lesions should be made in VL anterior to the VP representation of the corner of the mouth, thumb, or the index finger (33, 36). The lesion should be slightly more

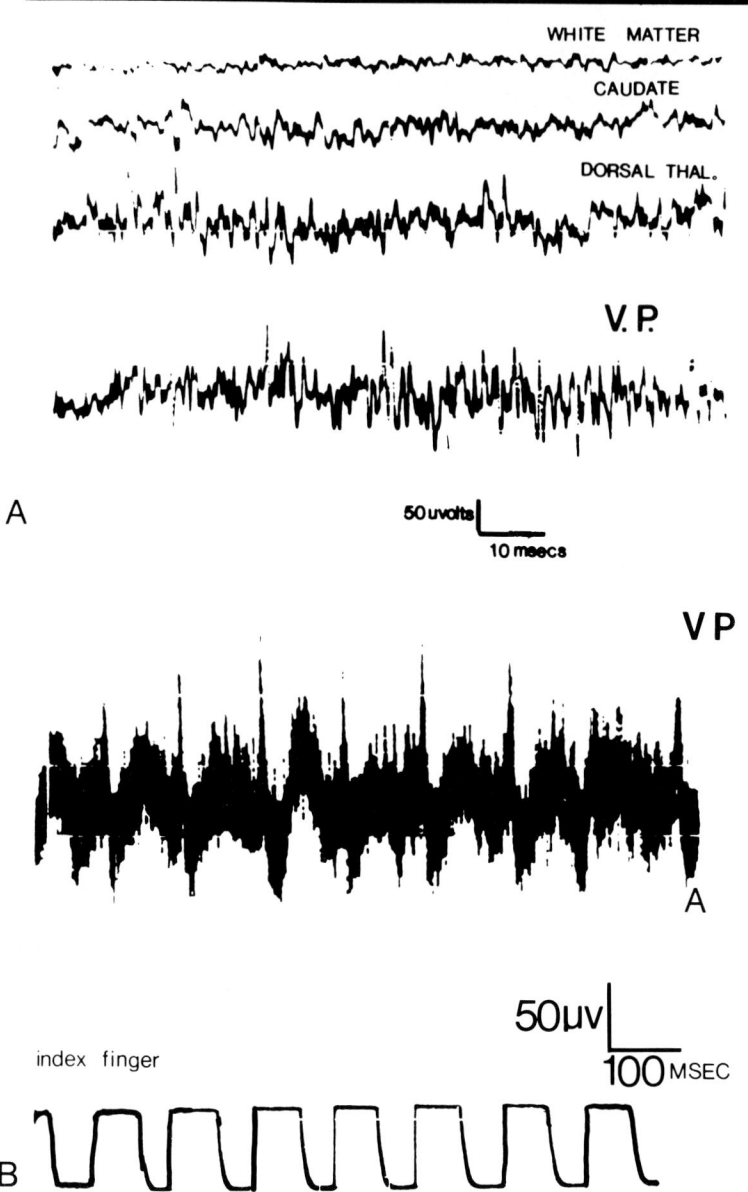

Figure 5.4. *A*) Electrical activity recorded as semimicroelectrode passes through subcortical white matter, caudate nucleus, dorsal thalamus, and VP. *B*) Unaveraged somatosensory- (150 mV) evoked responses with electrode within part of VP which corresponds to index finger. "Sawtooth" tracing indicates each touch of patient's contralateral index finger.

lateral for the treatment of lower extremity tremor (anterior to the VP representation of the fifth finger, Fig. 5.7). Radiofrequency lesions are made with a 1.1- to 1.6-mm diameter, 4-mm exposed temperature-monitored electrode. First a test lesion is made in which the electrode tip is heated to 42°C for 60 sec. The patient is then examined to assess the neurological effects of the lesion on tremor, strength, and coordination. Speech is carefully tested by a speech pathologist when the procedure is

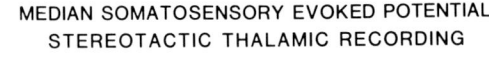

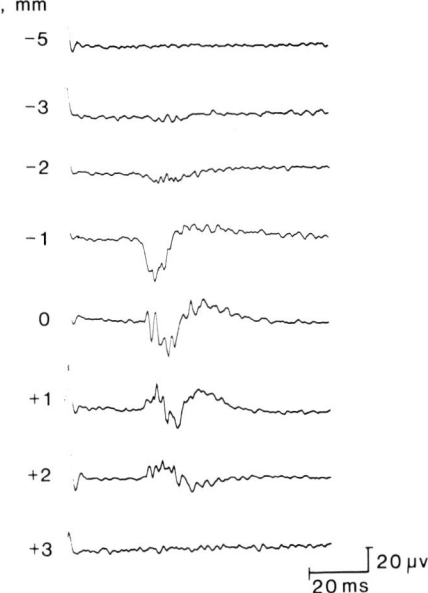

Figure 5.5. Averaged median nerve-evoked responses as semimicroelectrode passes within VP (negative numbers) toward the AC-PC line and into the subthalamic area (positive numbers). Note inversion of polarity as electrode passes out of thalamus into subthalamic regions.

being performed on the left side; the onset or worsening of dysarthria, perseveration, or disorientation, or the development of aphasic verbal errors, or increased verbal response latencies are particularly important signs of undesirable neurological sequelae. If no untoward effects have resulted from the test lesion, the electrode tip is then heated to 70 to 78°C for 60 sec. This generates a lesion approximately 4 mm in diameter and 4 to 5 mm in length.

RESULTS

Parkinsonian Tremor and Rigidity

There have been three major time periods in the surgical therapy for Parkinson's disease. The first period was that in which patients were operated on before sophisticated neurophysiological localization methods were generally available. Lesions were larger and the results may not have been as good as later became possible. The second time period to consider is that after the development of more precise localization methods but before the availability of L-dopa. The final time period comprises those patients operated on after L-dopa became available.

Most series claim between 70 to 90% success rate for the palliation of tremor associated with Parkinson's disease. However,

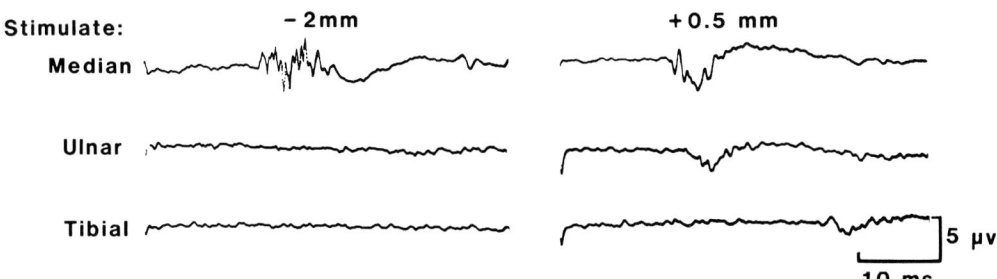

Figure 5.6. Averaged median and posterior tibial nerve-evoked responses from the electrode within VP and beyond. Note that in medial lemniscus, response from median nerve not only reverses in polarity, but response is recorded from contralateral posterior tibial nerve as well.

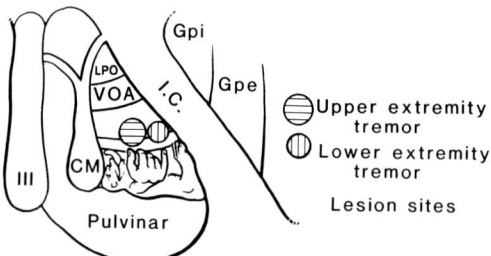

Figure 5.7. Drawing of horizontal section through the ventral thalamus showing the homuncular representation within VP and the desired laterality of lesion sites within VL.

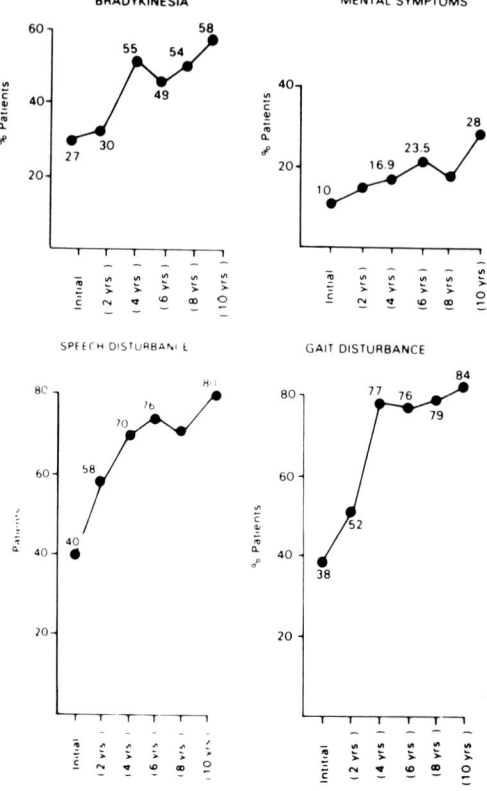

Figure 5.9. Percentage of patients in which bradykinesia, speech disturbance, gait dysfunction and mental symptoms were noted 2, 4, 6, 8, and 10 yr following a stereotactic thalamotomy. (Reprinted with permission from Kelly PJ, and Gillingham FG. *J Neurosurg* 53:332–337, 1980.)

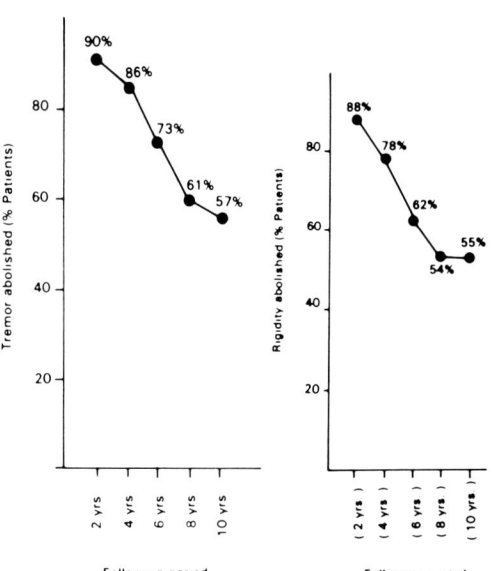

Figure 5.8. Percentage of patients having no contralateral tremor (*left*) and no contralateral rigidity (*right*) at 2 yr, 4 yr, 6 yr, 8 yr, and 10 yr following stereotactic thalamotomy with microelectrode recording control. (Reprinted with permission from Kelly PJ, and Gillingham FG. The long-term results of stereotactic surgery and L-dopa therapy in patients with Parkinson's disease: A ten-year follow-up study. *J Neurosurg* 53: 332–337, 1980.)

many of these series reporting these statistics are comprised of patients operated on prior to the availability of L-dopa. In a previously reported (38) retrospective study, we reviewed the extensive experience of Mr. F. John Gillingham of Edinburgh, Scotland. First, the short-term (2 yr) results on tremor and rigidity in patients treated during selected intervals during the three time periods listed above were evaluated, specifically patients operated on between 1957 and 1960, 1965 and 1967, and 1970 and 1976 were selected. During the early period, before sophisticated localization techniques were developed, 79% of the patients were relieved of tremor and 72% were relieved of rigidity. The group operated on between 1965 and 1967 fared best: tremor was abolished in 90%, and rigidity was abolished in 88% of the patients. The group operated on between 1970 and 1976 (the longer time period was necessary to accumulate a comparable number of patients) did not do as well as regards palliation of tremor and rigidity: 78% abolition of tremor and 71% abolition of rigidity. These "L-dopa failures" were usually operated later on in the course of their disease than patients operated on before the advent of L-dopa.

A longitudinal analysis based on biannual neurological examinations and activities of daily living (ADL) assessment was then undertaken in the subgroup who underwent surgery between 1965 and 1967. Ninety percent of the patients were free of contralateral tremor and 88% were free of rigidity when evaluated 2 yr postoperatively. However, as noted on subsequent examinations, tremor and rigidity recurred to a mild but nondisabling degree in some as indicated by Fig. 5.8. Then, tremor and rigidity were no longer the source for disability later on in the course of the disease in the majority of the patients. Figure 5.9 depicts the incidence of the other symptoms of Parkinson's disease. Bradykinesia, speech disturbance, gait dysfunction, and mental symptoms were not improved by surgery and affected an increasing number of individuals as the follow-up period progressed. The relative plateaus noted at 6, 8, and 10 yr reflect treatment with L-dopa (available in 1968 in the British Isles) and the death of the more severely affected individuals.

An ADL assessment was also performed on each of these patients every 2 yr utilizing the following scoring system: (*a*) class I, no significant slowing or difficulty produced by the symptoms of the disease; (*b*) class II, some difficulty and slowing of function produced by the disease (but the patient is still totally independent); (*c*) class III, moderate amount of difficulty produced by the disease (these patients require some part-time help to accomplish the ADL tasks); (*d*) class IV, the patient requires help with all tasks; or (*e*) class V, the patient is bedridden.

At the preoperative evaluation, as shown by the ADL scores, parkinsonian symptoms caused difficulty and slowing in the performance of activities of daily living in 41 of the 60 patients (Fig. 5.10). Two years following the first stereotactic procedure, most of the patients showed no slowing or difficulty in performing ADL tasks when compared with normal controls. However, at each subsequent biannual evaluation, progressively more patients declined into poorer levels of function due to contralateral tremor (34 patients underwent contralateral surgical procedures) and to progressive bradykinesia. L-Dopa was instituted in 42 of the 60 patients studied and was responsible for the relative plateaus in the functional decline. At the 10-yr follow-up evaluation, only 10 patients remained in ADL class I, 16 were in class II (independent), 10 had died, while the rest were in various stages of dependency. We concluded from this study that carefully performed stereotactic surgery can remove functional impairment due to tremor and rigidity and delay disability until the onset of bradykinesis which can be managed by L-dopa or carbidopa.

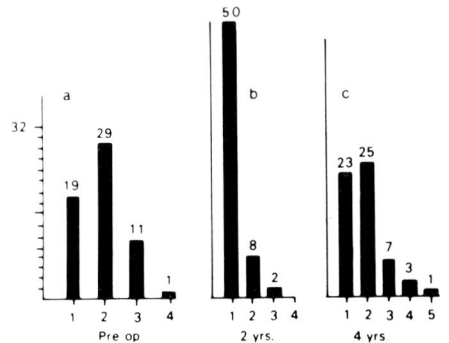
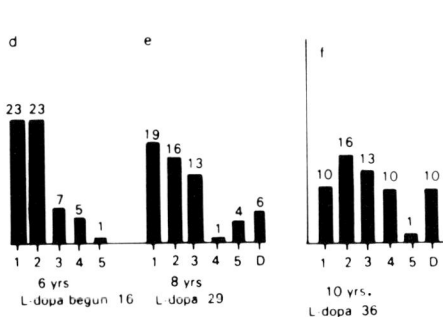
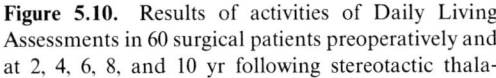

Figure 5.10. Results of activities of Daily Living Assessments in 60 surgical patients preoperatively and at 2, 4, 6, 8, and 10 yr following stereotactic thalamotomy. (Reprinted with permission from Kelly PJ, and Gillingham FG. *J Neurosurg* 53: 332–337, 1980.)

TABLE 5.1.
Summary of Procedures for Treatment of Movement Disorders

	Movement Disorder Abolished	Significant Improvement	Failure
Parkinson's	12	2	—
Intention tremor	4	—	—
Dystonia	—	1	1
Complex movement disorders	3	1	1
Essential tremor	1	—	1[a]

[a]Unable to get adequate neurophysiological localization; no lesion made.

Contemporary Experience

Unfortunately, few American centers do enough stereotactic thalamotomies for Parkinson's disease at present to make any definitive statements on the long-term effectiveness of modern stereotactic methods in the management of Parkinson's disease. Since August 1984, 657 stereotactic procedures have been performed at the Mayo Clinic. Most were for the biopsy and treatment of intracranial neoplasms. However, 27 procedures (16 left- and 11 right-sided) were performed for the treatment of various movement disorders as summarized in Table 5.1. No persistent postoperative major neurological deficits were noted in any of these patients. Neurological examinations performed 3 months postoperatively revealed the following: all of the 14 patients with Parkinson's disease had significant abolition of contralateral tremor with total absence of tremor in 12 and significant reduction of tremor in two. In the latter two patients, purposefully small (3 mm) lesions had been made in order to avoid worsening of the speech and gait problems that were already manifest in the advanced disease of these two individuals. All of the patients with intention tremor had complete abolition of tremor, and four of the five patients with complex movement disorders had abolition (three patients) or significant reduction (one patient) of the resting and intention tremor. Patients with tremor due to Parkinson's disease have represented a progressively increasing group of surgical candidates.

DISCUSSION

Carefully performed stereotactic surgery remains an option for selected patients with medically intractable tremor due to Parkinson's disease (25, 38). The best surgical candidates are patients whose symptoms remain unilateral and who do not develop midline symptoms in speech and gait disturbances. In our experience, the patients who have speech and gait disturbances and with more advanced Parkinson's disease have greater risk of complications from the surgery than those in whom gait, speech, and mental symptoms are absent. Bilateral surgical procedures are possible if the procedures are staged approximately 3 months apart (38, 40).

Patients are now being referred for surgery much later in the course of the disease than they were in the 1960s. Most now have bradykinesia and speech and gait problems associated with their more advanced parkinsonism. However, modern stereotactic surgery with CT and microelectrode control can result in more precise lesions, and a much greater chance for abolition of tremor and less risk than noted in the past.

The methodology described in this report is in part a modification of CT-based stereotactic procedures for intracranial tumors which have been described previously (32–35, 37, 39). Incorporation of stereotactic CT scanning into the data base for functional procedures provides the surgeon with information on the axial configuration of the third ventricle and on the laterality of the internal capsule. The neurophysiological portion of the procedure was modified from the original method described by Guiot et al. (25). Guiot's posterior-to-anterior approach was not practical for our stereotactic instrumentation. The methods for functional exploration from the coronal approach and lesion site determination was developed and proven in previous experience (33).

There exists a somatotopic organization within VL which reflects the homuncular arrangement of the body in VP and that the somatotory of the latter may be used to guide the placement of VL lesions. The electrophysiological findings of both cellular activity and summated activity support this hypothesis and identify the specific location of the microelectrode within the thalamus and specifically within VP. These methods allow more accurate calculation of the inferior border of the thalamus and the laterality of proposed lesion sites. Thus, smaller lesions may then be made in the subportion of VL corresponding to the upper or lower extremity with more selective control of tremor.

REFERENCES

1. Albe-Fessard D, Arfel G, Guiot G: Activities electriques caracteristiques de quelques structures cerebrales chez l'homme. Ann Chir 1185-1214, 1963.
2. Albe-Fessard D, Arfel G, Guiot G, Hardy J, Vourc'h G, Hertzog E, Aleonard P, Derome P: Derivations d'activities spontanees et evoquees dans les structures cerebrales profondes de l'homme. Rev Neurol 106: 89-105, 1962.
3. Albe-Fessard D, Guiot G, Lamarre Y, Arfel G: Activation of thalamocortical projections related to tremorgenesis. In Purpura, Y (ed): The Thalamus. New York, Columbia University Press, 1966, pp 237-253.
4. Alberts WW, Wright EW, Levin G, Feinstein B, Mueller M: Threshold stimulation of the lateral thalamus and globus pallidus. Electroenceph Clin Neurophysiol 13: 68-74, 1961.
5. Alexander GL, Szekely EG, Spiegel EA: Effect of stimulation of the pallidum on experimental segment tremor in the cat. J Neuropath Exp Neurol 19: 116-124, 1960.
6. Andrew J, Watkins ES: A Stereotactic Atlas of the Human Thalamus. Baltimore, Williams & Wilkins, 1969.
7. Austin B, Hayward W, Tasi C, Hill C: Stereotactic localization with midline bony landmarks and electrical stimulation. Conf Neurol 29: 230-237, 1967.
8. Bates J: Computer techniques in the analysis of electrophysiological data from the human thalamus. Conf Neurol 36: 310-311, 1974.
9. Bertrand C, Molina-Negro P, Martinez SN: Stereotactic targets for dystonias and dyskinesias: Relationship to corbicobulbar fibers and other adjoining structures. Adv Neurol 24: 395-399, 1979.
10. Bertrand C, Molina-Negro P, Martinez SN: Combined stereotactic and peripheral surgical approach in spasmotic torticollis. Appl Neurophysiol 41: 122-133, 1978.
11. Bertrand G, Hardy J: Computerized graphic study of the distribution, in the human thalamus, of neurones responding to tactile stimuli. Meeting of the World Society for Stereotactic and Functional Neurosurgery, Sao Paulo, 1977, p 40.
12. Bertrand G, Jasper H: Microelectrode recording of unit activity in the human thalamus. Conf Neurol 26: 205-208, 1965.
13. Bertrand G, Jasper H, Wong A: Microelectrode study of the human thalamus: Functional organization in the ventrobasal complex. Conf Neurol 29: 81-86, 1967.
14. Bravo GJ, Cooper IS: A clinical and radiological correlation of the lesion produced by chemopallidectomy and thalamectomy. J Neurol Neurosurg Psychiatr 22: 1-10, 1959.
15. Brierley JB, Beck E: The significance in human stereotactic brain surgery of individual variation in the diencephalon and globus pallidus. J Neurol Neurosurg Psychiatr 22: 287-298, 1959.
16. Broggi G, Angelini L, Bono R, Giorgi C, Nardocci N, Franzini A: Long term results of stereotactic thalamotomy for cerebral palsy. Neurosurgery 12: 195-202, 1983.
17. Bucy P: Cortical extirpation in the treatment of involuntary movements. Res Publ Assoc Nerv Ment Dis 21: 551-595, 1942.
18. Cooper IS: Dystonia: Surgical approaches to treatment and physiologic implications. In Yahr M (ed): The Basal Ganglia. New York, Raven Press, 1976, pp 369-384.
19. Cooper IS, Poloukhine N: Chemopallidectomy: a neurosurgical technique useful in geriatric parkinsonians. J Am Geriatr Soc 3: 839-859, 1955.
20. Dierssen G, Bergmann LL, Gioino G, Cooper IS: Hemiballism following surgery for Parkinson's disease. Arch Neurol 5: 627-637, 1961.
21. Emmers R, Tasker RR: The Human Somesthetic Thalamus. New York, Raven Press, 1975.
22. Fenelon F: Essais de traitment neurochirurgical du syndrome parkinsonien par intervention directe sur les voies extrapyramidales immediatement sous striopallidales (anse lenticulaire). Communication suivie de projection due film d'un des operes pris avant at apres l'intervention. Rev Neurol 83: 437-440, 1950.
23. Fukamachi A, Ohye C, Narabayshi H: Delineation of the thalamic nuclei with a microelectrode in stereotaxic surgery for parkinsonism and cerebral palsy. J Neurosurg 39: 214-225, 1973.
24. Guiot G, Brion S: Traitement des mouvements anormaux par la coagulation pallidale. Technique et resultats. Rev Neurol 89: 578-580, 1953.
25. Guiot G, Derome P, Jedynak P, et al: Permanence des indications de la chirurgie stereotaxique dans le treblement Parkinsonien et certains mouvements anormaux rebelles. Ann Med Intern 126: 295-296, 1975.
26. Guiot G, Hardy J, Albe-Fessard D: Delimitation precise des structures sous-corticales et identification des moyaux thalamiques chez l'homme par l'electrophysiologie stereotaxique. Neurochirurgie 5: 1-18, 1962.
27. Hassler R: The influence of stimulations and coagulations in the human thalamus on the tremor at rest and its physiopathologic mech-

anisms. In *Proc Sec Int Cong Neuropath* Amsterdam, 1955, 2: 627-642.
28. Hassler R, Riechert T: Indikationen und Lokalisationsmethode der gezielten Hirnoperationen. *Nervenarzt* 25: 441-447, 1954.
29. Hecaen H, Talairach J, David M, Dell MD: Coagulations limitees du thalamus dans les algies du syndrome thalamique. *Rev Neurol* 81: 917-931, 1949.
30. Horsley V: The Linacre lecture. The function of the so-called motor area of the brain. *Br Med J* 2: 125-132, 1909.
31. Jasper HH, Bertrand G: Thalamic units involved in somatic sensation and voluntary and involuntary movements in man. In Purpura Y (ed): *The Thalamus*. New York, Columbia University Press, 1966, pp 365-390.
32. Kall BA, Kelly PJ, Goerss SJ, Grieder G: Methodology and clinical experience with computed tomography and a computer-resident stereotactic atlas. *Neurosurgery* 17: 400-407, 1985.
33. Kelly PJ: Microelectrode recording for the somatotopic placement of stereotactic thalamic lesions in the treatment of parkinsonian and cerebellar intention tremor. *Appl Neurophysiol* 43: 262-266, 1980.
34. Kelly PJ, Alker GJ, Goerss SJ: Computer assisted stereotactic laser microsurgery for the treatment of intracranial neoplasms. *Neurosurgery* 10: 324-331, 1982.
35. Kelly PJ, Alker GJ, Kall B, et al: A method of CT-based stereotactic biopsy with arteriographic control. *Neurosurgery* 14: 172-177, 1984.
36. Kelly PJ, Derome P, Guiot G: Thalamic spatial variability and the surgical results of lesions placed with neurophysiological control. *Surg Neurol* 9: 307-315, 1978.
37. Kelly PJ, Earnest F, Kall BA, et al: Surgical options for patients with deep-seated brain tumors: computer-assisted stereotactic biopsy. *Mayo Clin Proc* 6: 223-229, 1985.
38. Kelly PJ, Gillingham FG: The long-term results of stereotactic surgery and L-dopa therapy in patients with Parkinson's disease: A ten-year follow-up study. *J Neurosurg* 53: 332-337, 1980.
39. Kelly PJ, Kall BA, Goerss S: Stereotactic CT scanning for the biopsy of intracranial lesions and functional neurosurgery. *Appl Neurophysiol* 46: 193-199, 1983.
40. Krayenbuhl H, Wyss OAM, Yasargil MG: Bilateral thalamotomy and pallidotomy as treatment for bilateral parkinsonism. *J Neurosurg* 18: 429-444, 1961.
41. Krayenbuhl H, Yasargil MG: Relief of intention tremor due to multiple sclerosis by stereotaxic thalamotomy. *Conf Neurol* 22: 368-374, 1962.
42. Meyers R: The modification of alternating tremors, rigidity and festination by surgery of the basal ganglia. *Res Publ Assoc Nerv Ment Dis* 21: 602-665, 1942.
43. Narabayashi H, Ohye C: Importance of microstereoencephalotomy for tremor alleviation. *Appl Neurophysiol* 43: 222-227, 1980.
44. Rumler B, Schaltenbrand G, Spuler H, Wahren W: Somatotopic array of the ventro-oral nucleus of the thalamus based on electrical stimulation during stereotactic procedures. *Conf Neurol* 34: 197-199, 1972.
45. Schaltenbrand G, Bailey P: *Introduction to Stereotaxis with an Atlas of the Human Brain*. Stuttgart, Thieme, 1959.
46. Spiegel EA, Wycis HT: *Stereoencephalotomy: Parts I and II*. New York, Grune & Stratton, 1952 and 1962.
47. Spiegel EA, Wycis HT: Ansotomy in paralysis agitans. *Trans Am Neurol Assoc* 78: 178-198, 1953.
48. Spiegel EA, Wycis HT, Marks M, Lee AJ: Stereotaxic apparatus for operations on the human brain. *Science* 106: 349-350, 1947.
49. Talairach J, David M, Tournoux P, Corredor H, Kvasina T: *Atlas d'Anatomie Stereotaxique*. Paris, Masson, 1957.
50. Tasker RR, Hawrylyshyn P, Rowe IH, Organ LW: Computerized graphic display of results of subcortical stimulation during stereotactic surgery. *Acta Neurochir* 24: 85-98, 1977.
51. Van Buren JM, Borke RC: *Variations and Connections of the Human Thalamus. 2. Variations of the Human Diencephalon*. New York, Springer, 1972.
52. Van Buren JM, MacCubbin DA: An outline atlas of the human basal ganglia with estimation of anatomical variation. *J Neurosurg* 19: 811-839, 1962.

Chapter 6

Stereotactic Methods in the Management of Pain

RONALD F. YOUNG, M.D.

INTRODUCTION

Considerable advances have been realized in recent years in the management of pain by stereotactic methods. Before the early 1970s, emphasis had been placed primarily on ablative stereotactic approaches. Advances in our understanding of the physiological and chemical mechanisms that allow the brain to modulate or suppress pain, led to an entirely different stereotactic technique, that of electrical stimulation via chronically implanted electrodes. Few neurosurgical therapeutic endeavors depend as heavily on a basic understanding of the anatomical, physiological, and chemical bases for disease as stereotactic treatment of pain. Thus, it is necessary to review our current understanding of the neural basis for pain, to serve as the groundwork for a discussion of specific neurosurgical stereotactic procedures for the treatment of chronic pain.

NEURAL BASIS FOR PAIN

Until 1965, the neurosurgical management of pain was based on the concept of a direct, one-way pain-conducting pathway from the periphery to the brain. A specific set of pain receptors, pain-conducting fibers in peripheral nerves, a specific pain pathway in the spinal cord and brainstem, specific thalamic nuclear relays, and a localized area of the cerebrum responding to pain were the basic elements in this construction (42). The receptors thought to transduce noxious or potentially tissue-damaging external stimuli into nerve action potentials were so-called "free" nerve endings, but studies identified a specific nociceptive receptor, the "delta-nociceptor," responsible for the transduction of at least some pain-related information. Small myelinated fibers in peripheral nerves, the A-delta and A-gamma fibers, and the small unmyelinated C-fibers were thought to carry pain-related neural information into the spinal canal via the dorsal spinal nerve roots. Following synapse in the dorsal horn of the spinal cord, secondary or tertiary neurons were thought to cross to the contralateral anterolateral quadrant of the cord and ascend, as the lateral spinothalamic tract. This pathway, thought to conduct information about pain and temperature sensation, was described as relaying to the ventro basal thalamic nuclei, specifically to the nucleus ventralis postero lateralis (VPL), information from the trunk and extremities (54). A homologous system in the trigeminal nerve and brainstem was felt to relay information from orofacial regions to the contralateral thalamic nucleus ventralis posteromedialis (VPM). Mehler (52), however, showed that as few as 25% of fibers in the lateral spinothalamic tract actually reached VPL. Many fibers were shown to leave the spinothalamic tract in the medulla, pons, and midbrain to synapse in the medially located brainstem reticular formation. A multisynaptic pathway was then postulated to extend into the medial thalamic nuclei, particularly the nuclei parafasicularis and centrum medianum (16). These medial relays were thought to relate possibly to the emotional accompaniments of pain, i.e., the "suffering," by way of connections with limbic lobe structures (30). Relays via VPL and

VPM were thought to relate to the spatial and temporal or "sensory" qualities of pain and were felt to project to specific cerebral regions, namely the anterior parietal cortex (6). In addition, the anterior and dorsomedial thalamic nuclei were felt to be involved in the emotional response to pain via thalamoprefrontal connections (13, 45).

Recent information, obtained with the horseradish peroxidase (HRP) and other tracer techniques, suggests that a number of other pathways may also be involved in pain perception. For instance, it appears that C-fibers carrying pain information synapse on lamina-1 neurons at the apex of the spinal dorsal horn without penetrating to deeper layers. Higher order neurons that ascend, probably in the spinothalamic tract, terminate in the nucleus submedius and centralis lateralis, located in the medial thalamus, inferior to nucleus parafasicularis and centrum medianum (38).

Jones and colleagues (39) presented anatomical and physiological evidence for a dorsally located spinothalamic tract, in the cat and monkey, situated in the dorsolateral quadrant of the spinal cord and conducting information to the thalamus. Although not confirmed yet in man, such a system could account for some of the hitherto unexplained outcomes following spinothalamic tractotomy (anterolateral cordotomy), such as persistent pain or minimal loss of pain and temperature sensation or unexpected location of lesions in the dorsolateral quadrant after successful relief of pain by percutaneous cervical cordotomy (54, 73). Thus, more recent information suggests that the afferent pain system is much more complex than a simple linear pathway from the periphery to the central nervous system. The stereotactic ablative approach to the treatment of chronic pain has been based on a general understanding of the pain perception system as outlined above. This approach has been based on the placement of permanent, destructive lesions in virtually all components of afferent pain system at spinal, brainstem, and cerebral levels.

In 1965 Melzack and Wall (53) proposed the gate hypothesis of pain, which incorporated, for the first time, the idea that pain could be modulated or suppressed via naturally present brain and spinal systems. Melzack and Wall postulated that activation of large myelinated nerve fibers could suppress pain and this idea led to the use of peripheral nerve and spinal cord stimulation to treat pain. Melzack and Wall also postulated a "central control" mechanism for pain suppression, but gave no specific details of such a system. In 1969 Reynolds (63) demonstrated that electrical stimulation of the midbrain periaqueductal gray (PAG) could induce analgesia. Subsequent studies by a number of investigators led to the description of a descending pain control system, incorporating structures in the brainstem, dorsolateral quadrant of the spinal cord, and spinal dorsal horn, activation of which could block or inhibit pain (10, 48, 85). The development of tolerance to the analgesic effect of PAG stimulation, the demonstration of cross-tolerance to exogenous opiates, and at least partial reversal of stimulation-produced analgesia (SPA) by the narcotic antagonist naloxone, gave rise to the hypothesis that endogenous opioid release accounted for analgesia incident to PAG stimulation (47).

Although some conflicting research data have been published, it is reasonably well accepted that SPA, which results from electrical stimulation of the PAG, depends on an endogenous opioid mechanism. Recent information also suggests that SPA, resulting from dorsal PAG stimulation, may be nonopioid in nature, whereas SPA from ventral PAG stimulation is mediated by endogenous opioids (19, 20). Adams, Richardson, and Hosobuchi pioneered the application of PAG and periventricular gray (PVG) stimulation to the treatment of chronic pain in man, via the stereotactic implantation of chronic stimulating electrodes (2, 35, 65, 66).

In a separate series of experiments, Gerhart et al. demonstrated that electrical stimulation in the thalamic sensory relay nuclei, i.e., VPL, could inhibit the firing of wide dynamic range lamina-5 neurons, in the dorsal horn of the spinal cord, when the neurons were activated by noxious stimuli (26, 27). Tsubokawa et al. (77) then reported that VPM stimulation suppressed neuronal hyperactivity seen in the cat trigeminal nucleus caudalis following trigeminal rhizotomy (77). The exact mechanism of such suppression is unknown but the inhibitory effect appears to be bilateral, at the spinal cord level, during unilateral VPL stimulation. Analgesia incident to VPL stimulation has not been demonstrated in an animal model. In fact, Aiko et al. (3) could not produce a reduction of withdrawal in the rat tail-pinch test with VPL stimulation (3). They reported that VPL stimulation increased local cerebral glucose utilization in VPL, VPM, substantia nigra, and sensory cortex, exclusively unilaterally and suggested that pain relief related to VPL stimulation may depend on inhibitory activity at the cerebral level rather than at the spinal cord level (3). Benabid and colleagues (12) demonstrated inhibition of responses to noxious stimuli in nucleus parafasicularis by VPL stimulation in an animal preparation and suggested a similar mechanism for pain suppression in man by VPL stimulation. Mazars et al. (49, 50) and Hosobuchi, Adams, and Fields (33) first described the relief of chronic pain in humans by electrical stimulation of the sensory thalamus (VPL and VPM).

STEREOTACTIC TREATMENT OF PAIN

For convenience, the discussion of the stereotactic treatment of pain will be divided into two general sections. The first will consider ablative or lesioning techniques and the second will consider stimulation techniques.

Ablative Lesions

The concept of ablative stereotactic lesions for the treatment of chronic intractable pain represents an effort to selectively interrupt the afferent pain system in an attempt to relieve pain but produce little or no interference with normal neurological function. Unfortunately, this goal has been achieved with only limited success. Recent reports on the ablative stereotactic approach for treating chronic pain are very few. The author's experience, and that of others, is that long-term pain relief following stereotactic ablative lesions is unusual and that pain recurrence within 3 to 6 months is common (75). The stereotactic ablative approach is, therefore, most useful for the treatment of pain due to malignant disease, when life expectancy is limited. The ability to carry out stereotactic procedures under local anesthesia also makes this technique particularly suitable for patients who cannot tolerate general anesthesia, due to the debilitating effect of malignancy.

Stereotactic ablative lesions are most useful for control of pain in the head and neck and at times in the upper extremities. Pain in the lower body and legs can usually be controlled with procedures such as percutaneous cordotomy, dorsal root ganglionectomy, median myelotomy, or chronic narcotic infusion into the spinal canal. Control of pain in the shoulder or arm by high cervical cordotomy may be difficult even when combined with cervical rhizotomy. In such patients, stereotactic procedures may prove useful. Some patients with intractable pain in the head and neck due to cancer may be successfully treated by trigeminal rhizotomy, medullary trigeminal tractotomy or upper cervical rhizotomy. Stereotactic ablative procedures offer a suitable and, at times, superior alternative to these procedures, particularly when patients are very ill due to cancer.

Ablative stereotactic lesions cannot be recommended enthusiastically for chronic pain not related to cancer. Hassler has recommended medial thalamotomy to treat pain due to the so-called "thalamic syndrome," but published results of such an approach are few (30). The author prefers stereotactic stimulation procedures for treatment of chronic pain of noncancerous origin.

Target Selection

Ablative stereotactic lesions have generally been placed in two conceptually different and, to a certain degree, physiologically different aspects of the afferent pain system. Lesions in the pontine and midbrain lateral spinothalamic tract as well as the thalamic nuclei VPL and VPM result in loss of pain and temperature sensation in the contralateral body or face (62, 75). VPL lesions, depending on exact size and location, may also lead to loss of proprioceptive and tactile sensation which, in spite of retained motor power, results in poorly functioning extremities. In addition, lesions in the pontine and mesencephalic spinothalamic pathway have a risk of producing injury to cranial nuclei, or other pathways, with the production of undesired neurological deficits (58, 72). Hitchcock et al. described 16 patients with pain in the upper body due to malignancies in whom excellent pain relief was obtained by stereotactic pontine spinothalamic tractotomy, in one patient for up to 4 yr (31). Twenty percent of Hitchcock's patients developed a transient hemiparesis, 15% facial weakness, and 7% cranial nerve palsies. To avoid the problems of undesired loss of normal sensation, stereotactic ablative lesions can be placed in certain medially located components of the afferent pain system, such as the mesencephalic reticular formation, the centrum medianum parafasicularis complex of the thalamus (67, 76, 83, 88), the pulvinar (24, 64), and the intralaminar nuclei of the thalamus (67). Nashold et al. (56, 59) and Amano et al. (7) have carefully studied the effects of recording, stimulating, and lesioning in the medial mesencephalic reticular formation. They (7, 57) and others (25) have reported successful relief of intractable pain in the head and neck due to malignancies with such an approach.

Watkins (83), as well as this author and his former colleague, Dr. Luciano Modesti (88), have reported successful relief, at times long-term, of intractable pain with lesions in the CM-PF complex. Such lesions produce little or no interference with normal neurological function. Lesions must usually be placed bilaterally and serial rf lesions about 6 to 8 mm in diameter produce the best results. The recommended target for these lesions is 18 mm posterior to the foramen of Munro (FM), 6 to 10 mm lateral to the midline, and 1 mm below the plane connecting the FM and the posterior commissure (PC). Our observation, based on autopsy specimens, has been that such lesions are most effective when placed in the inferior portion of CM-PF. In fact, such lesions may be effective on the basis of the ablation of the nucleus submedius or centralis lateralis, now known to receive input from unmyelinated fibers, rather than on the basis of the ablation of CM-PF.

Ablative lesions have also been placed in the thalamoprefrontal and limbic systems in an effort to deal with the emotional suffering that accompanies pain, rather than with the sensory aspect of pain. Thus, lesions have been placed in the anterior nucleus (8), medial dorsal thalamic nucleus, the prefrontal white matter, the cingulum (22, 23, 80) and amygdala among others (75). Such procedures are difficult to quantify as to their effects. The production of lesions large enough to reduce the suffering related to pain without producing a general blunting of all emotional responses is difficult. The author rarely recommends such an approach for pain due to malignancy, and virtually never recommends it for other types of pain.

Results and Complications

In spite of the many publications concerned with ablative stereotactic lesions for treatment of pain, there is little consensus concerning the long-term success of such procedures. Nashold indicates that mesencephalotomy will relieve central pain due to pathological processes such as thalamic syndrome, lateral medullary infarction, phantom limb pain, or postherpetic neuralgia in 50% of patients (57, 59). However, the follow-up on such patients is usually brief, and recurrent pain is frequent. Nashold believes stereotactic mesencephalotomy to be the treatment of choice for pain due to cancers of the head and neck where survival is likely to be less than 2 yr (59).

Complications of stereotactic mesencephalotomy have been reported in up to 37% of patients, with mortality rates of 3 to 5% (72, 82). The most common complication involves alterations in ocular motility such as tonic ocular deviation, retraction nystagmus, and diplopia (58). Postoperative dysesthesias were reported to occur very frequently after mesencephalotomy by Walker (82), but modern reports describe this complication in 5 to 28% of patients (59). Stereotactic lesions are most useful for treatment of so-called somatic or nociceptive pain. Central pain, characterized by complaints of burning dysesthesias and often accompanied by demonstrable sensory loss, respond less well. Tasker carried out an extensive review of ablative stereotactic procedures in the thalamus for treatment of somatic pain in 811 patients as reported in the literature and added 29 patients of his own (75). Pain relief was reported in 46 to 81% of patients with a mean of about 65 to 70%. Tasker also reviewed the published results of ablative stereotactic procedures in the thalamus and hypothalamus for treating dysesthetic pain in 145 patients and added a further 12 patients of his own (75). Relief was noted in only 22 to 26% of patients.

In summary, stereotactic ablative lesions may provide pain relief in about two-thirds of patients with somatic pain, but early recurrences are frequent and loss of normal sensory function and disabling dysesthesias are fairly frequent occurrences. Ablative lesions for treatment of central pain due to deafferentation are effective in less than 50% of patients.

Stimulation

In 1973 Hosobuchi *et al.* (32) in San Francisco and Mazars *et al.* (49) in Paris reported independently that electrical stimulation of the thalamic sensory relay nuclei could relieve pain due to deafferentation. Following elucidation of the descending opioid pain inhibitory system in animals, Adams and Hosobuchi *et al.* (2, 35, 34) as well as Richardson and Akil (65, 66) reported encouraging preliminary results of chronic electrical stimulation in the periaqueductal gray (PAG) and periventricular gray (PVG) in humans. The same groups reported evidence that pain relief in humans due to PAG-PVG stimulation was dependent on an endogenous opioid mechanism (2, 4, 34, 35). Subsequently, several authors have reported clinical results of brain stimulation for treatment of chronic pain (36, 37, 41, 43, 50, 51, 55, 69–71, 77–79, 81, 86, 87). Advantages of the stimulation technique include: (*a*) no intended damage to the nervous system nor alteration in neurological function; (*b*) the technique is reversible in that electrodes may be removed if pain relief is not obtained; (*c*) secondary pain syndromes, such as may occur after ablative procedures, do not occur with stimulation; and (*d*) stimulation depends upon activation of pain suppression systems that occur naturally in the brain.

Target Selection

The general hypothesis has been proposed that PAG-PVG stimulation results in the release of endogenous opioids and is effective for treatment of pain that can be demonstrated to be opioid responsive (37, 40, 86, 87, 89). Considerable conflicting data exist, however, indicating that previously described elevations in ventricular fluid concentrations of β-endorphin following PAG-PVG stimulations (4, 35) may be artifactual (21, 17). Likewise, the value of preoperative screening to determine that pain can be relieved by opioids (40, 37) remains unproven (87). Stimulation of the sensory thalamus has been recommended for treatment of pain related to deafferentation, as a result of injury to the peripheral or central nervous system. Several problems exist with this dichotomous hypothesis. First, determination that a patient's pain is opiate responsive, or due to deafferentation, may be difficult and the two pain types may coexist. Second, it is difficult to understand how the release of natural opioids can relieve pain when exogenous opiates are ineffective. Hosobuchi originally recommended preoperative screening of candidates for PAG-PVG stimulation with intravenous morphine in order to aid in selecting target sites for stimulation (37, 40). The author used this method originally but discontinued it, due to the poor correlation between pain relief and stimulation targets selected on this basis (86, 87). The author's current approach for unilateral pain is to place two electrodes, one in PVG and one in the sensory thalamus contralateral to the patient's pain (Figs. 6.1–6.3). Trial stimulation is then carried out via percutaneous extension leads and permanent electrode targets are selected on this basis. Selection of targets for electrode placement for bilateral pain is more difficult, since placement of four electrodes for trial stimulation carries increased risk. The author's usual approach for bilateral pain is to place an electrode in PVG and one in the sensory thalamus, contralateral to the side of the greater pain. If there is no preference as to side, electrodes are placed in the nondominant hemisphere. If contralateral but not ipsilateral pain relief occurs, then a second set of electrodes may be placed on the contralateral side at a sec-

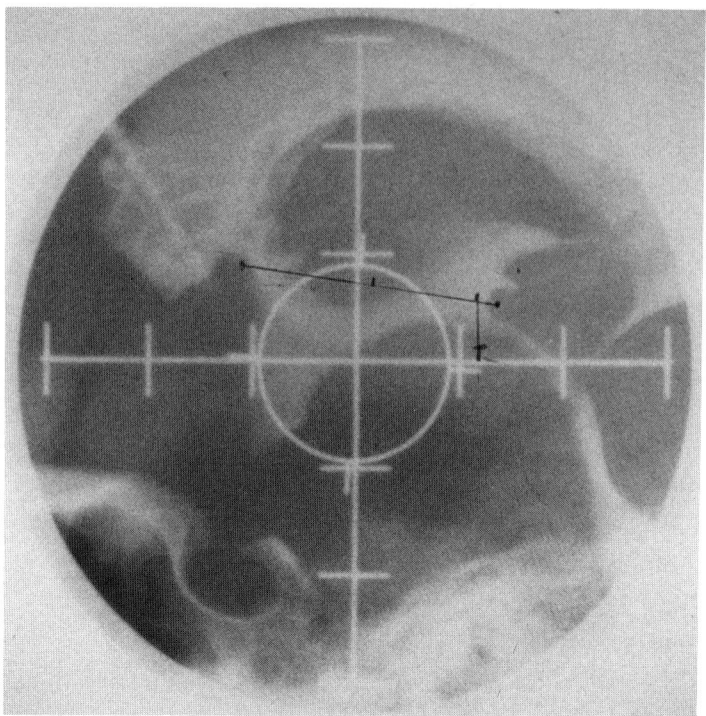

Figure 6.1. Lateral view of positive contrast ventriculogram obtained with Todd-Wells stereotactic apparatus. AC-PC line is shown with target points for PVG stimulation (2 mm anterior to PC) and VPL stimulation (5 mm below AC-PC line and 2 mm anterior to PC).

ond stereotactic procedure. The exact target for stimulation in PAG-PVG is somewhat controversial. A few studies of electrode locations have been reported in autopsy specimens of patients who died with implanted electrodes (11, 15, 28). Baskin et al. (11) recently suggested that stimulation in the ventral PAG at the level of the posterior commissure is the ideal target site. Boivie and Meyerson (15) suggested a target slightly more anterior in the PVG. The author has employed the PVG site suggested by Richardson in most patients (65, 66). This target is 10 mm posterior to the midcommissural line, 3 to 4 mm lateral to the midline and at the level of the commissural line in the horizontal plane (Figs. 6.1 and 6.2). Exact coordinates in an individual patient must be adjusted to the length of the commissural line and width of the third ventricle. The ideal site is about 1 to 2 mm anterior to the posterior commissure and within 1 to 2 mm of the third ventricular wall. At this site, patients usually experience a sensation of warmth or well-being during stimulation. At higher stimulation intensities patients may experience tachycardia, oscillopsia, diplopia, limitation of upward gaze, or a feeling of dizziness. In the author's experience stimulation more posteriorly, closer to the posterior commissure and in the PAG region, increases the incidence of such undesirable side effects at stimulation intensities required to provide pain relief (86, 87, 89). At both the PAG and PVG targets, periods of stimulation of 15 to 30 min may produce pain relief that lasts several hours.

Target sites for chronic sensory thalamic stimulation are selected on the basis of acute intraoperative electrical stimulation during electrode placement. Reference to standard atlases (68) provides a guide to initial trajectory, aimed at the portion of the VPL or VPM that corresponds to the region of the body in which the patient experiences pain (Figs. 6.1 and 6.2). For the leg, this region is about 10 mm posterior to the midcommissural line, 15 to 18 mm lateral to the

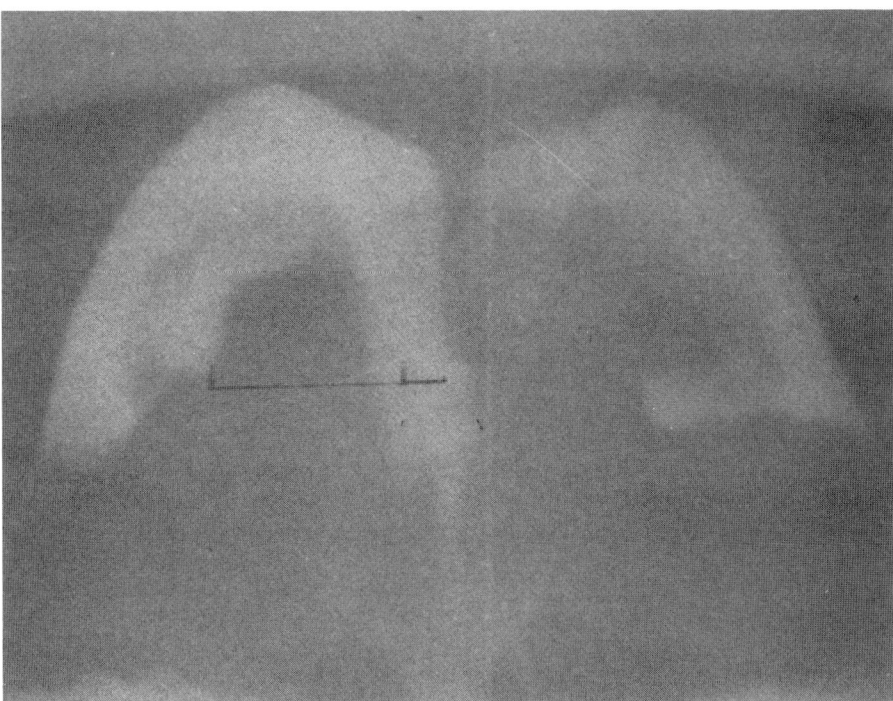

Figure 6.2. Anteroposterior view of positive-contrast ventriculogram obtained with Todd-Wells stereotactic apparatus. Target points are shown for PVG stimulation (just lateral to third ventricular wall) and for VPL stimulation (16.5 mm lateral to the midline).

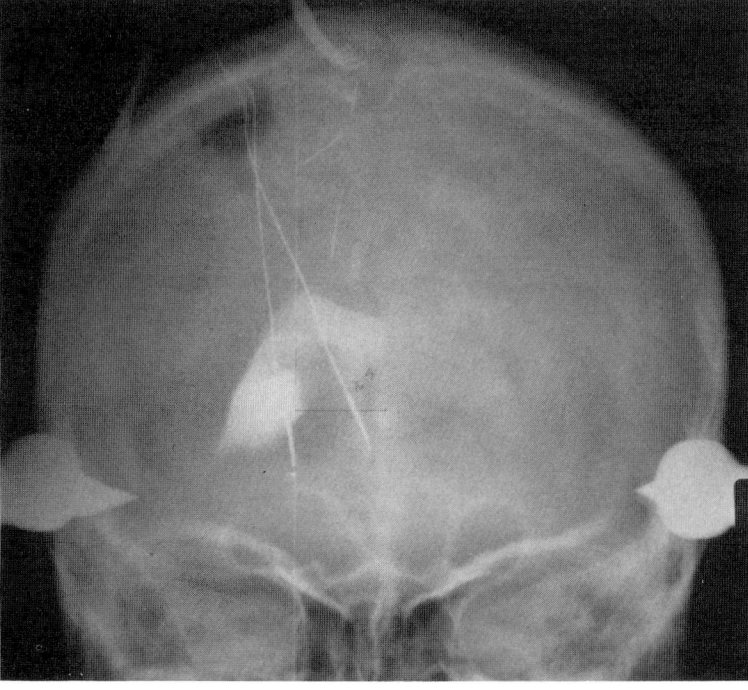

Figure 6.3. Anteroposterior view after insertion of stimulating electrodes in PVG and VPL.

midline, and 5 mm below the commissural plane. For the arm, the target is adjusted medially and superiorly and perhaps anteriorly. For the head and face, VPM is even more medial, anterior, and superior. As Hosobuchi has suggested, targets for sensory thalamic stimulation may not correspond to standard atlases and adjustments must be made for alterations in brain size, third ventricular and thalamic size, and locations on the basis of the results of stimulation (37). The ideal target produces a pleasant sensation of paresthesias or tingling in the distribution of the patient's pain, during low-intensity electrical stimulation.

Other targets, most notably the posterior limb of the internal capsule and the septal region, have been suggested for electrical stimulation to treat chronic pain (1, 33, 55, 60, 69). This author has rarely utilized internal capsular stimulation and has never used septal stimulation. The number of reported patients is too small to be able to comment on the efficacy of these possibly alternative stimulation sites.

Results

The author reviewed the results of electrical stimulation in a variety of brain target sites for treatment of chronic pain published in nine reports from 13 neurosurgical centers in the United States, Canada, Japan, and South Africa (87). These reports described successful pain relief in 396 of 698 patients (57%). Hosobuchi recently published the largest single series of patients (122) with chronic pain treated by electrical brain stimulation (37). He reported relief of pain in 50 of 65 patients (77%) with PAG stimulation and 44 of 76 patients (58%) with sensory thalamic stimulation (87). Overall, he reported pain relief in 94 of 122 or 77% of patients. In 1985, the author and his colleagues (87) reported greater than 50% pain relief in 72% of a group of 43 patients followed for a mean of 20 months and treated by both PAG-PVG and sensory thalamic stimulation. As with Hosobuchi, we found deafferentation pain more difficult to treat successfully with stimulation. At present, the author has implanted stimulating electrodes in 115 patients followed from 1 to 96 months (mean 38.6 months). Virtually complete pain relief has been achieved in one-third of patients, greater than 50% relief in another third, and less than 50% relief in another third. Narcotics use by these patients has decreased by 60% and 58% are able to carry on normal daily activities, unrestricted by pain.

Complications

The most serious complications of electrode implantation are intracranial hemorrhage and infection. Hosobuchi reported ventricular hemorrhage in three patients and intracranial hemorrhage in two patients with a total of two deaths (37). He also reported ventriculitis in one patient, subdural empyema in one patient, and subgaleal infection in four patients. In his series of 115 patients, the author has seen intraventricular hemorrhage in one patient and a small intracerebral hemorrhage in another patient (Fig. 6.4) with no deaths. In

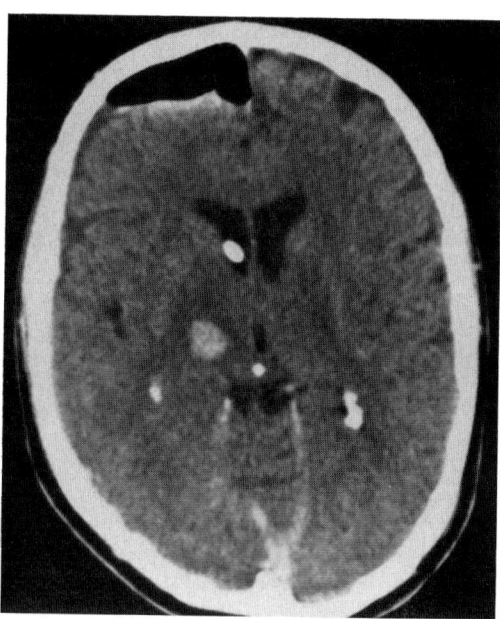

Figure 6.4. CT scan demonstrating hemorrhage into thalamus following electrode placement. Electrode was removed from thalamus, but a second electrode is visible in the PVG region near midline. Hemorrhage resulted in a "thalamotomy" effect with loss of pain and temperature sensation in contralateral upper limb and trunk, location of the patient's pain secondary to recurrent carcinoma of breast.

addition, two patients have experienced ventriculitis, two have experienced subgaleal infections, and two have experienced local subcutaneous infections at the site of implantation of the rf receiver in the subclavicular region. In four of the six patients with infections, removal of the electrodes was required, whereas in two patients, one with ventriculitis and one with subcutaneous infection, the processes were resolved with antibiotics. Combining the series of 122 patients reported by Hosobuchi (37) and the 115 patients treated by the author, there were seven intracranial hemorrhages in 237 patients (2.9%) with two deaths (0.84%). There were also 12 infections (5.1%). Less serious complications of electrode implantation for chronic stimulation include eye movement disorders, unintended motor stimulation, hardware malfunction, and pain at the site of implanted electrical connectors (37, 87, 89).

TECHNICAL CONSIDERATIONS

In most reports of stereotactic surgery for treatment of chronic pain, target localization has been based on delineation of third ventricular anatomy via air or positive-contrast ventriculography. Reference has then been made to standard stereotactic atlases for preliminary target localization. The importance of physiological parameters obtained from intraoperative recording and/or stimulation has been stressed in many reports (5, 18, 37, 74, 75,). The author has had limited experience with intraoperative recording but considerable experience with stimulation for target localization, and enthusiastically supports the use of these measures to improve target localization.

With the advent of computerized tomographic (CT) guidance systems for stereotactic neurosurgery, some reports have appeared describing such a technique for functional stereotactic neurosurgery (9, 14, 29, 44, 46, 61). For stereotactic diagnosis or treatment of intracranial lesions, the CT-stereotactic method is excellent, since the target is visible on the scan. Functional targets within the normal brain are less easily visualized. Likewise, the resolution limit of CT scanning makes visualization of the usual stereotactic reference points (i.e., AC and PC) difficult. The author has carried out stereotactic placement of electrodes for chronic stimulation of PVG and sensory thalamus using the Leksell stereotactic system (44) and CT guidance with the General Electric 9800 CT scanner. While generally satisfactory, the CT method does not allow radiographical confirmation that the intended target has been reached, unless the procedure can be carried out completely in the CT scan unit. Although some centers possess dedicated CT scanners for stereotactic surgery, such an arrangement is usually unavailable. Additionally, the artifact created by electrode tips on the CT scan makes exact localization difficult, even when intraoperative CT scanning is available.

Perhaps the problem of target localization will be improved by a stereotactic system that employs magnetic resonance (MR) imaging. Few reports of such an approach for functional stereotactic neurosurgery have appeared. The author's preliminary experience with this technique is too limited for a definitive comment, but it appears that target identification will be improved by this method compared with the CT method. Problems with confirmation that the intended target has been reached, however, have not been solved fully with MR localization.

CONCLUSIONS

Our ability to treat intractable pain depends on our understanding of the nervous system mechanisms responsible for pain perception. Stereotactic neurosurgery for treatment of pain has expanded substantially with the discovery of powerful pain modulatory systems. The treatment of pain by activation of natural inhibitory systems via stereotactically implanted stimulating electrodes rather than by destruction of normal nervous tissue represents a substantial step forward.

Recent technical advances in stereotactic systems such as the application of CT- and MR-guided systems have not substantially improved our ability to attain functional targets within the normal brain in the same way that they have improved our ability to deal with pathological lesions. Intraoperative recording and stimulation remain essential adjuncts to ascertain that the intended target has been reached for stereotactic treatment of chronic pain, whether by ablative or stimulation techniques.

REFERENCES

1. Adams JE, Hosobuchi Y, Fields HL: Stimulation of internal capsule for relief of chronic pain. *J Neurosurg* 41: 740–744, 1974.
2. Adams JE: Naloxone reversal of analgesia produced by brain stimulation in the human. *Pain* 2: 161–166, 1976.
3. Aiko Y, Shima F, Kato M, Kitamura K: Changes in local cerebral glucose utilization induced by electrical stimulation of the parafiscicular and VPL thalamic nuclei in rats. *Appl Neurophysiol* 48: 172–174, 1985.
4. Akil H, Richardson DE, Barchas JD, et al: Appearance of Betaendorphin-like immunoreactivity in human ventricular cerebrospinal fluid upon analgesic electrical stimulation. *Proc Natl Acad Sci USA* 75: 5170–5172, 1978.
5. Albe-Fessard D: Electrophysiological methods for the identification of thalamic nuclei. *Z Neurol* 205: 15–28, 1973.
6. Albe-Fessard D, Berkley KJ, Kruger L, Ralston HJ III, Willis WD Jr: Diencephalic Mechanisms of Pain Sensation. *Brain Res Rev* 9: 217–296, 1985.
7. Amano K, Kitamura K, Sano K, Sekino H: Relief of intractable pain from neurosurgical point of view with reference to present limits and clinical indications. A review of 100 consecutive cases. *Neurol Med Chir* (Tokyo) 16: 141, 1976.
8. Andy OJ: Successful treatment of long-standing hysterical pain and visceral disturbances by unilateral anterior thalamotomy. *J Neurosurg* 39: 252–254, 1973.
9. Asakura T, Uetsuhara K, Kanemaru R, Hirahara K: An applicability study on a CT-guided stereotactic technique for functional neurosurgery. *Appl Neurophysiol* 48: 73–76, 1985.
10. Basbaum AL, Fields HL: Endogenous pain control mechanisms: Review and hypothesis. *Ann Neurol* 4: 451–462, 1978.
11. Baskin DS, Mehler WR, Hosobuchi Y, Richardson DE, Adams JE, Flitter MA: Autopsy analysis of the safety, efficacy and cartography of electrical stimulation of the central gray in humans. *Brain Res* 371: 231–236, 1986.
12. Benabid AL, Henricksen SJ, McGinty JF, et al: Thalamic nucleus ventro-postero-lateralis inhibits nucleus parfasicularis response to noxious stimuli through a non-opioid pathway. *Brain Res* 280: 217–231, 1983.
13. Bertrand C, Martinez N, Hardy J: Frontothalamic section for intractable pain. In Knighton RS, Dumke PR (eds): *Henry Ford Hospital International Symposium.* Boston, Little Brown, 1966, pp 531–533.
14. Birg W, Mundinger F, Mohadjer M, Weigel K, Fuermaier R: X-ray and magnetic resonance stereotaxy for functional and nonfunctional neurosurgery. *Appl Neurophysiol* 48: 22–29, 1985.
15. Boivie J, Meyerson BA: A correlative anatomical and clinical study of pain suppression by deep brain stimulation. *Pain* 13: 113–126, 1982.
16. Bowsher D: Role of the reticular formation in responses to noxious stimulation. *Pain* 2: 361–378, 1976.
17. Dionne RA, Mueller GP, Young RF, et al: Contrast medium causes the apparent increase in beta-endorphin levels in human cerebrospinal fluid following brain stimulation. *Pain* 20: 313–321, 1984.
18. Donaldson ML: The properties of some human thalamic units. Some new observations and a critical review of the localization of the thalamic nuclei. *Brain* 96: 419–440, 1973.
19. Fardin V, Oliveras JL, Besson JM: A reinvestigation of the analgesic effects induced by stimulation of the periaqueductal gray matter in the rat. I. The production of behavioral side effects together with analgesia. *Brain Res* 306: 105–123, 1985.
20. Fardin V, Oliveras JL, Besson JM: A reinvestigation of the analgesic effects induced by stimulation of the periaqueductal gray matter in the rat. II. Differential characteristics of the analgesia induced by ventral and dorsal PAG stimulation. *Brain Res* 306: 125–139, 1984.
21. Fessler RG, Brown FD, Rachlin JR et al: Elevated beta-endorphin in cerebrospinal fluid after electrical brain stimulation; Artifact of contrast infusion? *Science* 224: 1017–1019, 1984.
22. Foltz EL, White L: Pain relief by frontal cingulumotomy. *J Neurosurg*, 1962, 19: 89, 1962.
23. Foltz EL, White LE Jr: Rostral cingulumotomy and pain relief. In Knighton RS, Dumke PR (eds): *Pain. Henry Ford Hospital International Symposium.* Boston, Little, Brown, 1966, p 469.
24. Fraioli B, Guidetti B: Effects of stereotactic lesions of the pulvinar and lateralis posterior nucleus in intractable pain and dysaesthetic syndromes of man. *Appl Neurophysiol* 38: 23–30, 1975.
25. Frank F, Sturiale C, Gaist G, Fabrizi AP, Frank-Ricci R: Stereotactic mesencephalic tractotomy in the treatment of pancoast syndrome. *Appl Neurophysiol* 48: 274–276, 1985.
26. Gerhart KD, Yezierski RP, Wilcox TK, et al: Inhibition of primate spinothalamic tract neurons by stimulation in ipsilateral or contralateral ventral posterior lateral (VPL) thalamic nucleus. *Brain Res* 229: 514–519, 1981.
27. Gerhart KD, Yezierski RP, Fang ZR, et al: Inhibition of primate spinothalamic tract neurons by stimulation in ventral posterior lateral (VPL) thalamic nucleus: Possible mechanisms. *J Neurophysiol* 49: 406–423, 1983.
28. Gybels J, Dom R, Cosyns P: Electrical stimulation of the central gray for pain relief in human autopsy data. *Acta Neurochir* (Suppl) 30: 259–268, 1980.
29. Hadley MN, Shetter AG, Amos MR: Use of the Brown-Roberts-Wells stereotactic frame for functional neurosurgery. *Appl Neurophysiol* 48: 61–88, 1985.

30. Hassler R: The division of pain conduction into systems of pain sensation and pain awareness. In Janzen R, Keidel WD, Herz A, Steichele C (eds): *Pain:. Basic Principles Pharmocology Therapy.* Stuttgart, Thieme, 1972, pp 98–112.
31. Hitchock E, Kim MC, Sotelo M: Further experience in stereotactic pontine tractotomy. *Appl Neurophysiol* 48: 242–246, 1985.
32. Hosobuchi Y, Adams JE, Rutkin B: Chronic thalamic stimulation for the control of facial anesthesia dolorosa. *Arch Neurol* 29: 158–161, 1973.
33. Hosobuchi Y, Adams JE, Fields HL: Chronic thalamic and internal capsular stimulation for the control of anesthesia dolorosa and dysesthesia of thalamic syndrome. In Bonica JJ (ed): *Advances in Neurology. International Symposium on Pain.* New York, Raven Press, 1974, 4: 783–787.
34. Hosobuchi Y, Adams JE, Linchitz R: Pain relief by electrical stimulation of the central gray matter in humans and its reversal by naloxone. *Science* 197: 183–186, 1977.
35. Hosobuchi Y, Ressier J, Bloom FE, et al: Stimulation of human periaqueductal gray for pain relief increases immunoreactive beta-endorphin in ventricular fluid. *Science* 203: 279–281, 1979.
36. Hosobuchi Y.: Combined electrical stimulation of the periaqueductal gray matter and sensory thalamus. *Appl Neurophysiol* 46: 112–115, 1983.
37. Hosobuchi Y.: Subcortical electrical stimulation for control of intractable pain in humans. *J Neurosurg* 64: 543–553, 1986.
38. Jones EG: Functional subdivision and synaptic organization of the mammalian thalamus. *Int Rev Physiol* 25: 173–245, 1981.
39. Jones MW, Hodge CJ Jr, Apkarian AV, Stevens RT: A dorsolateral spinothalamic pathway in cat. *Brain Res* 335: 188–193, 1985.
40. Judson BA, Himmelberger DU, Goldstein A: The naloxone test for opiate dependence. *Clin Pharmacol Ther* 27: 492–501, 1980.
41. Katayama Y, Tsubokawa T, Hirayama T, Yamamoto T: Pain relief following stimulation of the pontomesencephalic parabrachial region in humans. Brain sites for nonopiate-mediated pain control. *Appl Neurophysiol* 48: 195–200, 1985.
42. Kerr FWL, Casey KL: Pain. *Neurosci Res Progr Bull* 16: 1206, 1978.
43. Kuroda R, Nakatani J, Ioku M, Koshino K: Clinicoanatomical study of thalamic stimulation for pain relief. *Appl Neurophysiol* 48: 181–190, 1985.
44. Leksell L, Leksell D, Schjwebel J: Stereotaxis and nuclear magnetic reasonance. *Neurol Neurosurg and Psychiatry* 48: 14–18, 1985.
45. Martinez SN, Bertrand C, Molina Negro P, Perez-Calvo JM: Alteration of pain perception by stereotactic lesions of frontothalamic pathways. *Conf Neurol* 37: 113–118, 1975.
46. Matsumoto K, Shichijo F, Masuda T, Miyake H: Computer tomography-controlled stereotactic surgery. *Appl Neurophysiol* 48: 39–44, 1985.
47. Mayer DJ, Hayes RL: Stimulation-produced analgesia: development of tolerance and cross-tolerance to morphine. *Science* 188: 941–943, 1975.
48. Mayer DJ, Price DD: Central nervous system mechanisms of analgesia. *Pain* 2: 379–404, 1976.
49. Mazars GJ, Merienne L, Ciolocca C: Stimulations thalamiques intermittentes antalgiques. Note preliminaire. *Rev Neurol* 128: 273–279, 1973.
50. Mazars GJ, Merienne L, Ciolocca C: Treatment of certain types of pain by implantable thalamic stimulators. *Neurchirurgie* 29: 117–127, 1974.
51. Mazars, GJ: Intermittent stimulations of nucleus ventralis posterolateralis for intractable pain. *Surg Neurol* 4: 93–95, 1975.
52. Mehler WR: Central pain and the spinothalamic tract. In Bonica TJ, Albe-Fessard D (eds): *Advances in Neurology.* New York, Raven Press, 1974, pp 127–148.
53. Melzack R, Wall PD: Pain mechanisms; a new theory. *Science* 150: 971–979, 1965.
54. Moosy J, Sagone A, Rosomoff HL: Percutaneous radiofrequency cervical cordotomy; pathological anatomy. *J Neuropath Exp Neurol* 26: 118–123, 1967.
55. Namba S, Nakao Y, Matsumoto Y, Ohmoto T, Nishimoto A: Electrical stimulation of the posterior limb of the internal capsule for treatment of thalamic pain. *Appl Neurophysiol* 47: 137–148, 1984.
56. Nashold BS Jr, Wilson WP, Slaughter DG: Sensations evoked by stimulation in the midbrain of man. *J Neurosurg* 30: 14, 1969.
57. Nashold BS Jr: Extensive cephalic and oral pain relieved by midbrain tractotomy. *Conf Neurol* 34: 382, 1972.
58. Nashold BS Jr: Defects of ocular motility after stereotactic midbrain lesions in man. *Arch Opthalmol* 88: 245, 1972.
59. Nashold BS Jr: Brainstem stereotaxic procedures. In Schaltenbrand G, Walker AE (eds): *Stereotaxy of the Human Brain: Anatomical, Physiological and Clinical Applications.* New York, Thieme-Stratton, 1982, pp 475–483.
60. Nishimoto A, Namba S Nakao Y, et al: Inhibition of nociceptive neurons by internal capsule stimulation. *Appl Neurophysiol* 47: 117–127, 1984.
61. Olivier A, Peters T, Bertrand G: Stereotactic system and apparatus for use with magnetic resonance imaging, computerized tomography, and digital subtraction imaging. *Appl Neurophysiol* 48: 94–96, 1985.
62. Pagni CA, Maspes PE: The relief of intractable pain in malignant disease of the head and neck by stereotactic thalamotomy or sensory root lesions. In Janzen R, Keidel WD, Herz A, Steichele C (eds): *Pain: Basic Principles, Pharmocology, Therapy.* Stuttgart, Thieme, 1972, pp 202–204.
63. Reynolds DV: Surgery in the rat during electrical analgesia induced by focal brain stimulation. *Science* 164: 444–445, 1969.
64. Richardson DE, Zorub DS: Sensory function of the pulvinar. *Conf Neurol* 32: 165–173, 1970.
65. Richardson DE, Akil H: Pain reduction by electric brain stimulation in man. I. Acute administration in periaqueductal and periventricular sites. *J Neurosurg* 47: 178–183, 1977.
66. Richardson DE, Akil H: Pain reduction by electric

brain stimulation in man. II. Acute administration in periaqueductal and periventricular sites. *J Neurosurg* 47: 184, 1977.
67. Sano K: Intralaminar thalamotomy (thalamolaminotomy) and posteromedial hypothalamotomy in the treatment of intractable pain. *Prog Neurol Surg* 8: 50-103, 1977.
68. Schaltenbrand G, Wharen W: *Atlas for Stereotaxy of the Human Brain.* New York, Georg Thieme, 1977.
69. Schvarcz JR: Chronic stimulation of the septal area for the relief of intractable pain. *Appl Neurophysiol* 48: 191-194, 1985.
70. Siegfried J: Monopolar electrical stimulation of nucleus ventroposteromedialis thalami for postherpetic facial pain. *Appl Neurophysiol* 45: 179-184, 1982.
71. Siegfried J, Kuhner A, Sturm V: Neurosurgical treatment of cancer pain. *Rec Res Cancer Res* 89: 148-156, 1984.
72. Spiegel EA: Mesencephalotomy in treatment of intractable facial pain. *Arch Neurol Psychiatr* 69: 1, 1953.
73. Sweet WH: Craniospinal surgery for pain. *Audio-Visual Education in Neurosurgery (AVENS, 1973)* p 12.
74. Tasker RR, Organ LW, Hawrylyshyn P: The sensory organization of the human thalamus. *Appl Neurophysiol* 39: 137-154, 1977.
75. Tasker RR: Thalamic stereotaxic procedures. In Schaltenbrand G, Walker AE (eds): *Stereotaxy of the Human Brain: Anatomical, Physiological and Clinical Applications.* New York, Thieme-Stratton, 1982, pp 484-497.
76. Tsubokawa T, Morijiyama N: Followup results of centre median thalamotomy for relief of intractable pain. *Conf Neurol* 37: 280-284, 1975.
77. Tsubokawa T, Yamamoto T, Katayama Y, et al: Thalamic relay nucleus stimulation for relief of intractable pain. Clinical results and beta-endorphin immunoreactivity in the cerebrospinal fluid. *Pain* 18: 115-126, 1984.
78. Tsubokawa T, Katayama Y, Yamamoto T, Hirayama T: Deafferentation pain and stimulation of the thalamic sensory relay nucleus: Clinical and experimental study. *Appl Neurophysiol* 48: 166-171, 1985.
79. Turnbull IM, Shulman R, Woodhurst WB: Thalamic stimulation for neuropathic pain. *J Neurosurg* 52: 486-493, 1980.
80. Turnbull IM: Bilateral cingulotomy combined with thalamotomy or mesencephalic tractotomy for pain. *Surg Gynecol Obstet* 134: 958, 1972.
81. Turnbull IM, Graeb D, DaSilva V: Functional stereotactic neurosurgery with computerized tomographic guidance using the Brown-Roberts-Wells apparatus. *Appl Neurophysiol* 48: 93, 1985.
82. Walker AE: Relief of pain by mesencephalic tractotomy. *Arch Neurol Psychiatr* 48: 856, 1942.
83. Watkins ES: The place of neurosurgery in the relief of intractable pain. In Swerdlow M (ed): *Relief of Intractable Pain.* Amsterdam, Excerpta Medica, 1974, pp 21-58.
84. Whisler WW, Voris HL: Mesencephalatomy for intractable pain due to malignant disease. *Appl Neurophysiol* 41: 52-56, 1978.
85. Willis WD Jr: Central nervous system mechanisms for pain modulation. *Appl Neurophysiol* 48: 153-165, 1985.
86. Young RF, Feldman RA, Kroening R, Fulton W, Morris J: Electrical stimulation of the brain in the treatment of chronic pain in man. In Kruger L, Liebeskind JC (eds): *Advances in Pain Research and Therapy.* New York, Raven Press, 1984, Vol. 6: 289-303.
87. Young RF, Kroening R, Fulton W, Feldman R, Chambi I: Electrical stimulation of the brain in treatment of chronic pain. *J Neurosurg* 62: 389-396, 1985.
88. Young RF, Modesti LM: Stereotactic ablative procedures for pain relief. In Wilkins RH, Rengachary SS (eds): *Neurosurgery.* New York, McGraw Hill, 1985, pp 2454-2457.
89. Young RF, Brechner T: Electrical stimulation of the brain for relief of intractable pain due to cancer. *Cancer* 57: 1266-1272, 1986.

Chapter 7

Stereotactic Methods in the Management of Epilepsy

DENNIS D. SPENCER, M.D.

INTRODUCTION

Stereotactic techniques for human epilepsy are utilized to identify intracerebral targets thought to be seizure foci or pathways involved in the electrical propagation of a seizure. This chapter will discuss stereoelectroencephalography (SEEG) in the diagnosis of focal seizures, together with strategies of patient selection, and instrumentation techniques.

HISTORICAL REVIEW

The realization that some forms of epilepsy can originate from a single focus of hyperexcitable neurons introduced an exciting era in 19th century neuroscience (22). In the early 20th century, concurrent with the development of electroencephalography (EEG), abnormal sharp electrical potentials recorded from the human scalp were correlated with pathological substrates of epilepsy which when removed could abolish the seizure disorder. The early pioneers in epilepsy surgery also noted, however, the tremendous attenuation of the brain's tiny electrical signal by the overlying dura, skull, and scalp. Recording directly from the surface of the human brain, Penfield and Jasper measured at least a 10-fold amplitude difference (28). Although this small signal can be amplified, it is still contaminated with a variety of electrical potentials emanating from muscle and eye movement which frequently obscure a spontaneous ictal event. In addition, the magnitude of an electrical potential drops off rapidly as you move away from the primary generator, as scalp potentials can record only large synchronous neuronal activity (20). Because of the dipole effect noted by early scientists, where a field potential is generated by current flowing from a neuron membrane to its synapse, discharging neurons arranged around gyri and sulci may cancel each other's charge and present a distorted electrical position relative to the present recorders (19). These field problems are coupled with possible additional distortions when a subcortical structure (amygdala or hippocampus)(16) or a neocortical region distant to surface recording (medial or orbital frontal, medial occipital) is the initial generator and discharges along a preferred anatomical pathway to a distant site before emerging to the surface of the lobe in which it originated.

Depth electrode studies thus grew from the realization that epilepsy can originate deep in the brain's lateral convexity and that localization of many of these sites is difficult, if not impossible, from surface recording (42). As we trace the development of depth electrode recording in human epilepsy, however, we can find the same danger of distorting reality that scalp recordings demonstrated. A depth electrode records only a small field of local neurons or preferentially a pathway through which it is inserted. This emphasizes the need for us not to depend on a single technique or philosophy when confronted with an individual patient's seizure disorder. In fact, some of the first recordings of seizure-like activity from the depths were made by Spiegel and Wycis, who were studying electrical discharges prior to making lesions in the thalamus and hypothalamus for a variety of conditions, ranging from "grand mal and petit mal seizures" to schizophrenia and anxiety neurosis (43). They noted seizure discharges in the thalamus propagating to the cortex in the epileptics and postelectroshock schizophrenics they studied. Lesions made in the medial part of the lamina medullaris interna seemed to benefit two patients suffering from grand mal and petit mal seizures. Subsequent recordings and lesions made in various subcortical nuclei over succeeding years have not supported thalamic origination of generalized epilepsy, but these initial pioneering studies are emphasized to remind us to take care when interpreting depth electrical activity.

STEREOTACTIC SURGERY AS A THERAPEUTIC MODALITY

Stereotactic studies such as those described by Spiegel and Wycis prompted a sustained interest in seizure pathway spread and a variety of these pathways were subjected to stereotactic interruption (44). Field of Forel lesions were reported to reduce the incidence of generalized seizures by 50% in one study, but this has not been systematically pursued (54). Other regions whose partial ablation has not been particularly efficacious in seizures are the thalamus, pallidum, putamen, mesencephalic reticular system, and substantia nigra (27, 30, 49). The amygdala has been the most frequent structure lesioned and there have been reports of seizure control when a unilateral amygdala was proven by SEEG to initiate a seizure and was then ablated (17). In our experience, the amygdala is infrequently the source of a seizure disorder and the efficacy of this treatment needs better documentation.

Reports of subcortical recordings for localization, not intervention, in patients with epilepsy were provided by Brazier (7), Dodge et al. (14) and others (12). Dodge reported two patients whose definitive operation was planned by use of depth electrodes (14). Ajmone-Marsan and Van Buren reported in 1958 an additional group of six patients first studied with combined depth, subdural, and epidural electrodes. They never recorded spontaneous seizures but induced a variety of seizures with Metrazol (2). A major disadvantage of these early studies involved lack of precise localization.

Stereotactic atlases were developed based primarily on cerebral structures uniformly localizable with ventricular contrast, i.e., the temporal horns and the anterior and posterior commissure (47). The French team of Talairach, Bancaud and others, beginning in the 1950s have published extensively about "global" stereotactic methodology and pioneered the use of SEEG (3, 4, 45–48). Their work was followed in the 1960s by Crandall's detailed macro- and microelectrode studies of the temporal lobe and eventually led to a renewed interest in this technique (10, 11, 40). Today, a number of centers are demonstrating the efficacy of surgical treatment in medically intractable epilepsy (39). This renaissance of interest has coincided with improved invasive electrophysiological techniques and a tremendous growth in our ability to image the brain with computerized tomography (CT), magnetic resonance imaging (MRI), and positron emission tomography (PET).

STEREOTACTIC SURGERY AS A DIAGNOSTIC MODALITY

The need for depth electrode studies in medically intractable patients began when some centers perceived inadequacies in scalp EEG recording (1, 10, 11, 24, 31, 34). This reflected a desire to improve seizure control in the surgical patient (approximately 50–60% of patients were seizure-free in some series) and, in part, to provide an alternative approach to removing neocortex in an awake patient guided only by interictal spiking. This interictal spiking may or may not indicate that the underlying neocortex is part of the seizure focus. Rather, it may only indicate that this region of the brain is an epileptogenic zone to which a focus projects but may or may not be responsible for the spontaneous seizure. The strategy of chronic depth electrode recording over days was designed to better define, if possible, the actual zone of seizure onset such that a minimal amount of brain might be removed sparing more functional regions. To help establish the efficacy of depth electrode recording, Spencer, in 1981, tabulated the world literature comparing scalp EEG to depth electrode studies (38). This involved a collected series of 178 patients from 23 reports. The patients were grouped into one of five categories: (*a*) Scalp localization the same as depth localization; (*b*) Scalp localization different from depth localization (both localized); (*c*) Scalp not localized or multifocal, depth well localized; (*d*) Scalp localized, depth not localized or multifocal; or (*e*) Scalp and depth both not localized or multifocal. Table 7.1 catalogues these 178 patients into the appropriate categories. From an analysis of this table, one notes that depth electrodes could have altered the surgical plan in more than 50% of these patients. This study pointed out that when scalp localization alone was used, a surgical success rate of 67% could be predicted compared with an 85% success rate when both depth and scalp localization agreed. This fact, coupled with our own experience, prompts depth electrode utilization in more

TABLE 7.1.
Result of Depth Electrode Localization in 178 Patients

Category	Total Patients (%)
1	30
2	9
3	36
4	9
5	16

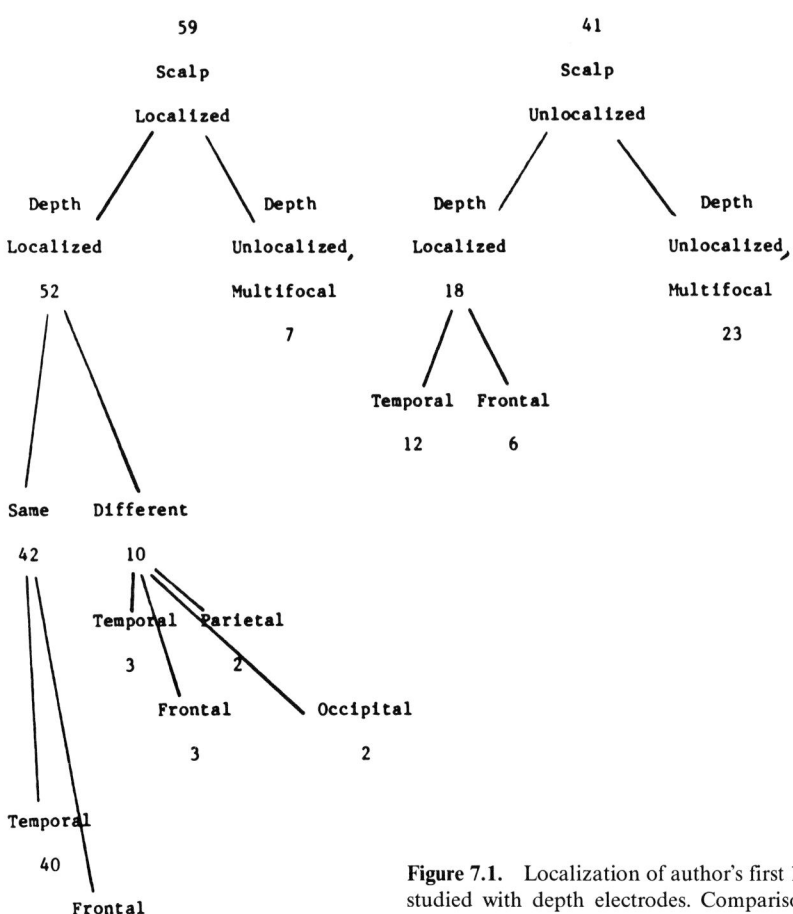

Figure 7.1. Localization of author's first 100 patients studied with depth electrodes. Comparison of scalp and depth localization illustrates change in treatment possible for these patients' pre- and postdepth study.

than 90% of our surgical candidates. Figure 7.1 illustrates our experience with depth electrodes and compares depth and scalp localization. In 29% of patients where the scalp recordings could be localized by the electroencephalographer, the eventual surgical treatment was altered because depth study was either multifocal or unlocalizable (12%), or was localized to a different cerebral lobe (17%). Conversely, when the scalp EEG could not be localized, depth recordings singled out one focus in 44% of cases. This represents 73% of our patients whose treatment was affected by the depth recordings. Concentrating on temporal lobe epilepsy, we have recently studied a group of patients with spontaneous seizures recorded by depth electrodes and subdural and scalp electrodes. The purpose of this study was to enumerate those patients with lateral versus medial temporal lobe ictal onset and to study the spread pattern within the temporal lobe and interhemispherically. In this small group of patients, 11 had unilateral temporal seizures with bilateral depth electrodes studying amygdala and hippocampus and subdural electrodes sampling lateral temporal lobe. Fifty-five seizures were recorded in these patients, four starting in neocortex and hippocampus simultaneously, and 51 in a single hippocampus. Most temporal lobe seizures in this study originate in hippocampus and spread initially to the ipsilateral neocortex. Twenty-four percent spread first to the contralateral hippocampus. These same depth studies pointed out that three patients had anterior-midhippocampus, three patients midposterior hippocampus, and four patients regional hippocampal ictal onset. A depth and neocortical survey such as this may then allow the surgeon to design a resection tailored to onset and spread data (36).

TIMING OF DEPTH ELECTRODES IN THE EVALUATION OF THE SURGICAL CANDIDATE

It should be emphasized that depth electrodes are but one part of the patient evaluation. There is controversy regarding when to use invasive monitoring in selecting surgical candidates and what form that monitoring should take. The following list compiled from several centers enumerates the major justifications for depth electrodes:

1. Patients with temporal lobe scalp ictal events but not clearly lateralized;
2. Patients with bilateral interictal spiking;
3. Patients with scalp ictal onset that conflicts with other localizing criteria (neuropsychological cognitive deficits, imaging, neurological exam, carotid amytal examination);
4. Patients with clinical seizures but normal EEG;
5. Patients with suspected extratemporal focus;
6. Patients with suspected unitemporal lobe ictal onset but lateral versus medial ictal onset is unclear or the anterior-posterior medial axis needs clarifying.

At Yale, the patient is introduced to the surgical program if he has suspected focal epilepsy that interferes with his life and has been treated with multiple medications over a period of years and has remained uncontrolled. The following phased workup is mandatory before depth electrodes or cortical excision is considered:

Phase I (noninvasive):
  A. History, physical, and neurological examination;
  B. Psychiatric evaluation;
  C. Neuropsychological testing;
  D. Visual fields;
  E. CT scanning;
  F. Prolonged 24-hr audiovisual EEG monitoring designed to capture three or more typical seizures;
  G. MRI scanning;
  H. *Conference I:*
     Discussion by neurologists, neurosurgeon, and neuropsychologist and decision to proceed for surgical evaluation.

Phase II:
  A. Angiogram to evaluate vessels for depth electrode placement;
  B. Carotid Amytal to establish speech dominance and memory adequacy;
  C. *Conference II:*
     Discussion of memory and language localization; Discussion of need for

depth electrodes, where they should be placed, and if combined subdural monitoring is warranted.

Phase III:
A. Depth electrodes with or without subdural electrodes;
B. Twenty-four hour EEG audiovisual monitoring requiring three or more ictal events;
C. *Conference III*
Discussion of depth and/or subdural localization and recommendations for surgical intervention.

Phase IV:
A. Surgical excision.

It should be noted that the evaluation stresses correlation of electrical events with functional deficits (neuropsychological evaluation) and the anatomical substrate (imaging abnormalities). Phase IV surgical intervention is usually performed under general anesthesia. The extent of any resection is defined three-dimensionally by the preceding phases, emphasizing the invasive monitoring. Under unusual circumstances, a lateral dominant focus may be identified, requiring language mapping under local anesthesia. Patients with a mass noted during phase I (CT and MRI) that correlates with functional deficits may have direct surgical intervention or may have subdural or combined subdural/depth studies to define the epileptogenic zone if the structural abnormality approximates a functional area that should be further defined (i.e., language or sensorimotor cortex) (35). If a structural abnormality is felt not to be a tumor nor clearly responsible for the patient's seizure disorder, then the placement of recording devices for invasive studies (phase III) is based on the additional phase I and phase II focal phenomena.

SELECTING TARGETS FOR INVASIVE STUDY

Table 7.2 lists some of the "focal phenomena" identified in phase I and II. Each abnormality in the six categories examined is individually analyzed regarding a specific anatomical region defined by that phenomenon. This region will then be subject to invasive scrutiny by either a depth or subdural electrode. Consideration is given to each phenomenon listed regarding the invasive survey.

The focal patterns of higher cortical function tested by the neuropsychological examination are still evolving but those noted here have been statistically significant localizers of functional deficit when correlating structural abnormalities and cognitive dysfunction in age-matched groups of patients on our neurosurgical service.

Our experience indicates that left frontal lesions most significantly impair new learning and praxis, while right frontal lesions most significantly affect attention and problem solving. A low performance intelligence quotient (PIQ) index is common in patients with right frontal lesions. In general, one temporal lobe processes information encoded verbally and in the other temporal lobe, information is otherwise encoded. Lesions in the verbal temporal lobe are associated with dysfluency or frank aphasia and verbal information adequately recalled immediately deteriorates rapidly. Lesions in the nondominant temporal lobe are associated with impaired perception of faces and angular line displacement and perhaps contribute to the melodic quality of speech. The verbal intelligence quotient (VIQ) index of the Wechsler Adult Intelligence Scale may reliably differentiate left versus right temporal disease. The posterior aspects of either hemisphere contribute significantly to visual perception and construction, stereognosis, and manual dexterity. Lesions in the left or right parietal area can lower the PIQ. Our data, however, suggest that left parietal lesions impair performance verbally processed, and the right parietal lobe impairs judgment regarding angular line displacement, spatial location, and identification of nonspeech sounds.

The imaging category in Table 7.2 does not refer to space-occupying mass lesions thought to be tumors which are usually approached surgically after phase II. The abnormalties listed are atrophic lesions, ventricular or hemisphere asymmetries, and MRI signals not seen with CT and not felt to be tumors.

Category III in Table 7.2 stresses what the Paris group has long championed in their

TABLE 7.2
Phase I and II Prestereotactic Focal Phenomena

Cerebral Lobe	Neurological Examination 1	Scalp EEG Ictal, Interictal 2	AV-Monitored Peri-ictal Behavior 3	Neuropsychological Testing 4	Amytal Memory 5	Imaging Abnormalities 6
Frontal	Unilateral motor deficit Nonfluent aphasia	$FP_{1,2}$ $F_{3,4}$ $F_{7,8}$ $C_{3,4}$	Early tonic activity Rapid spread Complex partial status Sexual automatisms Fencer posture Leg automatisms Vocalization Rapid return to consciousness	Poor new learning Inflexible problem solving Poor self-monitoring Impaired attention on left Low PIQ on right	Memory usually intact	Atrophy Frontal horn dilatation MRI^+
Temporal	Superior visual field cut Fluent aphasia	$F_{7,8}$ $T_{5,6}$ $T_{3,4}$	Sometimes initial stare Prolonged upper extremity automatism Confusion postictal Vertigo Auditory hallucination Deja vu Jamai vu Visual hallucination Postictal aphasia Aggression	Left Poor verbal retention Dysfluent Right Face and angle imperception Good VIQ	Inadequate memory unilateral or bilateral	Temporal horn assymetry Uncal herniation MRI^+
Parietal	Inferior visual field cut Fluent aphasia Stereognostic deficit	$P_{3,4}$	Hemibody tingling aura spread from medial parietal to temporal or frontal lobe	Impaired visual perception, construction, stereognosis, manual dexterity and abstract reasoning Low PIQ Left and right same but right more auditory perception	Memory usually preserved	MRI^+
Occipital	Visual field crosses meridian	$O_{1,2}$ $T_{5,6}$	Unformed visual hallucinations Eyes pulling or moving Eye blinking, loss of vision Spread to temporal lobe and mimics temporal lobe seizure	Not specific	Memory preserved	Dilated occipital horn MRI^+

"global, whole brain, three-dimensional" stereotactic approach to depth electrode studies (3). They feel it is critical to correlate the observed behavior during the ictal and peri-ictal period with abnormal electrical activity and pathological brain structures. This analysis of peri-ictal behavior is termed "semiology." Clues regarding the anatomical substrate may be present when the patient can report his aura. For instance, a complex partial seizure beginning with tingling or twitching in one hand before loss of contact would point to the parietal and frontal-lateral neocortex, respectively, as the seizure source. In the cases of occipital foci, we have observed contralateral flashing lights or a sensation of eye pulling or blinking at the onset of a seizure (53). Other lobar localization may necessitate observing the entire seizure. We have noted frontal lobe seizures to be explosive, having early tonic motor signs which spread rapidly, terminate abruptly, and are associated with sexual automatisms and episodes of complex partial status (41, 51, 52). Temporal lobe seizures may have a great deal of overlap with extratemporal complex partial seizures but are the most common source of complex partial seizures which some feel begin frequently with staring, prolonged automatisms, and lengthy postictal confusion (13).

Wieser has extended this concept of electroclinical correlation even further with very specific hypothesis regarding psychomotor epilepsy (50). He details in his book what he considers reproducible seizure types isolated by depth electrodes to five specific components of the limbic system. He chose to scrutinize this system because of its low convulsive threshold. These five constellations are summarized briefly.

Temporobasal-Limbic Type

This, he feels, is the most distinct type of psychomotor seizure involving emotional behavior and integration of emotional processes with other various functions such as somatic and autonomous functions and changes in memory, learning, and coding of experiences. The neuroanatomical substrate is felt to be the hippocampal formation with secondary involvement of the amygdala and propagation to the regioretrosplenialis and cingulate gyrus.

Temporal Pole Type

Recordings of ictal events in the medial and lateral temporal polar cortex and adjacent to the amygdala correlate with irregularities of respiration, heart rate, and pupillary change, a progressive alteration in consciousness, staring, oroalementary automatisms and deja vu.

Frontobasal-Cingulate Type

This includes the cingulate gyrus and frontoorbital basal cortex. It is associated with a gesticulatory complex, severe confusion, and sudden loss of consciousness, bilateral lower limb movement, trunk movement, staring, changing facial expression, change in respirations and heart rate with pupillary dilatation and, finally, verbal and oroalementary automatisms.

Opercular Type

Operculum and insula events are associated with auditory hallucinations, nausea, aphasia, an intact warning, upper limb and head movement, and somesthetic hallucination.

Posterior Neocortical Temporal Type

This is primarily extralimbic with dense afferents to entorhinal cortex, and is associated with aphasia, staring, vestibular hallucinations, visual hallucinations, and unilateral upper limb exploratory movements.

The author has not listed these findings in the detail outlined in Wieser's book, but there is still overlap and imprecision in using these electroclinical categories and describing an individual patient's seizure disorder. This is, however, an important step in attempting to correlate reproducible behavior patterns with a three-dimensional electroanatomical image. The following case is a simplified example of how we use localizing phenomena vis à vis contributions by Penfield, Bancaud and Talairach, Wieser, and others in our six categories of phases I and II in an attempt to continue collecting important correlative data and to provide the best localization for the individual patient.

A right-handed patient has complex partial seizures suspected to be temporal lobe with predominantly right temporal interictal spiking and an obscure ictal scalp recording. Neuropsychological testing might reveal equal verbal and visual spatial IQs but verbal memory might be more affected on formal testing and dominant hemisphere memory poorly demonstrated on the intracarotid amytal test. The patient's seizure behavior observed during monitoring could reveal a suggestion of dysphasia in his postictal confusion state (8).

Although one would be very suspicious of a dominant temporal lobe seizure disorder, the right temporal lobe's contribution must be resolved and, if the focus is solely within the left temporal lobe, is it predominantly medial or lateral. Bitemporal electrode placement to study both hippocampi and the left temporal neocortex would be designed to answer these questions. Thus, the phase I focal phenomena are studied to create a three-dimensional function anatomical picture of the patient's brain solely to guide a stereotactic electrical survey, keeping in mind that stereotactic surgery as it relates to epilepsy includes surface neocortical and subcortical structures.

STEREOTACTIC TECHNIQUES

At any given center, when a decision has been made to study subcortical, medial, and lateral cortical regions in a patient with epilepsy, the methodology may be quite variable. In February 1986, the first international gathering of a group of physicians and scientists involved in the surgical treatment of medically intractable seizures took place in Palm Springs, California. This provides for us the most recent procedural data in stereotactic technique as it is applied in epilepsy. Those techniques represent the "state-of-the-art," and are summarized below.

Flanigin and Smith reported on the technique used for implantation at the Medical College of Georgia (15). They concentrated on placement for suspected temporal lobe epilepsy using bony targets within a stereotactic operating room with fixed mounted x-ray tubes for AP and lateral images. Their placement is performed on awake patients with local anesthesia using the floor-mounted Todd-Wells stereotactic instrument modified by Crandall, Flanigin, and Wells. The UCLA hollow screw technique described by Crandall is used in a modification here with a parasagittal placement of Schryver-type six-stranded Teflon-coated stainless steel wires 0.003 inches in diameter. The targets for the vertex placement are usually the amygdala, anterior hippocampus, inferior temporal cortex, and parahippocampal gyrus. The advantage of a vertex location is felt to be the security of the electrode anchors and the ability to record the depth EEG during and after temporal lobe resection.

The technique used by Munari at Hopital St. Anne in Paris reflects the philosophy of Talairach and Bancaud who began stereo EEG recording in epilepsy many years ago (21). Again, this group stresses stereo EEG methodology as a method to verify clinical observations and to provide an electrical, spatial, and temporal description. They reported on 300 investigations carried out between 1974 and 1985; 225 were performed for partial epilepsy and not related to a tumor, and 45 studies to define the epileptogenic zone around a tumor. Behavior during a seizure dictated the structure to be studied. For example, the group at St. Anne's would explore Heschel's gyrus in patients whose auras consist of an auditory hallucination. Munari uses the Talairach apparatus and atlas. A lateral approach with multicontact electrodes allows study of both lateral cortex and the medial cortex or subcortical structure. Stereotactic stereoscopic arteriography and ventriculography are employed to localize the targets in the intracranial space. Through the various grids in the Talairach frame, holes are placed laterally in the bone, and flexible electrodes of 0.8 mm in diameter are introduced. The electrode contacts vary between 5 and 20 in number, the length of each contact 2 mm spaced 1.5 mm apart. In only 30% of cases do they explore both sides of the brain, feeling that lateralization can be selected preoperatively. Fifty-two percent of their explorations were limited to the right hemisphere. As in other institutions, the frontal and temporal lobes are the most frequently explored. The percentage of electrodes per lobe breaks down to 33% in the frontal lobe, 31% in the temporal, 17% in the parietal, 10% in the central, and 6% occipitally. A major difference in St. Anne's depth electrode studies is the percentage of acute versus chronic depth electrode explorations. Approximately 70% of their last 300 cases were explored acutely relying on the immediate interictal spiking data to resolve the issue of the epileptogenic zone. Even their chronic explorations were generally terminated within the first day after sufficient interictal data had been accumulated.

At the Hopital Notre Dame in Montreal, Talairach's stereotactic frame is also used but has been modified by Bouvier and his co-workers (6). They believe that this frame has the advantages of bony fixation, the ability to reposition it, and the possible use of both orthogonal and nonorthogonal approaches. Again, the stereoarteriography and ventriculogram are performed and the placement of the electrodes is performed under general anesthesia in much the same manner as at St. Anne's. The electrodes used at Notre Dame are constructed in collaboration with the Biomechanical Department of the Universite Lauval, Quebec, Canada, and are constructed of poly vinyl chloride (PVC) tubing of 1.4 mm diameter carrying between 4 to 15 stainless steel contacts.

Over the past few years, the physicians and scientists at Montreal Neurological Institute have taken advantage of the computer and the newer imaging devices of digital subtraction angiography (DSA), magnetic resonance imaging (MRI), and position emission tomography (PET), and have devised an original stereotactic apparatus that is compatible and allows overlap of all these images and permits an orthogonal insertion of depth electrodes based on these computerized imaging systems (23–26). Their procedure is carried out in two stages. Stage 1 involves the stereotactic localization using the appropriate images, and stage 2 involves the implantation of the electrodes, usually carried out a few days following stage 1. The frame of this apparatus is lightweight and takes advantage of the Talairach orthogonal approach or the arc sphere approach of Leksell. It is constructed of an aluminum base with removable plastic bridges; a base ring supports four vertical plastic rods made of polyamide-imide. It is nonmagnetic, nonconductive, and, therefore, compatible with MRI and CT. Stereotactic digital angiography is performed with the frame affixed to the patient's head. Computer program permits display of fiducial markers on the frame for calculation of distances, surfaces, and angles; optimal arterial and venous structures can be superimposed and target selection performed with a pointer. The patient is then taken to the MRI suite. In the majority of cases, the MRI is carried out without the frame, but the information is integrated in the stereotactic data using the DSA stereotactic coordinates. In this instance, the corpus callosum becomes a common landmark for the MRI and DSA studies with superposition of the images taken from both modalities. PET slices demonstrating poor anatomical resolution but good metabolism data can be generated and superimposed on the previous studies and provide better anatomical localization of these metabolic changes. The patient is then brought to the operating room and the orthogonal approach is used exclusively. Two types of electrodes are commonly used at Montreal Neurological Institute (MNI), one commercially available and the second homemade stainless steel wires with nine recording sites located 5 mm apart. These electrodes are left in for chronic recording of spontaneous seizures.

Two systems of depth electrode implantation are utilized at Yale University (33). At the West Haven Veterans Administration Epilepsy Unit, we use depth electrodes that have been modified from those initially constructed by Ray (29). A no. 24 stainless steel needle stock has 180.0035-inch laminated wires jigged around its diameter. They are 90% platinum and 10% iridium. There are 18 evenly spaced platinized contacts measuring 0.075 mm. The electrodes are semirigid and range in length from 50 to 110 mm. They are placed using CT- and MRI-identified intracranial structures and bony landmarks using the modified Todd-Wells frame with a predominantly parasagittal placement, as seen in Fig. 7.2 (32, 37). Preoperative angiography is always performed to detail arteriovenous anatomy. The parasagittal placement is designed to study predominantly the medial structures of the temporal, frontal, occipital, and parietal lobes. A common electrode survey for us is illustrated in Fig. 7.3 and involves two posterior temporal electrodes, each inserted through the respective mesial occipital lobes and along the length of the hippocampus coming to rest anterior to the amygdala. These two electrodes are often complemented by two medial-frontal electrodes which will survey the cortex anterior to the cingulate gyrus and into the orbital frontal region. Figure 7.4 illustrates an electrode placement strategy based on phase I and II phenomena pointing to overlapping deficits in posterior frontal, temporal, and occipital lobes. In this case, ictal events began in the right occiput and spread rapidly into both the frontal and temporal lobes. A cuneus hamartoma was found at surgery. Whenever the preoperative phase I and II focal phenomena point to a possible lateral cortical source, flexible homemade, seven-contact subdural electrodes are placed through large burr holes for neocortical study. This electrode placement system is further checked for accuracy by a postoperative computer technique based on the stereotactic atlas of Talairach and Szikla (48). The AP and lateral operative x-rays taken in the frame are used. The positions of the external auditory meatus, the bony sulcus of the transverse sinus, and the tuberculum sella are used to transform each electrode location into the standardized proportional coordinate system. A reconstruction illustrating target plus trajectories in sagittal and frontal views is depicted in Fig. 7.5. If the patient's prestereotactic data are strongly suggestive of just one lobe, then additional electrodes may be inserted here or the lateral subdural electrodes will be added. In some instances, only regionalization or lobar localization is possible during the first implantations, and the patient comes back for subsequent invasive survey with more detailed depth and subdural arrays. The advantages of this system are three-fold. First, the large number of contacts allows a systematic survey along the length of low

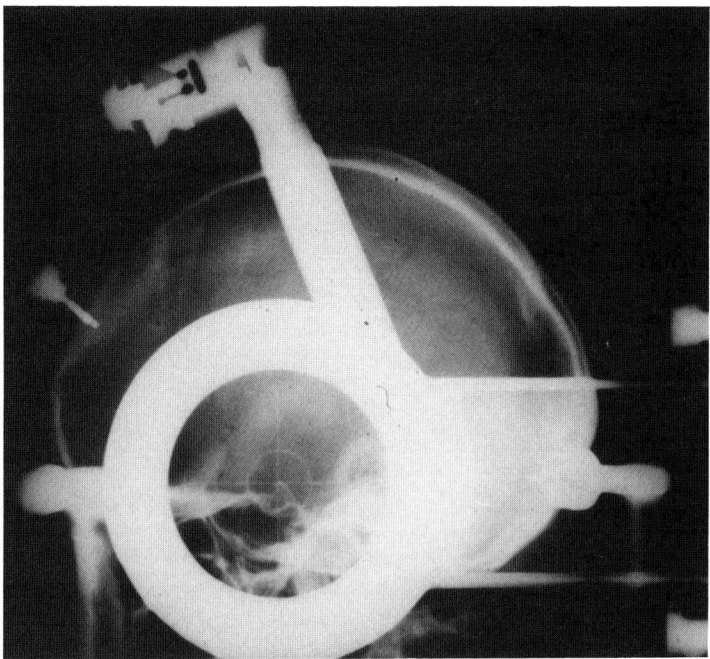

Figure 7.2. Modified Todd-Wells stereotactic frame in position for parasagittal anterior hippocampal placement, which will also study frontal lobe en passant.

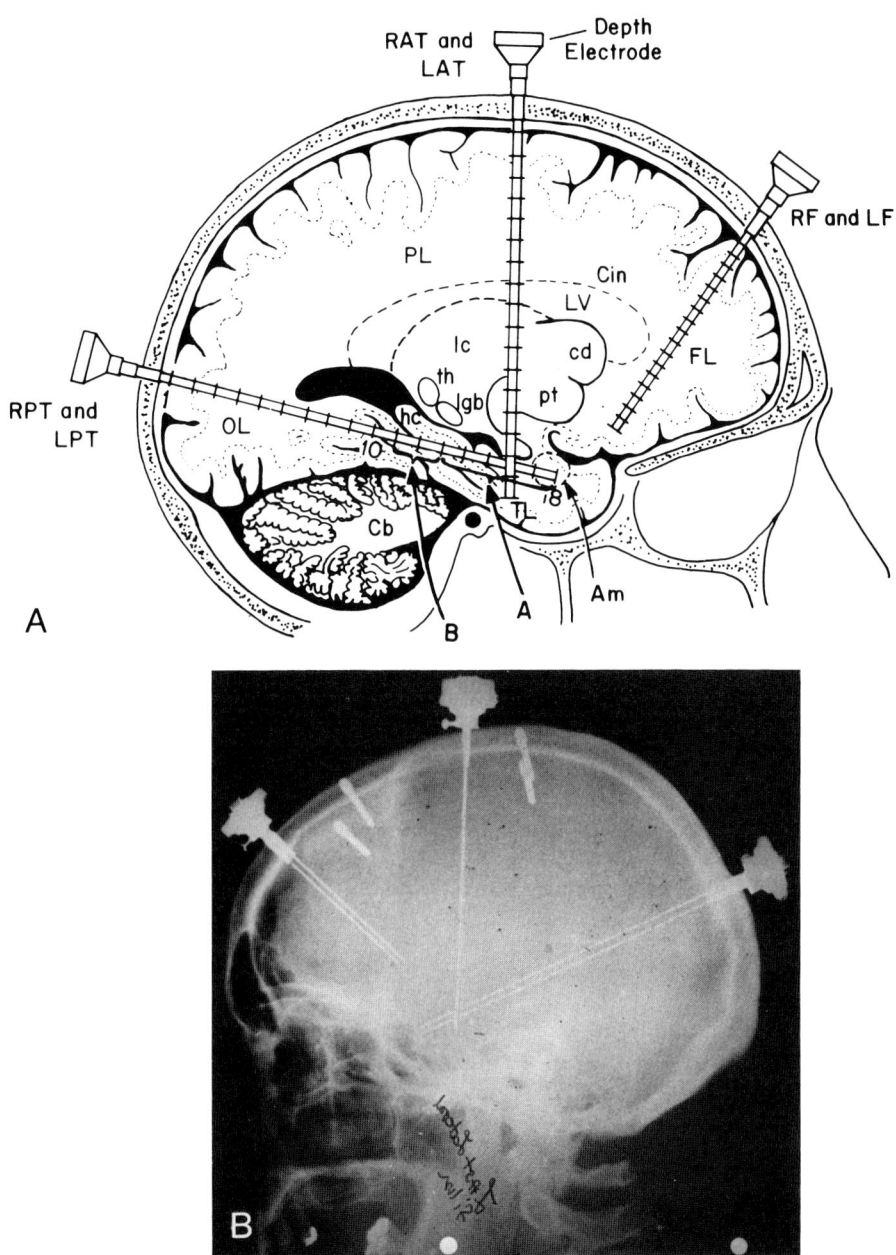

Figure 7.3. *A*) Depiction of one electrode grouping at the West Haven Veterans Administration Epilepsy Unit. *RF, LF*, frontal electrodes; *RAT, LAT*, frontotemporal electrodes; *RPT, LPT*, occipitotemporal hippocampal electrodes; *AM*, amygdala; *A*, brackets common location for anterior to mid-hippocampal ictal events; *B*, brackets position of mid- to posterior hippocampal events. *B*) Postimplantation lateral skull x-ray of the array portrayed in Fig. 7.2.

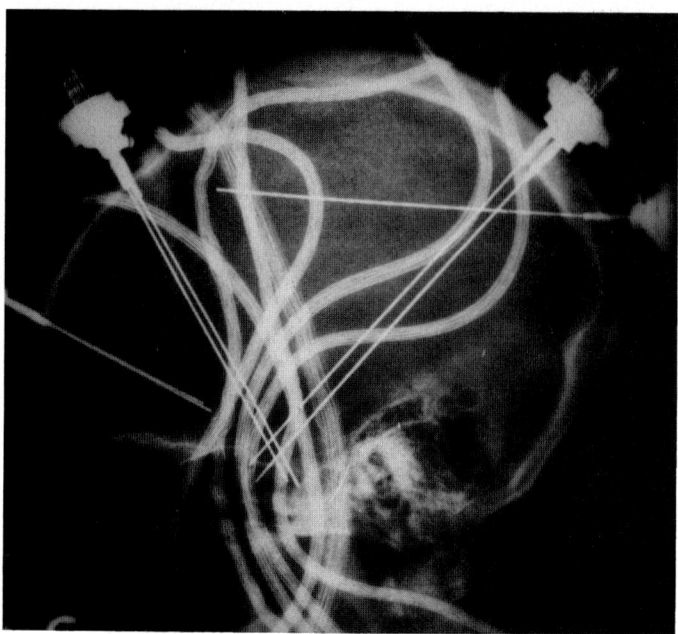

Figure 7.4. Electrode array for patient whose preoperative workup shows frontal, temporal, and occipital phenomena which need to be studied.

seizure threshold medial cerebral tissue, such as the hippocampus, supplementary motor region, and cingulate gyrus. Second, the large number of contacts can be recorded simultaneously by our 64-channel computerized monitoring system and provides a way to study seizure spread. Figure 7.6 is a 64-channel depth EEG illustrating the initial ictal regional discharge in the left hippocampus of an implanted surgical candidate. Finally, the small size of the electrodes minimizes electrode tract injury. In general, the risk of electrode implantation throughout the world is minimal. There has been approximately a 2 to 3% incidence of hemorrhage in our and most other series. Mortality is much less and has been 0 at our center. Others report no mortality or less than 0.5%.

Most recently, the authors have begun to take advantage of the detailed imaging available from the 1.5 Tesla General Electric Magnetic Resonance instrument (32, 37). Using the Brown-Roberts-Wells (BRW) stereotactic system adapted for use with the MRI head coil, one can now, with far more accuracy than most other stereotactic methods, place electrodes in easily identified subcortical structures picking the targets in axial, coronal, and sagittal planes. This localizing system allows the points of interest to be calculated from any slice reconstruction (9). The BRW MRI localizer is a cubical array of N-type units in three orthogonal planes (see Cosman *et al.* (9) for a detailed description of the frame and system). The localizer is scanner-independent and any target can be calculated where the rods and diagonals are cut by the scan plane. The head ring, head posts, and skull screws are made of anodized aluminum, the localizer constructed of polycarbonate with tubular channels generally filled with petroleum jelly, and all of these materials are nondistorting in magnetic fields from 0.1 to 1.5 Tesla. For purposes of creating more appropriate anatomical delineation of cortical and subcortical targets, particularly within the temporal lobe, we have altered the typical CT angle on the MRI instrument by extending the head and thus creating an axial plane in a more anatomically correct manner along the length of the hippocampus and temporal horn (Fig. 7.7). Targets may be chosen from axial, coronal, or sagittal cuts as noted in Fig. 7.8, and the coordinate data

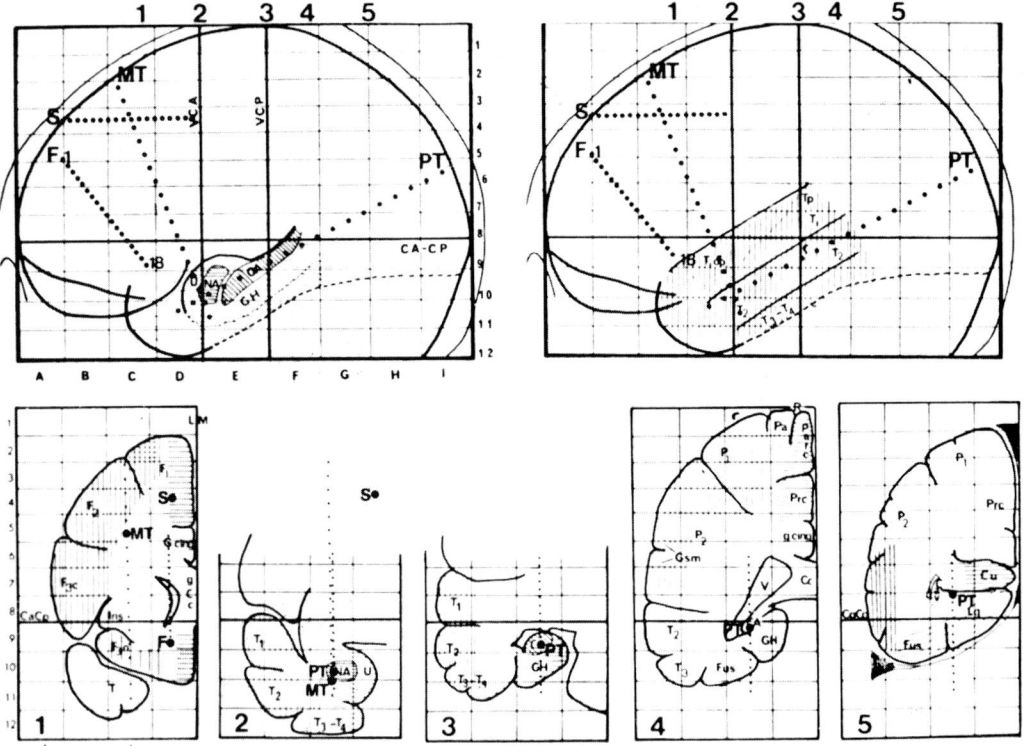

Figure 7.5. Stereotactic localization of recording sites. *MT*, parasagittal frontotemporal electrode studying frontal neocortex, orbital cortex, insula, and amygdala; *S*, parasagittal frontal electrode studying anteriormedial frontal lobe and directed toward the supplementary motor region; *F*, parasagittal anteriomedial electrode directed toward the subcallosal medial orbital region; *PS*, posterior medial parietal frontal directed through the posterior cingulum to supplementary motor area; *PT*, posterior medial occipital temporal along length of hippocampus directed toward amygdala; *VCA*, anterior commissure vertical line; *VCP*, posterior commissure vertical line; *CA-CP*, anterior commissure-posterior commissure line; *GH*, hippocampal gyrus; *NA*, amygdala.

taken from the MRI software entered into an off-line computer and used to calculate an approach to the targets. The subsequent placement of the electrodes takes place in the operating room using the routine BRW CT system components. Entry point for each electrode is flexible allowing the authors to continue parasagittal placement based on the angiographical location of blood vessels, or an orthogonal approach may be used as well. The electrodes used in this system are made by the Straumann Institut, Waldenburg, Switzerland. They are essentially the same electrode reported by Comte, Siegfried and Wieser, but are modified for our use with more contacts and longer lengths (8). They consist of helically wound stainless steel wires with 1-mm external diameter, and cylindrical contacts with a real surface area of 3.8 mm. They are flexible and can be introduced with a guiding stylet using the BRW frame.

In summary, human epilepsy is one of the singular diseases of the central nervous system to demand stereotactic concepts to help explain its pathogenesis. It is a disorder that may originate in a myriad of cortical and/or subcortical structures; it is a bioelectrical phenomenon that necessitates sophisticated electrophysiological analysis in three dimensions and spreads rapidly to involve other brain regions that may confound localization.

The stereotactic approach to this disease then begins long before depth electrodes are inserted and involves a detailed analysis of

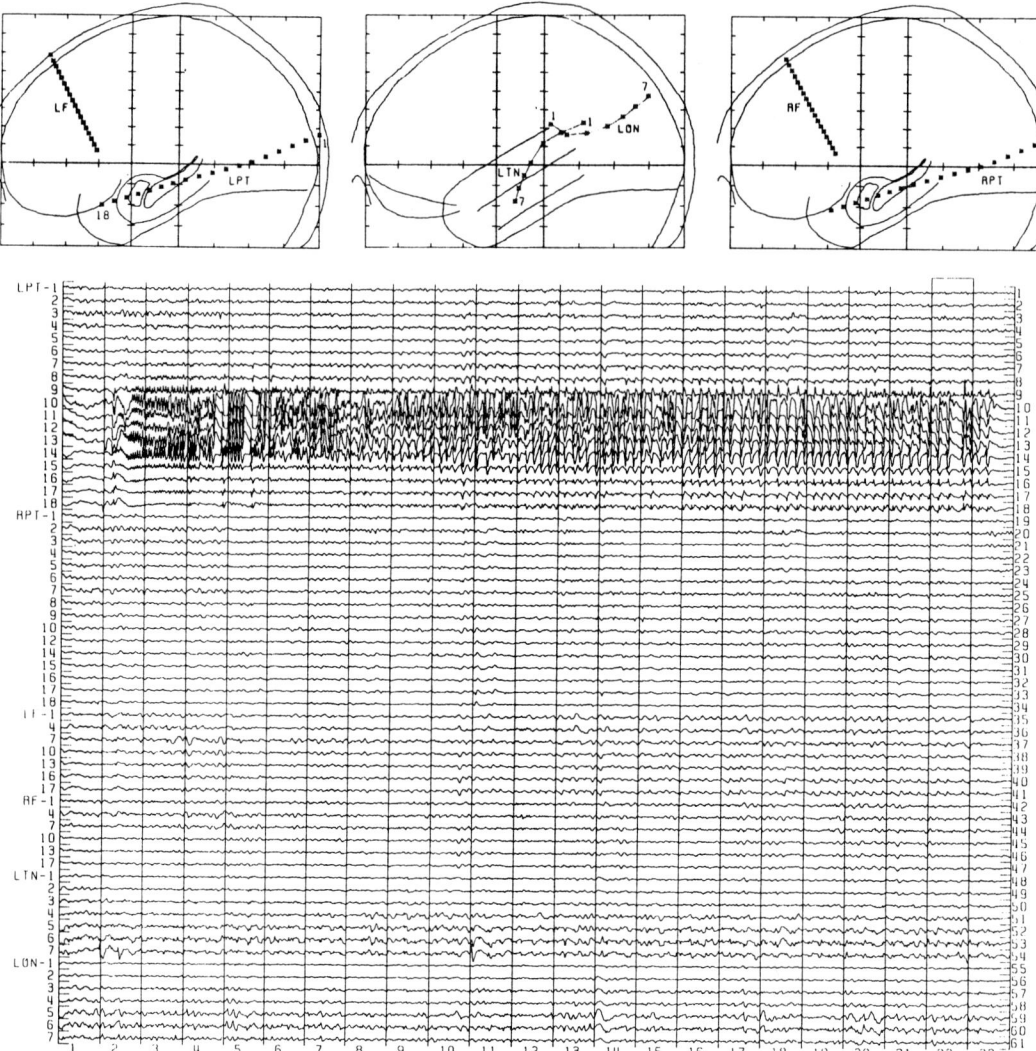

Figure 7.6. Sixty-four computerized simultaneous channels are used to illustrate regional onset of seizure in patient's left hippocampus preceding ictal behavior. Cartoon sketches above 64 stereo EEG array depict relationship of each contact point with appropriate intracerebral structure. Contact 1 for each electrode is proximal at cortical surface. Contact 18 is most distal point. Stereo EEG is shown with abscissa in seconds and ordinate denotes each contact point. *LPT*, left posterior occipital temporal hippocampal electrode; *RPT*, right posterior occipital temporal hippocampal electrode; *LF*, left mesial orbital frontal electrode; *RF*, right mesial orbital frontal electrode; *LTN*, left temporal neocortical subdural electrode; *LON*, left parietal occipital neocortical subdural electrode. Onset of this seizure is seen simultaneously in LPT sites 10 through 14 indicating regional hippocampal onset.

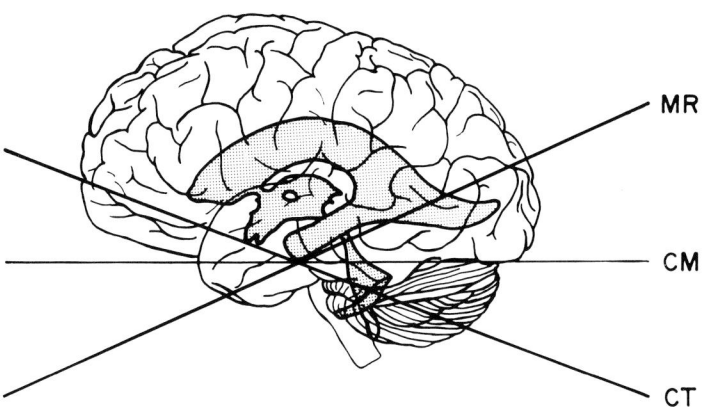

Figure 7.7. MR line illustrates that by extending head, axial slice is parallel with temporal horn. *MR*, extended head position; *CM*, canthomeatal line; *CT*, typical CT head position designed to decrease irradiation of corneas.

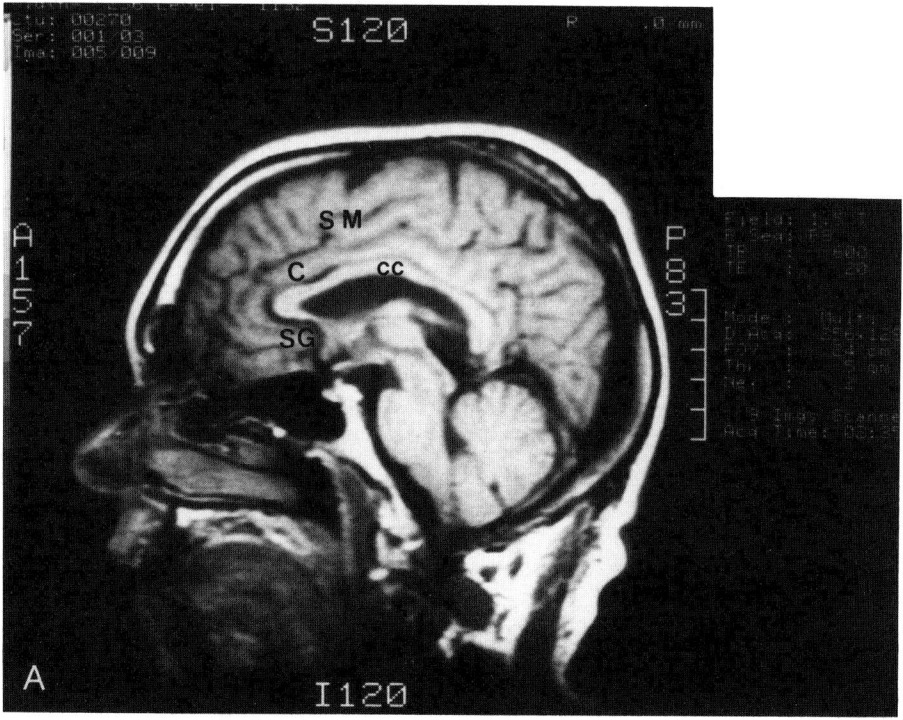

(continued)

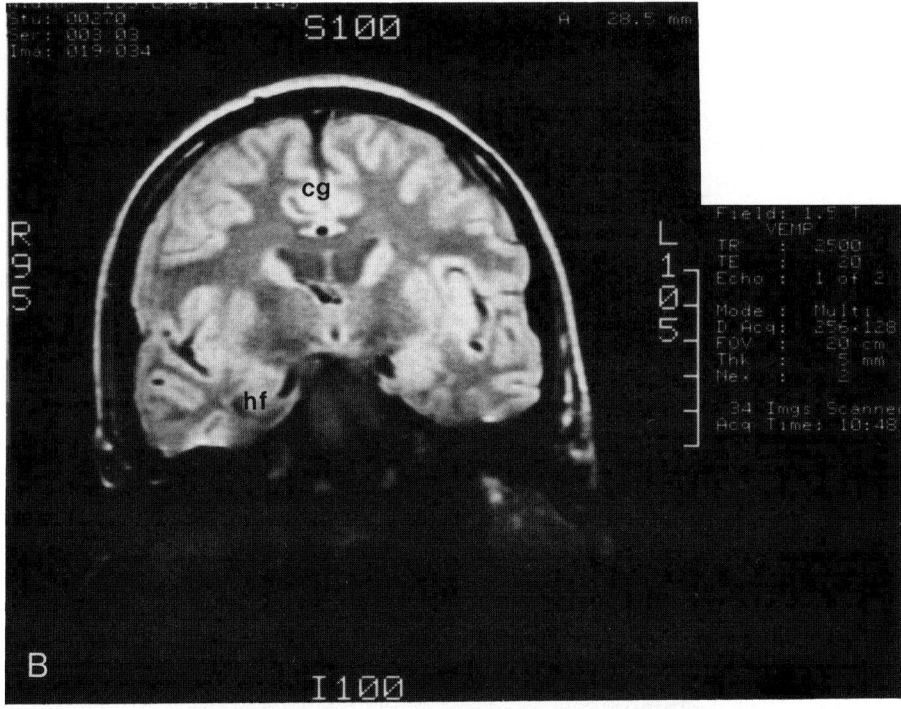

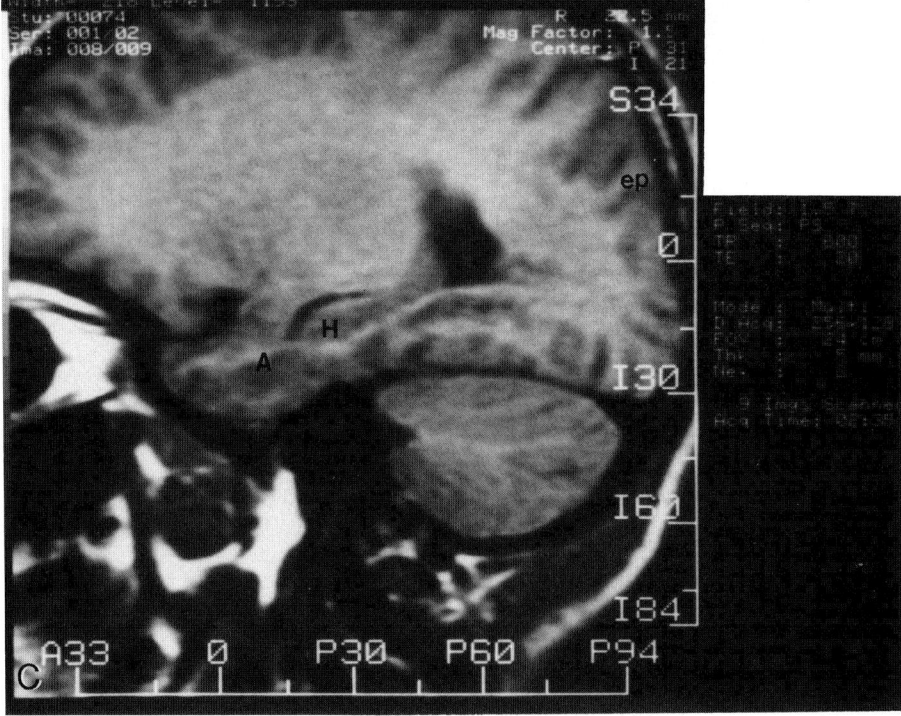

Figure 7.8. *A, B,* and *C,* Photographs of a General Electric 1.5 Tesla MR image used for depth electrode placement. Detailed anatomy allows precise electrophysiological study.

each patient to isolate focal epileptogenic phenomena using scalp EEG, neurological exam, scrutiny of the behavioral seizure, cognitive testing, and imaging. A three-dimensional anatomical concept of each patient's proposed possible seizure foci should then determine electrode type and placement such that each hypothesis can be tested.

The efficacy of cortical resection for epilepsy has been well established. We have been limited, however, in our ability to localize and characterize the epileptogenic focus or zone. We can, however, look forward to the growth of our electrophysiological monitoring and imaging capability (18). The computerized coupling of the two should allow us to define more precisely the relationship of electrophysiology and anatomy and their impact on metabolism. Stereotactic surgical management of medically intractable epilepsy is at the threshold of an exciting new era.

REFERENCES

1. Ajmone-Marsan C: Depth electrography and electrocorticography. In Aminoff MJ (ed): *Electrodiagnosis in Clinical Neurology.* New York, Churchill-Livingstone, 1980, pp 167–196.
2. Ajmone-Marsan C, Van Buren JM: Epileptiform activity in cortical and subcortical stuctures in the temporal lobe of man. In Baldwin M, Bailey P (eds): *Temporal Lobe Epilepsy.* Springfield, IL, Charles C. Thomas, 1958, pp 78–108.
3. Bancaud J: Stereoelectroencephalography. In *Handbook of Electroencephalography and Clinical Neurophysiology.* Amsterdam, Elsevier, 1975, Vol. 10B: pp. 3–45.
4. Bancaud J, Talairach J, Schaub C, Bonis A, Szikla G, Colomb D: Stereotactic functional exploration of the epilepsies of the supplementary areas of the mesial surface of the hemisphere. *Electroenceph Clin Neurophysiol* 14: 788, 1962.
5. Bickford RG: Application of depth electroencephalography in some varieties of epilepsy. Electroenceph. *Clin Neurophysiol* 8: 526–527, 1956.
6. Bouvier G, Saint-Hilaire J, Giard N, Lesage J, Cloutier L, Beique R: Depth electrode implantation at Hopital Notre-Dame, Montreal. In Engel J (ed): *Surgical Treatment of the Epilepsies.* New York, Raven Press, 1987, pp 589–593.
7. Brazier AB: Depth recordings from the amygdaloid region in patients with temporal lobe epilepsy. *Electroenceph Clin Neurophysiol* 8: 532–533, 1956.
8. Comte P, Siegfried J, Wieser HG: Multipolar hollow-core electrode for brain recordings. *Appl Neurophysiol* 46: 41–46, 1983.
9. Cosman ER, Heilbrun MP, Wells TE: A magnetic resonance imaging (MRI) localizer for determining stereotaxic targets in axial, sagittal, or coronal scan planes. In Apuzzo MLJ (ed): *Surgery of the Third Ventricle.* Baltimore, MD, Williams & Wilkins, 1986.
10. Crandall PH: Developments in direct recordings from epileptogenic regions in the surgical treatment of partial epilepsies. In Brazier MAB (ed): *Epilepsy: Its Phenomena in Man.* New York, Academic Press, 1973, pp 288–314.
11. Crandall PH, Walter RD, Rand RW: Clinical applications of studies on stereotactically implanted electrodes in temporal lobe epilepsy. *J Neurosurg* 0220: 827–840, 1963.
12. Delgado JMR, Hamlin H: Surface and depth electrography of the frontal lobes in conscious patients. *EEG Clin Neurophysiol* 8: 371–384, 1956.
13. Delgado-Escueta AV, Walsh GO: The selection process for surgery of intractable complex partial seizures. Surface EEG and depth electrography. In Ward AA, Penry JK, Purpura D (eds): *Epilepsy.* New York, Raven Press, 1983, pp 295–326.
14. Dodge HW, Bailey A, Bickford RG, Petersen MC, Sem-Jacobsen CW, Miller RH: Neurosurgical and neurologic application of depth electrography. *Proc Mayo Clin* 28: 188–191, 1953.
15. Flanigin HF, Smith JR: Depth electrode implantation at the Medical College of Georgia. In Engel J (ed): *Surgical Treatment of the Epilepsies.* New York, Raven Press, 1987, pp 609–612.
16. Gloor P, Vera CL, Sporti L: Electrophysiological studies of hippocampal neurons. I. Configuration and laminar analysis of the "resting" potential gradient, of the main-transient response to perforant path, fimbrial and mossy fiber volleys and of "spontaneous" activity. *Electroenceph Clin Neurophysiol* 15: 353–378, 1963.
17. Hood TW, Siegfried J, Wieser HG: The role of stereotactic amygdalotomy in the treatment of temporal lobe epilepsy associated with behavioral disorders. *Appl Neurophysiol* 46: 19–25, 1983.
18. Kelly PJ, Kall BA, Goerss S, Earnest F: Present and future developments of stereotactic technology. *Appl Neurophysiol* 48: 1–6, 1985.
19. Lorente de No R: Action potentials of the motoneurons of the hypoglossus nucleus. *J Cell Comp Physiol* 29: 207–287, 1947a.
20. Morris HH, Luders H: Electrodes. In Gorman J Ives JR, Gloor P (eds): *Long-term Monitoring in Epilepsy,* (EEG Suppl. No. 37). Elsevier Science Publ, 1985, pp 3–26.
21. Munari C: Depth electrode implantation at Hopital Sainte Anne, Paris. In Engel J (ed): *Surgical Treatment of the Epilepsies.* New York, Raven Press, 1987, pp 583–586.
22. O'Leary JL, Goldring S: *Science and Epilepsy: Neuroscience Gains in Epilepsy Research.* New York, Raven Press, 1976.
23. Olivier A, Bertrand G, Peters T: Stereotactic systems and procedures for depth electrode placement: technical aspects. *Appl Neurophysiol* 46: 37–40, 1983.
24. Olivier A, Gloor P, Quesney IF, Anderman F: The

indications for and the role of depth electrode recording in epilepsy. *Appl Neurophysiol* 46: 33-36, 1983.
25. Olivier A, Marchand E, Peters T, Tyler J: Depth electrode implantation at the Montreal Neurological Institute and Hospital. In Engel J (ed): *Surgical Treatment of the Epilepsies.* New York, Raven Press, 1987, pp 595-600.
26. Olivier A, Peters T, Bertrand G: Stereotactic system and apparatus for use with magnetic resonance imaging, computerized tomography, and digital subtraction imaging. *Appl Neurophysiol* 48: 94-96, 1985.
27. Osawa T: Surgical treatment of epileptic convulsion. In *Research of Epilepsy.* Tokyo, Igaku Shoin, 1952, pp 175-178.
28. Penfield W, Jasper H: *Epilepsy and the Functional Anatomy of the Human Brain.* Boston, Little, Brown & Co, 1954.
29. Ray CD: A new multipurpose human brain depth probe. *J Neurosurg* 24: 911-921, 1966.
30. Sano K: Upper mesencephalic reticulotomy. *Psychiatr Neurol Jpn* 63: 363-372, 1961.
31. Soloway SS, Williamson PD, Spencer DD, et al: Surgery for epilepsy: Role of depth electroencephalography. *Conn Med* 44: 70-75, 1980.
32. Sostman HD, Spencer DD, Gore JC, et al: Preliminary observations on magnetic resonance imaging in refractory epilepsy. *Mag Res Imag* 2: 301-306, 1984.
33. Spencer DD: Depth electrode implantation at Yale University. In Engel J (ed): *Surgical Treatment of the Epilepsies.* New York, Raven Press, 1987, pp 603-607.
34. Spencer DD, Spencer SS: Surgery for epilepsy. *Neurol Clin* 3: 313-330, 1985.
35. Spencer DD, Spencer SS, Mattson RH et al: Intracerebral masses in patients with refractory partial epilepsy. *Neurology* 34: 432-436, 1984.
36. Spencer DD, Spencer SS, Williamson PD, et al: Access to the posterior medial temporal lobe structures in the surgical treatment of temporal lobe epilepsy. *Neurosurgery* 15: 667-671, 1984.
37. Spencer DD, Spencer SS, Williamson PD, et al: Nuclear magnetic resonance imaging in refractory epilepsy patients. *Epilepsia* 25: 650, 1984.
38. Spencer SS: Depth electroencephalography in selection of refractory epilepsy for surgery. *Ann Neurol* 9: 207-214, 1981.
39. Spencer SS: Surgical options for uncontrolled epilepsy. In Porter RJ, Theodore WH (eds): *Neurologic Clinics.* WB Saunders, 1986, vol 4, pp. 669-695.
40. Spencer SS, Spencer DD, Williamson PD, et al: The localizing value of depth electroencephalography in 32 refractory epileptic patients. *Ann Neurol* 12: 248-253, 1982.
41. Spencer SS, Spencer DD, Williamson PD, et al: Sexual automatisms in partial complex seizures. *Neurology* 33: 527-533, 1983.
42. Spencer SS, Williamson PD, Bridgers SL, et al: Reliability and accuracy of localization by scalp ictal *EEG Neurology* 35: 1567-1575, 1985.
43. Spiegel EA, Wycis HT: Thalamic recordings in man with special reference to seizure discharges. *EEG Clin Neurophysiol* 2: 23-27, 1950.
44. Spiegel EA, Wycis HT, Freed H: Thalamotomy: neuropsychiatric aspects. *NYJ Med* 49: 2273-2274, 1949.
45. Talairach J, Bancaud J: Stereotaxic approach to epilepsy. *Prog Neurol Surg* 5: 297-354, 1973.
46. Talairach J, Bancaud J: Stereotactic exploration and therapy in epilepsy. In Vinken PJ, Bruyn GW (eds): *Handbook of Clinical Neurology vol. XV The Epilepsies.* Amsterdam, North-Holland, 1974, pp 758-782.
47. Talairach J, Bancaud J, Bonis A, Szikla G, Tournoux P: Functional stereotactic exploration of epilepsy. *Conf Neurol* 22: 328-330, 1962.
48. Talairach J, Szikla G: Application of stereotactic concepts to the surgery of epilepsy. *Acta Neurochirurgica* S30: 35-54, 1980.
49. Wada T: Thalamotomy for epileptic patient. In *Research of Epilepsy.* Tokyo, Igaku Shoin, 1952, pp.192-202.
50. Wieser HG: *Electroclinical Features of the Psychomotor Seizure.* Stuttgart, New York, Gustave Fischer Verlag, 1983.
51. Williamson PD, Mattson RH, Spencer SS, et al: Complex partial status epilepticus: A depth electrode study. *Ann Neurol* 18: 647-654, 1985.
52. Williamson PD, Spencer DD, Spencer SS, et al: Complex partial seizures of frontal lobe origin. *Ann Neurol* 18: 497-504, 1985.
53. Williamson PD, Spencer SS, Spencer DD, et al: Complex partial seizures with occipital lobe onset. *Epilepsia* 22: 247-248, 1981.
54. Yoshii N: Follow-up study of epileptic patients following Forel-H-Tomy. *Appl Neurophysiol* 40: 1-12, 1977-1978.

Chapter 8

Special Stereotactic Techniques: Trigeminus Stereoguide for Trigeminal and Glossopharyngeal Neuralgia

LAURI LAITINEN, M.D.

INTRODUCTION

Hartel's (4) free-hand technique from 1914 is still the dominating technique for percutaneous introduction of a therapeutic probe through the foramen ovale. In most cases, the technique is easy, but even in the most experienced hands, it sometimes is difficult and time-consuming to find the foramen. Kirschner (6) was the first who designed a guiding instrument to facilitate the procedure. I have, since 1984, used a fully stereotactic instrument for the percutaneous treatment of trigeminal and glossopharyngeal neuralgias (9). The instrument, the trigeminus stereoguide, has now been used in 217 patients and will be described here.

METHOD

The basal frame of the trigeminus stereoguide is illustrated in Fig. 8.1. It consists of a rectangular frame of duraluminum, three skull pins for bony fixation, a nasion support, and two ear bars. The ear bars, with a millimeter scale, have 10-mm long lead pins inside their tips. For mounting of the frame on the patient's head, a hanging brace of nylon is fixed at the four corners of the frame. On each side of the frame, a rectangular slide component permits insertion of a cylinder component with a 90° arc and an electrode carrier.

Mounting of the Frame

The patient is given premedication 15 min before surgery. The patient's hair is washed with a medical shampoo. The frame is mounted on the sitting patient. The hanging brace is adjusted so that the ear bars can be approximately positioned against the external auditory meati, but not so deep in the meati that pressure is experienced. The nasion support is pressed against the bridge of the nose. The skull pins are screwed into the scalp, where local anesthesia is applied. To avoid a shift of the ear bars at the meati, the screws are tightened in turns; first the posterior screws are tightened simultaneously, then the frontal screw, then the posterior screws again, etc., until the frame becomes rigidly fixed to the skull. If the patient experiences pain at the meati, the ear bars can be withdrawn by a few millimeters, after which the locking nuts are tightened. The millimeter position of the ear bar on the side of surgery is recorded. The hanging brace is removed.

Radiography

Radiography of the skull is carried out on a conventional x-ray table. An axial radiograph is taken with the x-ray beam perpendicular to the frame (Fig. 8.2). An interaural line is drawn between the lead pins. The

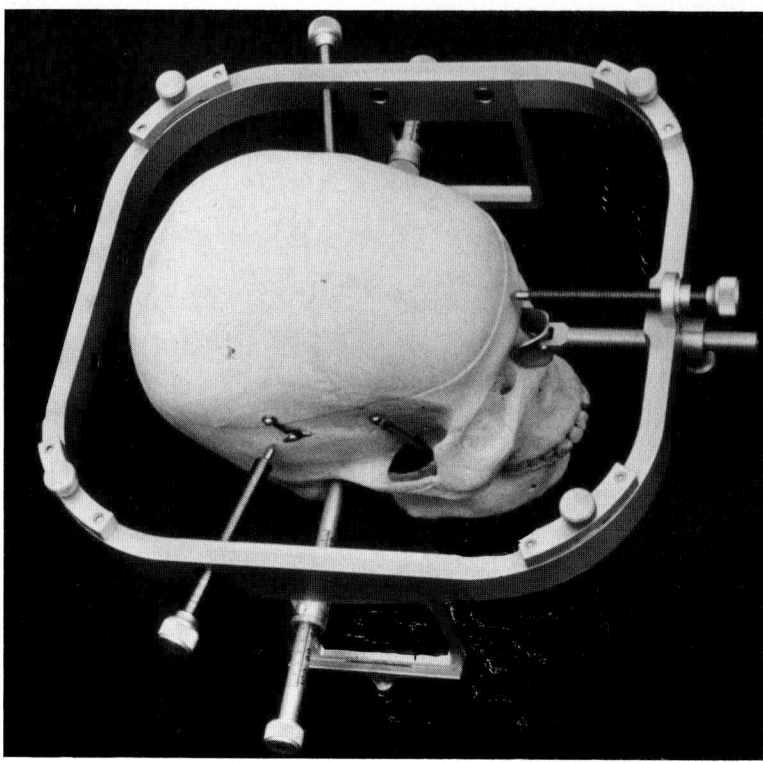

Figure 8.1. Base ring of the trigeminus stereoguide.

length of the lead pins indicates the magnification coefficient of the picture. A desired part of the foramen ovale is marked. The choice depends on the location of the pain and/or the method of treatment. If the mandibular division will be thermocoagulated, the target should be marked in the posterolateral part of the foramen. If the maxillary division is aimed for coagulation, or any division for glycerol/balloon treatment, an anteromedial part of the foramen is chosen as the target. The foraminal target is projected onto the interaural line. The distance is the y coordinate. The distance between the projection point and the lead pin is the inner part of the x coordinate. Its outer part is recorded from the ear bar. The sum of the inner and the outer part is the final x coordinate.

The ear bars are removed and a lateral radiograph is taken with the central x-ray beam going through the ear bar holes of the frame (Fig. 8.3). A line is drawn through the ear bar hole parallel to the frame. The distance between the floor of the middle fossa and the aural-nasion line is the z coordinate. (the film-focus distance is so chosen that the magnification coefficient is 1.2.)

Surgery

The depth of the probe to be used is determined on a stand for the cylinder component and the 90° arc (Fig. 8.4). The arc with a cylinder ring is positioned on the cylinder according to the x coordinate and locked. A rectanglular component is positioned on the frame according to the y coordinate and locked. The cylinder component is mounted to the rectangular component according to the z coordinate and locked (Fig. 8.5). The target at the foramen ovale now coincides with the midpoint of the spherical system of the cylinder component and the 90° arc and will be reached from any bone-free direction when the probe is advanced to the depth as measured on the stand. We routinely go to a depth level of 10 to 12 mm behind the target, without stopping at the

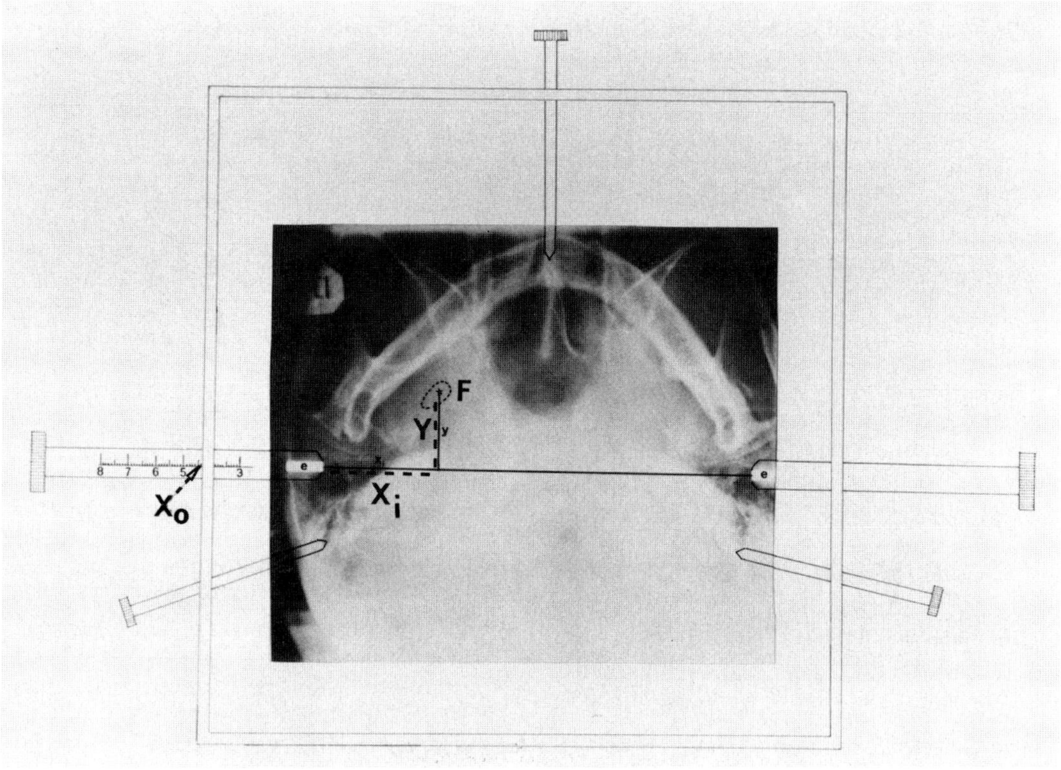

Figure 8.2. Axial radiograph showing the lead pins (*e, e*) at the tips of the ear bars. Target in the foramen ovale (*F*) is projected onto the interaural line. Its distance from the interaural line is the y coordinate. The x coordinate is the sum of the inner (xi) and outer (xo) components of the laterality of the target from the outer wall of the frame.

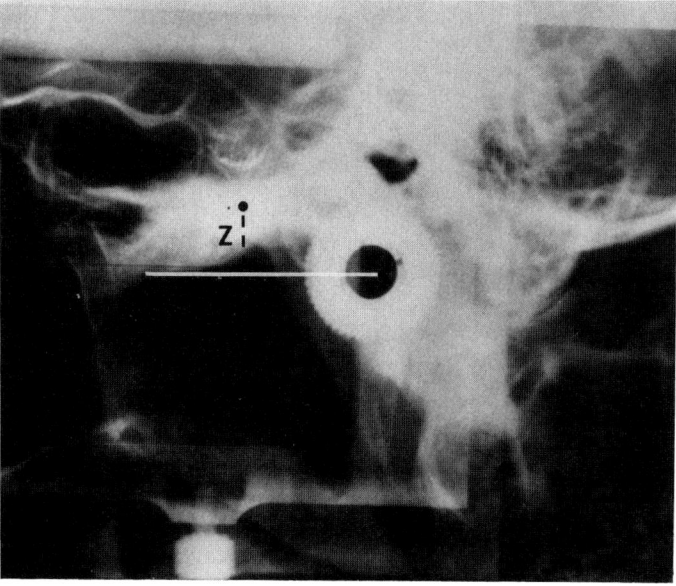

Figure 8.3. Lateral radiograph showing the distance between the floor of the middle fossa and the aural-nasion line (z coordinate).

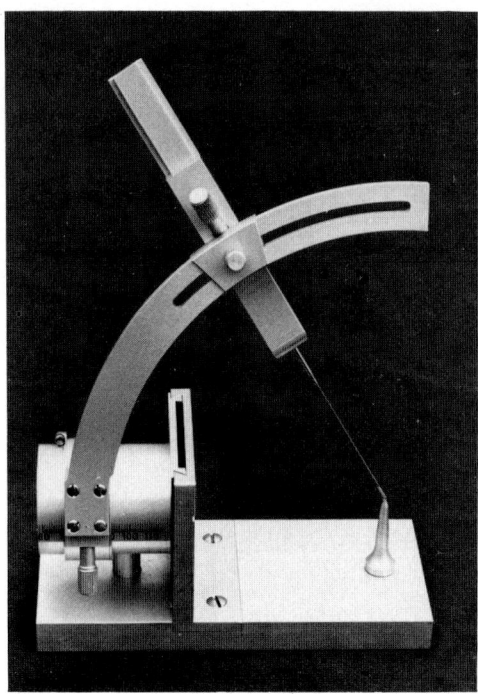

Figure 8.4. Cylinder-arc stand, where cone tip coincides with midpoint of spherical system of trigeminus stereoguide, is used for determination of depth of electrode.

foramen level. The final depth is chosen by means of impedence recording, which is an excellent way to corroborate that the probe tip lies in the cerebrospinal fluid (CSF).

Electrical stimulation is additionally needed for exact placement of the electrode, before thermocoagulation is carried out. The effects of coagulation are tested carefully. For this purpose, we use an electronic stimulator, called Isal Sensimeter 1412 (2). When glycerol treatment is used, CSF leakage from the cannula indicates the final depth level. The size of the cisterna semilunaris is measured by injecting contrast medium under fluoroscopy. After glycerol injection the sitting patient must keep the head in a maximal anteflexed position for 1 hr, after which the frame is detached.

When *glossopharyngeal neuralgia* is treated the frame is rotated around the interaural axis so that the nasion support points toward the front just above the eyebrows. The radiography is performed as described before. The pars nervosa of the foramen jugulare is reached from a submandibular approach, just medial to the internal carotid artery so that the X nerve will not be affected, either during electrical stimulation or during thermocoagulation.

RESULTS

In 217 patients treated through November 1986, the foramen ovale was always reached without a need for changing the stereotactic coordinates. In several patients, a bony ridge just below the foramen necessitated a change of the angle of the approach. Then the foramen was penetrated. When graded electrocoagulation with electrical sensimetry was used the whole procedure took approximately 40 min. The glycerol treatment took approximately 30 min. In this technical report the clinical results of the treatment will not be given.

DISCUSSION

In 1933, the German surgeon Kirschner (6) designed an instrument for percutaneous treatment of trigeminal neuralgia. He, among many others, had previously used Hartel's (4) free-hand technique, but he found that in several patients the puncture of the foramen ovale was difficult. His new instrument was not stereotactic in a proper sense; it was based on the fairly constant anatomical relationship of the foramen to the midline of the skull and to the interaural-nasion plane. It was used without radiography. Kirschner reported that with help of the new instrument, the foramen ovale was found in 75% of cases. Kirschner's instrument was widely used for decades by many neurosurgeons. Hartel's free-hand technique was reintroduced in 1974 by Sweet and Wepsic (19), who began to use controlled thermocoagulation.

Kirschner's trigeminal instrument played an important role for the development of stereotactic neurosurgery. When Lars Leksell designed his stereotactic frame in 1949 he had Kirschner's apparatus as a model. When Waltregny (23) and Laitinen (9) described their stereotactic frames for trigeminal surgery, an historical circle had been closed.

Those neurosurgeons who often perform percutaneous trigeminal surgery feel safe

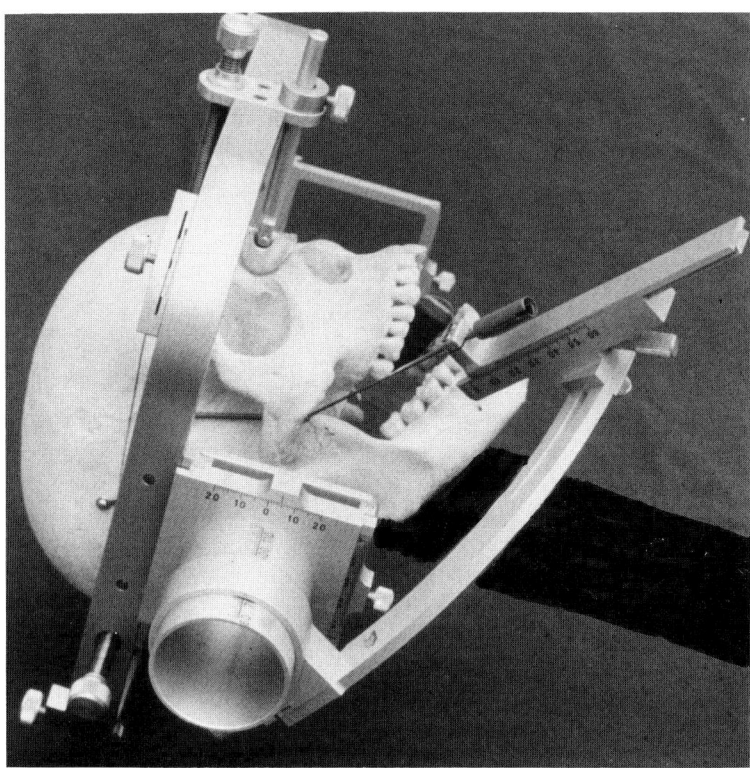

Figure 8.5. When cylinder component with a 90° arc electrode carrier is mounted to frame according to x, y, and z coordinates, electrode introduced from any bone-free direction will hit target point in foramen ovale.

with the free-hand technique of Hartel (10, 11, 16, 17, 19–22), but even they may have problems. Dr. Melker Lindquist, a neuroradiologist at the Karolinska Sjukhuset in Stockholm, said in a personal communication that in 10% of cases it is difficult and time-consuming to find the foramen ovale. Complications are not infrequent when free-hand technique is used, and several cases of death have been reported (3, 7, 8, 14, 18). Some of the fatalities may have been due to extensive electrocoagulation, but a repeated puncture of the internal carotid artery has been reported as a cause of death (11). Carotid cavernous fistulas and ischemic strokes have been observed after free-hand puncture of the foramen ovale (1, 12, 15). Sometimes the probe aimed at the foramen ovale had passed through the foramen jugulare (20). All this shows that the free-hand puncture is not safe. In the majority of cases it is easy, but it causes unnecessary pain and suffering to the patient; it definitely diminishes the chances of an optimal placement of the probe; and thus, it increases the risks of surgery.

The trigeminus stereoguide has been used by us in 217 patients. In all of them the foramen ovale has been reached directly, without a need for altering the stereotactic coordinates of the target. Not only has it been easy to find the foramen, but it also has been possible to place the probe from a desired direction and through a strictly selected part of the foramen so that the probe inside the Meckel's cavum directly hits a desired division of the V nerve fibers. The surgical procedure was reported by the patients to be less painful than previous interventions with the free-hand technique. The procedure takes 30 to 40 minutes. In some patients, a bony ridge below the foramen was found. But it could be avoided easily by slightly changing the introduction angle of the probe.

As soon as the target has been reached the probe is locked at the electrode carrier, which facilitates neurophysiological research of tic douloureux.

The trigeminus stereoguide has also been used in two patients with glossopharyngeal neuralgia. When the frame is mounted to the head, it is rotated around the interaural axis so that the nasion support lies at the level of the front, just above the eyebrows. The foramen jugulare is visualized in an axial radiogram, and its coordinates can be determined. The pars nervosa of the foramen is approached from below the mandible, just medial to the internal carotid artery. In the two patients so far operated on neither electrical stimulation of the petrous ganglion nor its thermocoagulation gave vagal responses. Such side effects are common when a lateral is used (5, 13, 20). The clinical effect in both of our patients has been good for more than 30 months.

Our experience with the trigeminus stereoguide is positive. It has made percutanous surgery easy and accurate. It has diminished the intraoperative suffering of the patients and improved the clinical results. No complications have been noticed.

REFERENCES

1. Galp HZ, Kanpolat Y, Ter B: Carotid-cavernous fistula following percutaneous trigeminal ganglion approach. *Clin Neurol Neurosurg* 82: 269–272, 1980.
2. Hariz IM, Laitinen LV: Mesures quantitatives p-et postoratoires de la sensibili cutan dans le tic douloureux. *Neurochirurgie* 32: 433–439, 1986.
3. Hensell V: Ist die Elektrokoagulation des Ganglion Gasseri auch heute noch berechtigt? *Chirurgia* 28: 544–548, 1957.
4. Hartel F: Die Behandlung der Trigeminusneuralgie mit intrakraniellen Alkoholeinspritzungen. *Dtsch Zeitschr Chir* 126: 429–552, 1914.
5. Isamat F, Fern E, Acebes JJ: Selective percutaneous rhizotomy in essential glossopharyngeal neuralgia. *J Neurosurg* 55: 575–580, 1981.
6. Kirschner M: Die Punktionstechnik und Elektrokoagulation des Ganglion Gasseri. Ueber "gezielte" Operationen. *Arch Klin Chir* 176: 581–620, 1933.
7. Klar E: Ueber die Erfahrungen mit der Elektrokoagulation bei der Trigeminusneuralgie an der Heidelberger Chirurgischen Universitsklinik. Langenbecks *Arch Klin Chir* 294: 713–723, 1960.
8. Kubanyi E: Sur le traitement de la nralgie du nerf trijumeau par l'ectro-coagulation intracranienne du ganglion de Gasser (d'aps 301 cas). *Lyon Chir* 41: 681–689, 1946.
9. Laitinen LV: Trigeminus stereoguide: An instrument for stereotactic approach through the foramen ovale and foramen jugulare. *Surg Neurol* 22: 519–523, 1984.
10. Latchaw JP Jr, Hardy RW Jr, Forsythe SB, et al: Trigeminal neuralgia treated by radiofrequency coagulation. *J Neurosurg* 59: 479–484, 1983.
11. Nugent GR, Berry B: Trigeminal neuralgia treated by differential percutaneous radiofrequency coagulation of the Gasserian ganglion. *J Neurosurg* 40: 517–523, 1974.
12. Rish BL: Cerebrovascular accident after percutaneous rf thermocoagulation of the trigeminal ganglion. *J Neurosurg* 44: 376–377, 1976.
13. Salar G, Ori C, Iob I, et al: Selective percutaneous thermolesions of the ninth cranial nerve by lateral cervical approach: Report of eight cases. *Surg Neurol* 20: 276–279, 1983.
14. Seeger VW: Genuine und symptomatische Trigeminusneuralgie. *Dtsch Med Wochenschr* 88: 171–175, 1963.
15. Sekhar LN, Heros RC, Kerber CW: Carotid-cavernous fistula following percutaneous retrogasserian procedures. *J Neurosurg* 51: 700–706, 1979.
16. Siegfried J, Hood T: Current status of functional neurosurgery. In Krayenbuhl H (ed): *Advances and Technical Standards in Neurosurgery*. Wien, Springer-Verlag, 1983, vol 10, pp 19–79.
17. Sindou M, Keravel Y: Thermocoagulation percutane'e du trijumeau dans le traitement de la ne'vralgie faciale essentielle. *Neurochirurge* 25: 166–172, 1979.
18. Sunder-Plassmann P: Ergebnisse der Elektrokoagulation des Ganglion Gasseri bei Trigeminusneuralgie. *Zentralbl Chir* 66: 2234–2236, 1939.
19. Sweet WH, Wepsic JG: Controlled thermocoagulation of trigeminal ganglion and rootlets for differential destruction of pain fibers. *J Neurosurg* 39: 143–156, 1974.
20. Tew JM: Percutaneous rhizotomy in the treatment of intractable pain. In Schmidek HH, Sweet WH (eds): *Current Techniques in Operative Neurosurgery*. Orlando, Grune & Stratton, 1977, pp 409–426.
21. Thiry S, Hotermans JM: Traitement de la névralgie essentielle du trijumeau par stéréotaxie et électrocoagulation partielle sélective du ganglion de Gasser. *Neurochirurgie* 20: 55–60, 1974.
22. Van Loveren H, Tew JM, Keller JT, et al: A 10-year experience in the treatment of trigeminal neuralgia. *J Neurosurg* 57: 757–764, 1982.
23. Waltregny AJM: A stereotactic frame for trigeminal ganglionectomy. *Appl Neurophysiol* 45: 516–517, 1982.

Chapter 9

Special Stereotactic Techniques: Stereotactic Lesions of the Spinal Cord and Pons for Pain

EDWARD R. HITCHCOCK, M.D.

INTRODUCTION

Stereotactic spinal surgery—not to be confused with percutaneous cordotomy, which uses simple aiming techniques—directs a percutaneous electrode to a cervical cord target using a stereotactic instrument fixed to the skull and with the neck in full flexion.

Unfortunately, target identification by anatomical landmarks and evoked potentials is less reliable than identification by stimulation in the conscious patient. The first spinal stereotactic procedure was performed by Rand et al. (24) who inserted a cryoprobe via Cl-2 interlamina space *against* the anterolateral cord quadrant. Independently, Crue (5) and Hitchcock (7) performed stereotactic cordotomies by a posterior route; Crue used the Cl-2 approach using the Todd-Wells apparatus, and Hitchcock penetrated the atlantooccipital space using a specially designed spinal stereotactic instrument.

The lower cranial nerves and the large first dentate ligament give relative fixity to the medulla and first two cervical segments. Fixation is greater with full-neck flexion when the cord has a smooth outline, although the anteroposterior (AP) diameter is reduced by 20% (22). Fixation of the instrument to the operating table with full-neck flexion greatly reduces movement and distortion. A clear coronal cord outline is difficult to achieve even with open mouth views and the use of contrast medium, but the odontoid peg can be confidently used as the midline landmark. The lateral target is chosen in relation to the "equatorial line" on the sagittal cord outline or to the anterior or posterior cord borders if the targets (arm area of spinothalamic tract or trigeminal tract) are closer. Some distortion is almost inevitable because of the difficulty in penetrating the tough pia even with very sharp electrodes. Electrode penetration posteroanteriorly produces less distortion than the lateral approach although, due to adhesion between pia and electrode, the cord may be deflected anteriorly. The original chosen target point may thus appear some millimeters short of the calculated position. The posterior approach for lateral targets, however, induces greater torsion than the lateral approach (Fig. 9.1). The rapid functional changes of tracts within very short distances demand the use of an electrode holder capable of fine adjustments in tenths of a millimeter to permit recognition of the electrode track. The accuracy of laterality using the posterior approach is within 1 mm, although the depth may deviate up to 5 mm (average 2 mm) indicating cord distortion and the need for electrophysiological recognition before lesion making. A particular response can be due to stimulation at any one of a number of different sites and

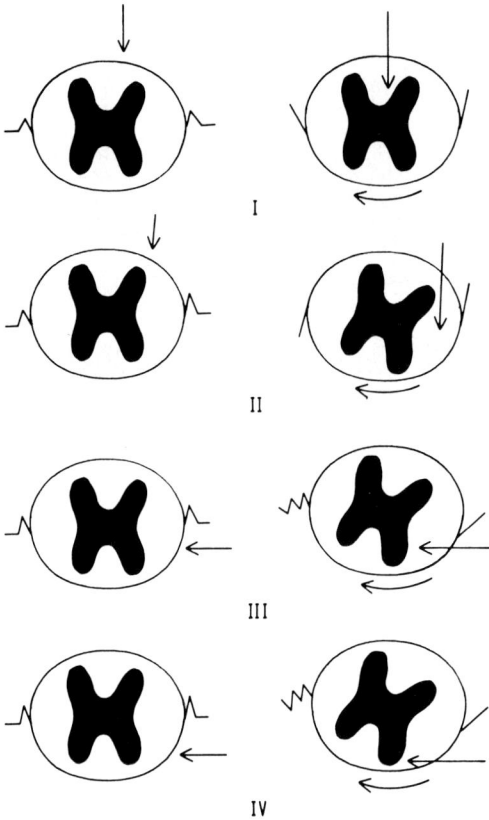

Figure 9.1. Torsion of cervical cord by medial (I) and lateral (II) posterior routes. The cord twists on its stretched dentate anchors. There is greater torsion by equatorial (III) or anterior (IV) lateral routes.

repeated testing at different depths is essential. Suitable fine-stimulating and temperature-recording electrodes are now available which have replaced the original tungsten wire electrodes. A technique of fast deep cord penetration and withdrawal to the target should be used to reduce pia/electrode adhesion. For upper body analgesia, spinothalamic tractotomy by the posteroanterior approach is most suitable, with the lateral approach being reserved for lower body analgesia.

The absolute values of impedence vary with the electrode size, but like others, we have invariably found increases in passing from cerebrospinal fluid (CSF) to cord contact and a further increase on cord penetration.

The exact situation of the ascending and descending tracts making up the bulk of the cord is uncertain, and there may be considerable individual variations. Taren et al. (31) and Zlatos and Cierney (33) have given gross and detailed measurements which are useful guides. The most consistent method of determining electrode position is by stimulation. In lateral tracks a shocklike sensation is experienced in the ipsilateral arm or face with penetration of the fasciculus cuneatus or the trigeminal tract. With further penetration and stimulation at low frequencies, there is movement in the ipsilateral arm or leg as the corticospinal tract is traversed. With further advance into the spinothalamic tract stimulation at 50 Hz produces an unpleasant or warm sensation in the contralateral arm or leg. The change from ipsilateral sensory responses to contralateral responses is usually very distinct.

With more medial penetration, tingling, movement, or shocklike sensations are experienced in one or both legs as the electrode penetrates fasciculus gracilis. With deeper penetration, sensations are often experienced in the more distal portions of the leg and often in one or other arm, suggesting that the somatotopic organization of posterior column fibers is with the distal extremities directed centrally. In the central portion of the cord with stimulation at low frequencies, there may be coughing or apnea, and at higher frequencies, nausea or truncal burning sensation. Central stimulation often produces indescribable but characteristic widespread unpleasant sensation.

A rf lesion is made in a stepwise manner until acceptable anesthesia is produced and sensation and motor power are tested frequently to ensure that analgesia is adequate and that no paresis or incoordination occurs. Patients tolerate these procedures extremely well under local anesthesia with appropriate premedication.

STEREOTACTIC SPINOTHALAMIC TRACTOTOMY

The technique has been fully described elsewhere (10, 12). The stereotactic frame is applied to the head with full neck flexion and fixed to the operating table with the patient in the sitting position. A water-soluble contrast medium is introduced into the cisterna magna and anteroposterior and lateral radiographs are taken. The target in the anterolateral position of the cord is marked on the film, 3 mm lateral and 3 to 4 mm anterior to the equatorial line for upper body analgesia and 5 mm lateral and 1 mm anterior to the equatorial line for lower body (Fig. 9.2). The cordotomy electrode is introduced via an outer needle through the atlantooccipital membrane posteriorly or for lateral approaches through the C1-2 interspace. Aided by impedance measurements and stimulation, an incremental series of rf lesions is made with examination of sensory and motor function at each step.

As a result of stereotactic surgical experience, the traditional concept of the spinothalamic fibers as laminated dermatomal layers has been replaced by a more complex concept. The general pattern of lower body fibers lying posteriorly and upper body fibers anteriorly has been confirmed many times. It is also evident that functionally important areas, such as the hand, occupy major areas. A "spinothalamic homonculus" and "posterior column homonculus" have been described (10, 12) and these concepts have received support from other workers (18, 25, 32). It is useful to have a simple functional map of the high cervical cord which helps in the recognition of electrode position and trajectory (Fig. 9.3). Experience with the results of open cordotomies has indicated that the spinal pathways of respiration and micturition bear a somatotopic relationship to the spinothalamic tract. The respiratory fibers are closely related to the cervicothoracic fibers (13), while micturition fibers lie close to the sacral fibers (14).

The opportunity of making selective lesions is of particular importance in young

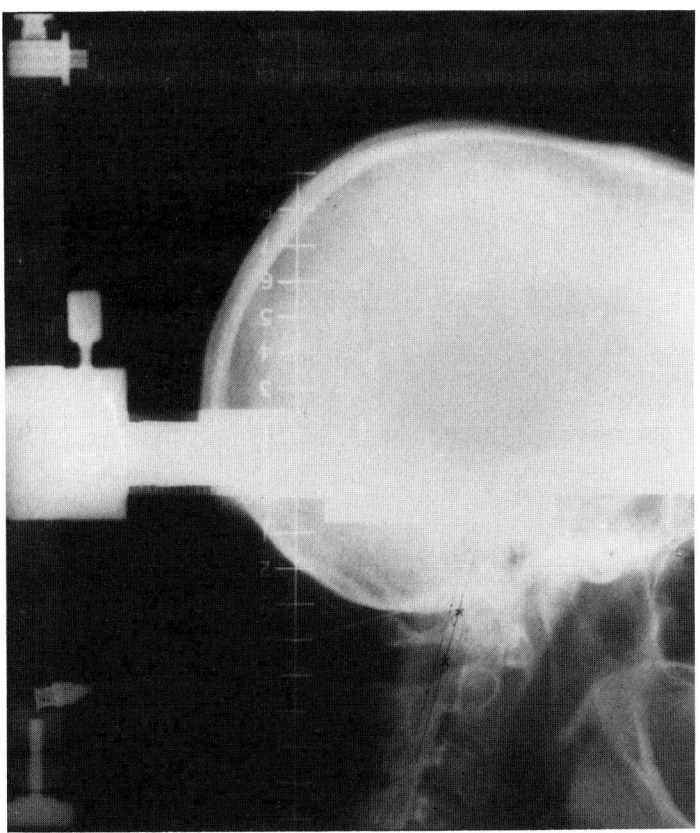

Figure 9.2. Two spinothalamic coordinates are marked with crosses halfway between the "equatorial line" and cord's anterior margin.

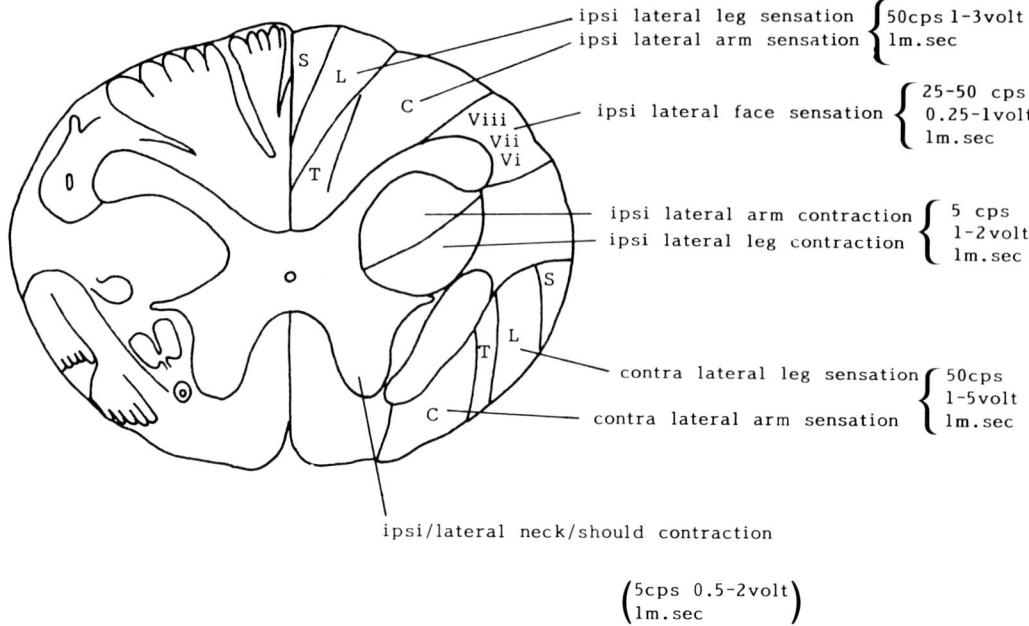

Figure 9.3. A simple functional map of C1-2 cord displaying posterior column and spinothalamic homonculi.

patients in avoiding sensory disabilities in an uninvolved limb. Against this must be set the relative low availability of expertise and the lengthier procedure, which may be taxing for sick patients. If injury to the respiratory pathways is feared, then neither percutaneous nor stereotactic cordotomy procedures should be attempted. Instead, a stereotactic pontine tractotomy, mesencephalotomy, or some other procedure should be used. Both percutaneous and stereotactic cordotomy require cooperation and oriented patients, while invasive cervical tumors, cervical spine deformity, or infection are contraindications.

Results

Both percutaneous and stereotactic cordotomies give excellent initial pain relief. Most series contain many terminal patients so that pain relief must be assessed on a decreasing number of survivors over 1 yr. In my own series (10), of the 90% who achieved grade 1 to 2 initial pain relief, this decreased progressively to 88% at 6 months and 80% in 9 months, remaining static at 1 yr and 1+ yr. Using a spinal stereotactic technique, Schvarcz (25) was able to obtain high levels of analgesia without any respiratory disorders and suggested that the stereotactic procedure had fewer contraindications than percutaneous cordotomy.

STEREOTACTIC TRIGEMINAL TRACTOTOMY AND NUCLEOTOMY

Sjoquist's (29) procedure of medullary trigeminal tractotomy open exposure was refined by Hosobuchi and Rutkin (17) using a microscope and a rf electrode. It is still a major procedure performed under general anesthesia, and the localizing value of patient response to stimulation is lost.

A stereotactic rf procedure was devised (4, 9) destroying the tract and nucleus via the atlantooccipital membrane. The "caudal" dermatome of the trigeminal tract is 3 mm anterior to the posterior aspect of the cord and 6 mm from the midline at the first cervical segment. More rostral dermatomes are located more laterally and anterior, while the intermedius, glossopharyngeal, and vagal components of the tract lie more posteriorly and medially.

The target point is determined using the coordinates already quoted, and the fine electrode introduced via an external needle through the occipitoatlantal space. Placement of the tip within the trigeminal tract is invariably followed by the complaint of ipsilateral facial pain and the electrode tip is then advanced or retracted, as determined by the patient's responses. A rf lesion is made in incremental steps testing analgesia, power, and coordination at each step. If central face or mucosal analgesia cannot be achieved, the electrode should be withdrawn and reinserted at a higher level.

Extensive analgesia in both head and neck dermatomes demonstrates the extensive overlap of sensory fibers within the caudal part of the trigeminal spinal nucleus. It is important to note that if the lesions are too medial and placed within an already crossed lateral spinothalamic tract and ventral secondary trigeminal ascending tract, contralateral analgesia of body and face may be produced, although such sensory losses are produced only by a lesion in the low medulla.

The procedure has been particularly useful in postherpetic neuralgia (15). Deafferentation pain may be due to hyperexcitable neuronal pools within the substantia gelatinosa or its homologue, the trigeminal nucleus. Radiofrequency destruction of this nucleus destroys these pools removing both hyperesthesia and deep background pain. Nashold *et al.* (20) accepted this concept as the basis for dorsal root entry zone lesions. Schvarcz (27) reported that of eight patients with postherpetic neuralgia, seven had either a reduction or removal of burning pain. Later (28), he reported 104 stereotactic nucleotomies that he advocated for central facial pain including anesthesia dolorosa. In my own series, there has been no operative mortality, but *transient* mild paresis or ataxia is common, and dysesthesia occurred in one patient for several weeks.

Pain relief was grade 1 to 2 until death in 47%, but 40% had grade 4 to 5 recurrent pain. The best results were for patients with pain due to malignancy, with 66% achieving grade 1 to 2 relief until death, and only 22% with grade 4 to 5 recurrence.

Stereotactic trigeminal tractotomy and nucleotomy have been used for a wide variety of facial pains including that due to malignancy, postherpetic neuralgia, atypical facial pain anesthesia dolorosa, and also for trigeminal neuralgia. Although the procedure has been used for trigeminal neuralgia, in general it should be limited to patients with oropharyngeal and head malignancy or selected cases of atypical facial pain or facial deafferentation pain.

CENTRAL CORD LESION (CCL)

Cervical myelotomy was attempted by Putnam (23) in 1934 and advocated to relieve intractable pain in arms and shoulders, especially if this was bilateral. Cervical commissurotomy should therefore be an ideal procedure for bilateral shoulder, arm, or upper chest pain which are, admittedly, uncommon.

Stereotactic Cervical Myelotomy (CCL)

CCL was introduced in 1970 and gave excellent results (8). Apart from the expected upper limb analgesia, pain sensation was also disordered in the lower parts of the body, suggesting interruption of a central multisynaptic pathway. There may be bizarre sensory losses (Fig. 9.4) with retention of initial pinprick sensation with loss of

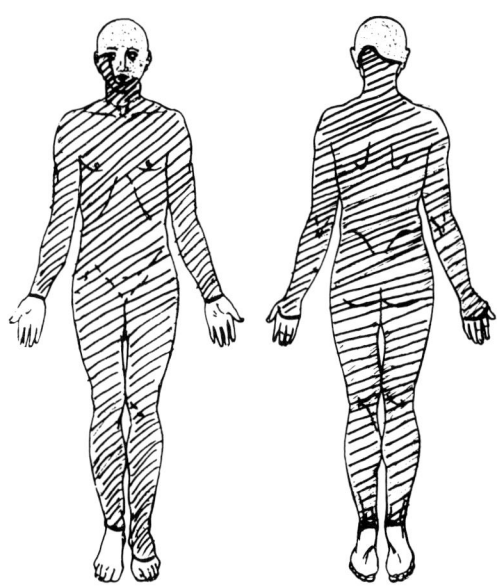

Figure 9.4. Extensive analgesia with extremity and vertex sparing produced by a single C1-2 central cord lesion.

"second" pain, and the sensory losses closely resemble those found in syringomyelia.

It is possible that injury to the posterior column and the associated bundles of C fibers may disturb conduction of slow impulses conveying burning diffuse pain from large body areas, while the destruction of the anterior commissure, which consists largely of A-delta fibers, interrupts conduction of localized sharp pain. This combined injury may thus account for the superiority of myelotomy over cordotomy, which interrupts predominantly A-delta fibers. Moreover, experimental work supports the concept of a multisynaptic grey pathway projecting to the ventral periaqueductal grey and into the hypothalamus (19). Cook and Kawakami (3) studied 25 cases of commissural myelotomy and concluded that even without sensory loss, pain relief can be obtained. They have argued that the central cord lesion interrupts pathways entering, within, or leaving the spinothalamic complex.

The procedure is the same as that of stereotactic spinothalamic tractotomy with a central cord target. Several points are chosen along the anterior and posterior margin of the cord image and a line is drawn down the cord halfway between them. This is assumed to demarcate the central canal. A suitable point is chosen along this line that will allow the passage of the electrode through the occipitocervical interval. When impedence measurement indicates cord contact, the electrode is partly withdrawn and then rapidly pushed through the cord. If the trajectory is correct, lower limb sensations are reported, but if arm or face sensations are produced the electrode should be withdrawn and a more appropriate angle chosen. With small electrode advances and stimulation, leg and perineal sensations are recorded and with further advances bilateral arm sensations. Physiological verification of position by stimulation is vital because the cord is pushed anteriorly by the electrode up to 5 or 6 mm. The central cord is reached approximately 2 mm after leg or bilateral arm sensations have ceased. At central cord, whole body paresthesia and frequently an unpleasant central chest and abdominal sensation are recorded. Small incremental lesions are made up to 75°C for 30 seconds.

Sourek (30) has commentated on the rapid fading of analgesia but preservation of analgesic effect after lumbosacral myelotomy, and this has been my own experience with cervical myelotomy (12). After 3 months, 64% of patients were still relieved of pain and one patient remained pain free for more than 5 yr. There has been no operative mortality, but 10% of patients had a few days postural gait disorder. Of 19 patients with neoplastic pain followed for more than 4 yr or until death, eight remained pain free without analgesics or further analgesic procedures; five needed weak analgesics. Schvarcz (26) achieved good results in 45 patients and later obtained excellent pain relief in 78% of 75 patients with malignancy (28).

Papo and Luongo (21) stated that the procedure was useful in cases of upper body pain with poor respiratory function and short life expectancy. Their immediate results in 10 patients were excellent, but six patients had pain recurrence, and they were disappointed with their open procedure performed by laminectomy and insertion of electrode. The patient response is vitally important for the successful performance of CCL. They were, however, unable to achieve this.

Cervical myelotomy is less successful with somatic leg pain but has excellent results with truncal pain, including pelvic and perineal pain. In general, the procedure has been used for those with bilateral pain, especially pelvic pain. Cook and Kawakami (3), apparently unaware of the stereotactic method, considered that, although ineffective for pelvic malignancy for other bilateral malignancies, open commissural myelotomy had many advantages.

Eiras et al. (6) used a simple percutaneous technique to perform cervical myelotomy and confirmed the good results of the stereotactic procedures in 12 patients with malignancy.

STEREOTACTIC PONTINE TRACTOTOMY

At pontine levels, autonomic and spinothalamic tracts become even more separated so that theoretically high analgesic levels can be achieved without affecting micturition or respiration.

Pontine spinothalamic tractotomy produces deep analgesia, but in a restricted region containing many complex tracts and cranial nerve nuclei, precise and refined stereotactic techniques are essential. The technique was first described in 1973 (11), with the results in seven patients. At that time, no stereotactic coordinates were available for the spinothalamic tract at that level. Examination of various anatomical atlases gave approximate values, and several brainstems were carefully prepared, sectioned, stained, and measured. Since the closest radiologically viable structure was the floor of the fourth ventricle, a system of coordinates was established for the spinothalamic tract and trigeminal tract throughout

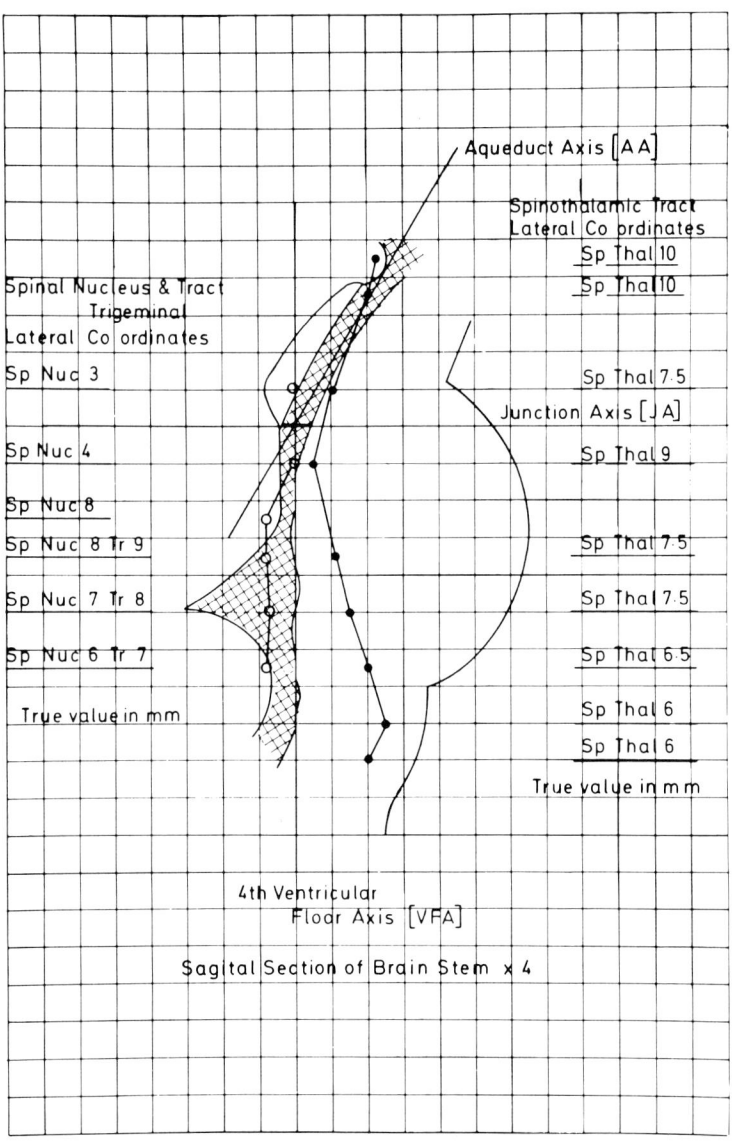

Figure 9.5. Brainstem coordinates of spinothalamic and trigeminal tracts in relation to fourth ventricular line and fastigial line.

the pons. The relationship of the fastigium to the fourth ventricle is not constant, but it provides a useful and well defined landmark. The rostrocaudal extent of the structures was therefore measured in relationship to a line drawn from the fastigium at 90° to the floor of the fourth ventricle (the fastigial line, Fig. 9.5).

The stereotactic frame is applied to the head and the fourth ventricle is filled with radiopaque, water-soluble medium via a frontal burr hole. The target is then marked on the lateral film and, the coordinates having been established, a posterior fossa burr hole is made on the opposite side to the pain and an electrode advanced to target. Electrical stimulation produces responses appropriate to the structures traversed and serve to confirm a satisfactory trajectory.

The procedure is less complex and difficult than it might appear, but it does require precise instrumentation and some knowledge of pontine anatomy. It is very dependent upon good patient cooperation and is not suitable for patients who are unable to cooperate or obtunded. Our experience with the procedure is still limited to 20 patients, but more patients have been accepted for this procedure in recent years. Barbera *et al.* (2) have also reported good results in five patients, and they continue to use the method. Two of their patients had deafferentation pain from brachial plexus destruction and obtained good relief. Schvarcz has also used the procedure with success (personal communication).

The atlas reproduced here (16) is a comparatively crude guide to a very complex region of the brainstem, and with further experience, it now appears that the lateral coordinate should be approximately 1 mm more medial. Unfortunately, a more detailed and precise brainstem atlas (1) fails to depict the 10 mm area around the fastigial plane, and the simpler atlas continues to be useful. The single operative death (mortality 5%) must be seen against the hazards of attempting other definitive analgesic procedures in a patient with an exceptionally severe respiratory inadequacy. For such patients, the risks cannot be greatly reduced, even by pontine tractotomy.

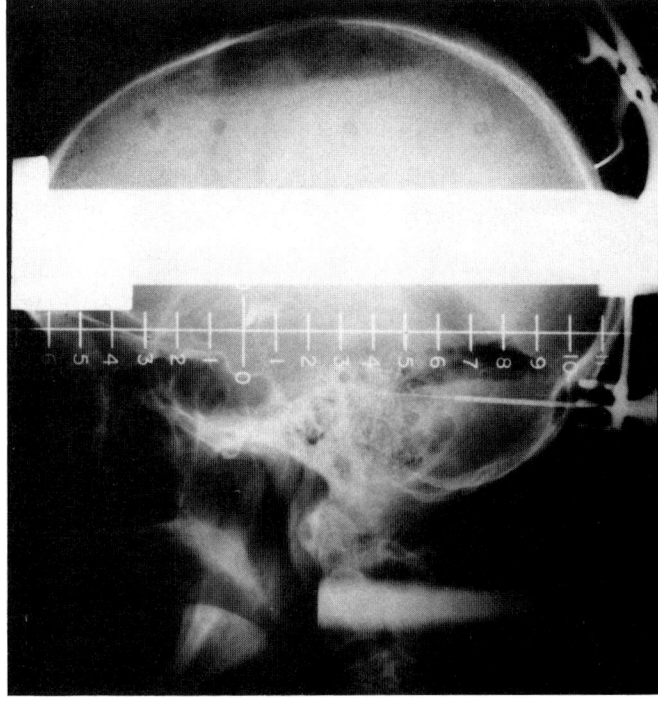

Figure 9.6. Electrode traversing pons.

REFERENCES

1. Afshar F, Watkins ES, Yap JC: *Stereotactic Atlas of the Human Brainstem and Cerebellar Nuclei.* New York, Raven Press, 1978, pp 80-88.
2. Barbera J, Barcia-Salorio JL, Broseta J: Stereotaxic pontine spinothalamic tractotomy. *Surg Neurol* 11: 111-114, 1979.
3. Cook AS, Kawakami K: Commissural myelotomy. *J Neurosurg* 47: 1-6, 1977.
4. Crue BL, Todd EM, Carregal EJM, Kilham O: Percutaneous Trigeminal tractotomy. *Bull L A Neurol Soc,* 32: 86, 1967.
5. Crue BL, Todd EM, Carregal EJA: Posterior approach for high cervical percutaneous radiofrequency cordotomy. *Conf Neurol* 30: 41-52, 1968.
6. Eiras J, Garcia J, Gomez J, et al: First results with extralaminescal myelotomy. *Acta Neurochir* (Suppl.) 304: 1980.
7. Hitchcock E: Stereotactic spinal surgery: A preliminary report. *J Neurosurg* 31: 386-392, 1969.
8. Hitchcock E: Stereotactic cervical myelotomy. *J Neurol Neurosurg Psychiatr* 33: 224-230, 1970.
9. Hitchcock E: Stereotactic trigeminal tractotomy. *Ann Clin Res* 2: 131-135, 1970.
10. Hitchcock E: Electrophysiological exploration of the cervico-medullary region. In Somjen G (ed): *Neurophysiology Studied in Man. International Congress Series.* Amsterdam, Excerpta Medica, 1971, pp 237-245.
11. Hitchcock E: Stereotaxic pontine spinothalamic tractotomy. *J Neurosurg* 39: 746-752, 1973.
12. Hitchcock E: Stereotactic spinal surgery. In *Neurological Surgery.* Proceedings of the Sixth International Congress of Neurological Surgery. Amsterdam/Oxford, Excerpta Medica, 1977, pp 271-280.
13. Hitchcock E, Leece B: Somatotopic representations of the respiratory pathways in the cervical cord of man. *J Neurosurg* 27: 320-329, 1967.
14. Hitchcock E, Newsome D, Salama M: The somatotopic representation of the micturition pathways in the cervical cord of man. *Br J Surg* 61: 395-400, 1974.
15. Hitchcock E, Schvarcz JT: Stereotactic trigeminal tractotomy for post-herpetic facial pain. *J Neurosurg* 37: 412-417, 1972.
16. Hitchcock E, Sotello MG, Kim MC: Analgesic levels and technical method in stereotactic pontine and spinothalamic tractotomy. *Acta Neurochir* 77: 29-36, 1985.
17. Hosobuchi Y, Rutkin B: Descending Trigeminal tractotomy. Neurophysiological approach. *Acta Neurol* 25: 115-125, 1971.
18. Illingworth RD, Molina-Negro P: Spontaneous and electrically evoked activity in the anterolateral column of the spinal cord in dogs. *J Neurosurg* 40: 58-64, 1974.
19. Kerr FWL, Lipman HH: The primate spinothalamic tract as demonstrated by anterolateral cordotomy and commissural myelotomy. *Ad Neurol* 4: 147-156, 1974.
20. Nashold BS, Ostdahl RH: Dorsal root entry zone lesions for pain relief. *J Neurosurg* 51: 59-69, 1976.
21. Papo I, Luongo A: High cervical commissural myelotomy in the treatment of pain. *J Neurol Neurosurg Psychiatr* 39: 705-710, 1976.
22. Penning L: *Functional Pathology of the Cervical Spine.* Excerpta, 1968.
23. Putnam PH: Myelotomy of the commisure. A new method of treatment for pain in the upper extremities. *Arch Neurol Psych* (Chicago), 32: 1189-1193, 1934.
24. Rand RW, Baner RO, Smart CR, et al: Experience with percutaneous stereotaxic cryocordotomy. *Bull LA Neurol Soc* 30/3: 142-147, 1965.
25. Schvarcs JR: Spinal cord stereotactic surgery. In Sano K, Ishii S (eds): *Recent Progress in Neurological Surgery.* Amsterdam, Excerpta Medica, 1974, pp 234-241.
26. Schvarcz JR: Stereotactic extralaminal myelotomy. *Neurosurg Psychiatr* 39: 53-57, 1976.
27. Schvarcz JR: Postherpetic craniofacial dysaesthesiae. Their management by stereotactic trigeminal nucleotomy. *Acta Neurochir* 38: 65-72, 1977.
28. Schvarcz JR: Spinal cord stereotactic techniques re trigeminal nucleotomy and extralamniscal myelotomy. *Appl Neurophysiol* 41: 99-112, 1978.
29. Sjoquist O: Studies on pain conduction in the trigeminal nerve. *Acta Psychiatr Neurol* (Suppl.) 17, 1938.
30. Sourek K: Mediolongitudinal myelotomy. *Prog Neurol Surg* 8: 15-34, 1977.
31. Taren JA, Davis R, Crosby EC: Target physiologic corroboration in stereotaxic cervical cordotomy. *J Neurosurg* 30: 569-584, 1969.
32. Tasker RR: The merits of percutaneous cordotomy over the open operation. In Morley TP (ed): *Current Controversies in Neurosurgery.* Philadelphia, WB Saunders, 1976, pp 496-501.
33. Zlatos J, Cierny G: Statistical model map of the spinal cord and its use. *Appl Neurophysiol* 38: 225-239, 1975.

Chapter 10
Special Stereotactic Techniques: Stereotactic Radiosurgery

DAN G. LEKSELL, M.D.

INTRODUCTION

Stereotactic radiosurgery by means of a Cobalt 60 Gamma Unit has been used in the treatment of a variety of intracranial disorders since 1968. The number of indications for this surgical modality has increased considerably since its introduction, and particularly since 1974, when stereotactic localization could be based on computerized tomography (CT). Today, many patients have been treated in Stockholm, and the radiosurgical principle has gained widespread acceptance. This chapter will present a historical review and a brief technical description of stereotactic radiosurgery. Some of the clinical indications are also highlighted, and possibilities for the future are outlined.

Definition

The term stereotactic radiosurgery is synonymous with the delivery, in a single session, of a high dose of ionizing radiation to a preselected and stereotactically localized intracranial volume of normal or pathological tissue. The dose is delivered by means of numerous evenly distributed and very precisely collimated narrow beams of ionizing radiation. The dose-profile (Fig. 10.1) illustrates the steep gradient, i.e., rapid reduction of dose at the periphery of the field of radiation. The resulting lesions are therefore very sharply circumscribed (Fig. 10.2) (50). Structures adjacent to the target volume receive very little radiation. This technique has little to do with conventional radiotherapy, which is based on the biological difference in radiosensitivity between normal and pathological tissues. Furthermore, the commonly available equipment for conventional radiotherapy does not fulfill the stipulated requirements on mechanical precision and reproducibility which are required for radiosurgical purposes.

Stereotactic radiosurgery is a technique used for noninvasive destruction of a variety of intracranial targets. It was introduced by Leksell in 1951 (23). He had designed his stereotactic instrument in 1949 (Fig. 10.3) (22), and the basic principle of this instrument, with the target in the center of a semicircular arc (Fig. 10.4), was easily adapted also for crossfiring of a target with narrow beams of ionizing radiation.

It appeared feasible to destroy precisely, by the administration of a single heavy dose of radiation, any deep structure in the brain, without opening of the skull. The first tentative experiments were aimed at interrupting intracerebral pathways in functional disorders such as chronic obsessive-compulsive states (30). Conventional x-rays were used, and the results were promising. Subsequently, and in collaboration with the physicists Liden and Larsson, the source of radiation was replaced by a synchrocyclotron (18, 32, 33). The proton beam was excellent for this purpose, but the cyclotron itself was too clumsy. A linear accelerator was also used, but it soon became apparent that, in order to find a sufficiently precise and reliable radiation delivery system, further work was needed.

Two independent investigations were made in order to establish the requirements to be applied to a clinical unit for radiosurgical applications (19, 36). These studies resulted in a large number of requirements that would have to be met during design and construction work. Standards for stereotactic radiosurgery were thus established. The goal was to find a solution that could be used in the environment of a hospital that could be handled by the surgeon himself,

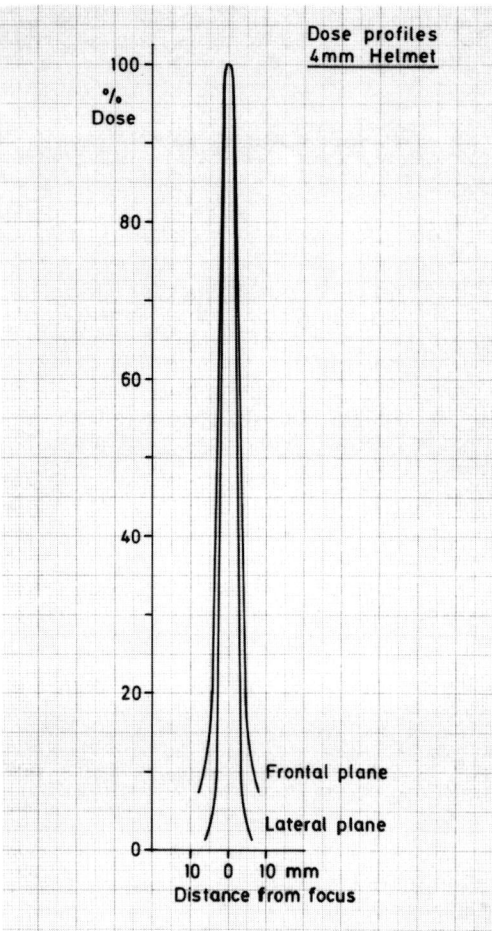

Figure 10.1. Dose profile obtained with 4 mm collimator alternative.

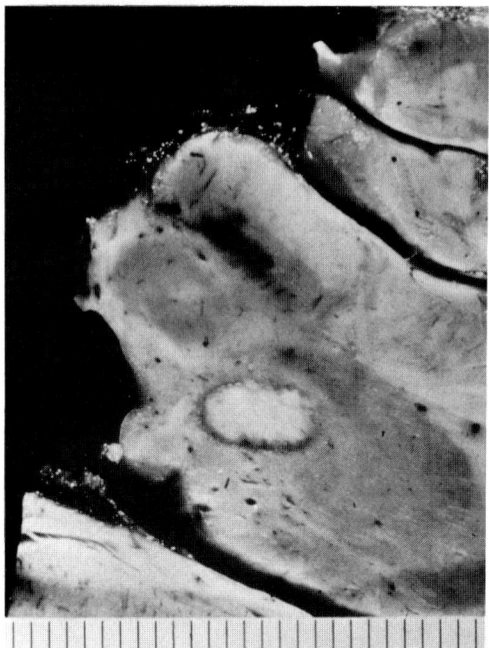

Figure 10.2. Gammathalamotomy in patient treated for intractable cancer pain (scale in millimeters).

without a large team of assistants. The combined technical and radiophysical properties of the apparatus also had to ensure a high degree of precision at the target, where the requirements had been set to ±-0.1 mm. The first stereotactic Cobalt 60 Gamma Unit was installed in a private hospital in Stockholm in 1968 (Fig. 10.5).

Technically, the Gamma Unit consists of a heavily shielded central body containing about 200 sources of Cobalt 60 (Fig. 10.6) (26). The sources are radially distributed over a segment of a sphere, and the beams are individually collimated toward a common point, located in the center of a final collimator helmet. The size of the point of beam intersection can be varied by the exchange of collimator helmets. Standard collimator sizes are 4, 8, 14, and 18 mm, and their use, singly or in combination, allows lesions of any size and shape to be obtained. A stereotactic three-dimensional dose-planning system is used to obtain a lesion configuration that closely matches the shape of the target volume to be irradiated (2). In addition, single-beam channels can be plugged if a particular structure in proximity with the target must be protected.

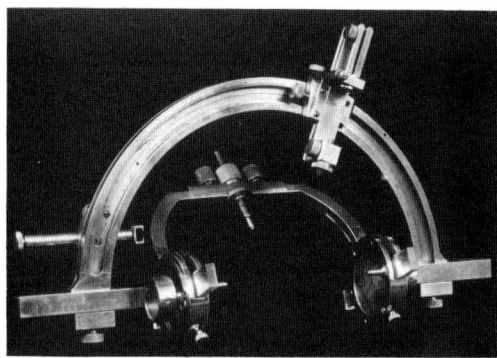

Figure 10.3. First version of Leksell stereotactic instrument.

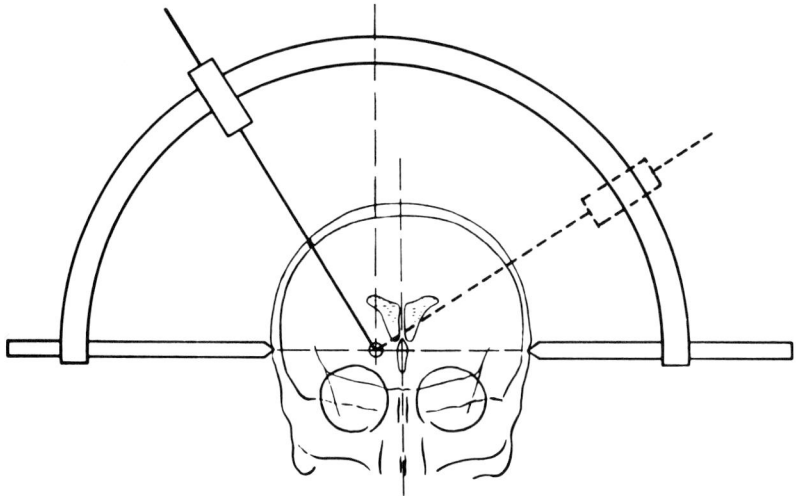

Figure 10.4. Arc principle by which target always lies in center of semicircular arc.

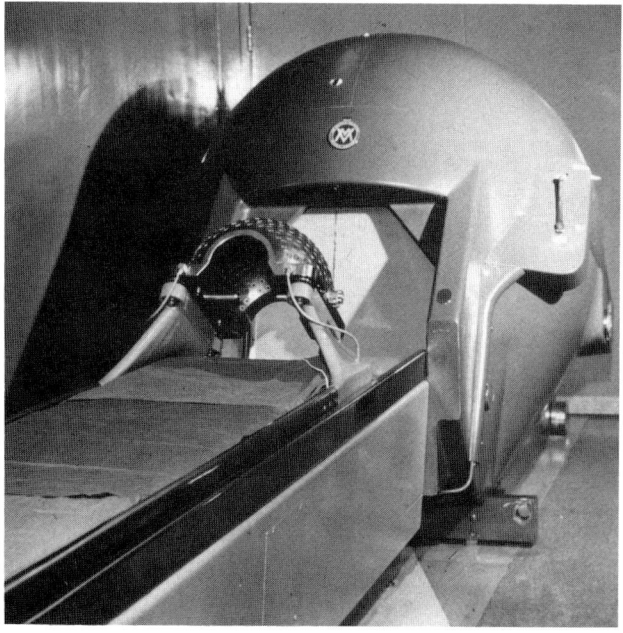

Figure 10.5. Gamma Unit.

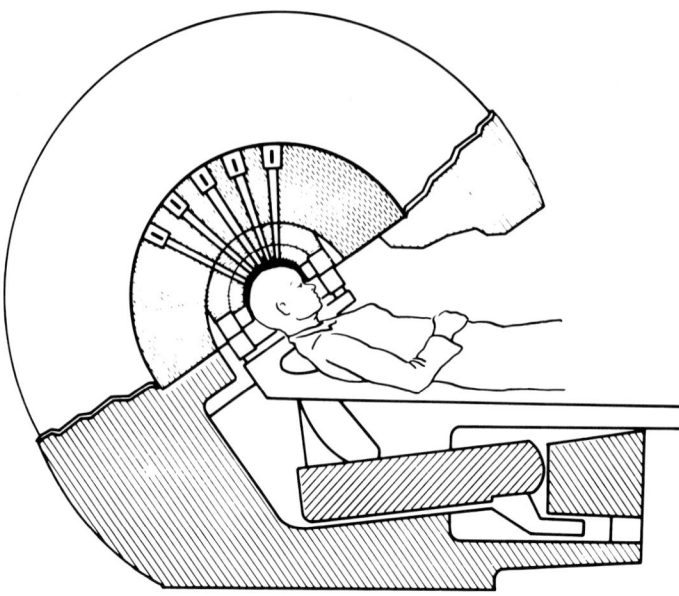

Figure 10.6. Sectional diagram of Gamma Unit illustrating principle of cross-firing of target with multiple beams of ionizing radiation.

Neuroimaging at this time was still based mainly on conventional x-ray techniques and the first Gamma Unit was designed for treatment of functional disorders; the lesions were disc-shaped, and it was also called the "Gamma Knife." However, it was soon used in some tumors and arteriovenous malformations as well. The results were good, but the disc-shaped dose distributions were not optimal for these indications. The first unit had proved to be a cost-effective alternative, and a second Gamma Unit, with more suitable spherical fields of radiation, was therefore ordered by the Karolinska Hospital (49). Its installation coincided with the introduction of computerized tomography (CT), and the stage was set for a period of intense work in establishing a series of suitable indications for radiosurgery. Today, more than 1300 patients have been treated in Stockholm. The various conditions that have been approached radiosurgically are listed in Table 10.1.

TABLE 10.1
Stereotactic Radiosurgery 1968–1986

Functional	
Intractable pain	83
Trigeminal neuralgia	63
Parkinsonism	6
Psychoneurosis	30
Epilepsy	1
Tumor	
Pituitary adenoma (nonsecreting)	38
Prolactinoma	6
Cushing/Nelson	137
Acromegaly	41
Craniopharyngioma	37
Pineal tumor	25
Meningioma	45
Acoustic tumor	177
Various	69
Vascular	
Arteriovenous malformation (AVM)	537
Arterial aneurysm	6
Various	10
Total number of procedures	1311

STEREOTACTIC LOCALIZATION

The varying nature of the targets requires a flexible approach to the localization. The stereotactic instrument used for the determination of target coordinates therefore has to be compatible with all imaging techniques that may be of interest in radiosurgery. Conventional x-rays with angiography or enchephalography are still useful in some cases. Short-distance exposures are used, and magnification is corrected by means of a simple manual, geometrical or graphical, localizational technique (1, 10). A stereophotogrammetric technique can also be used and makes the distance between focus and target irrelevant. Such a technique may also be valuable for localization of individual vessels from angiograms in radiosurgery of AVMs. A stereotactic software program is incorporated in a small computer. Target coordinates read directly off the films are fed into the microcomputer, which calculates the correct x, y, and z instrument coordinates.

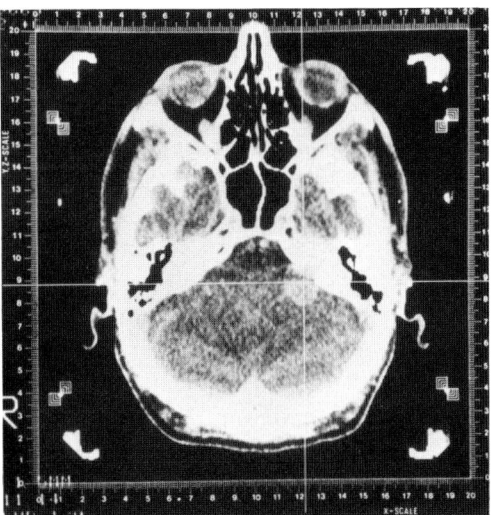

Figure 10.7. Manual CT localization of acoustic tumor. Film and coordinate scale are superimposed on viewing box. A cross-line ruler over target immediately identifies its x, y, and z coordinates.

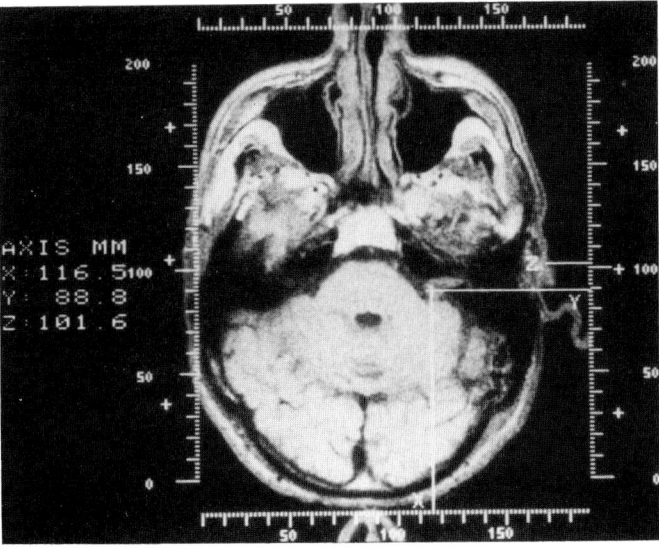

Figure 10.8. Dedicated stereotactic CT and MR localization software applied to a case with an acoustic tumor to be treated in Gamma Unit.

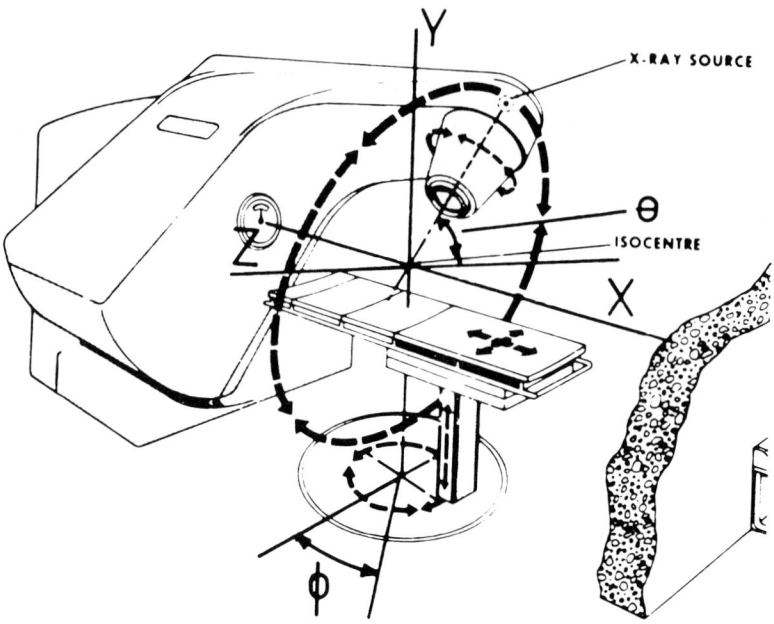

Figure 10.9. Mechanical basis for radiation delivery with a linear accelerator.

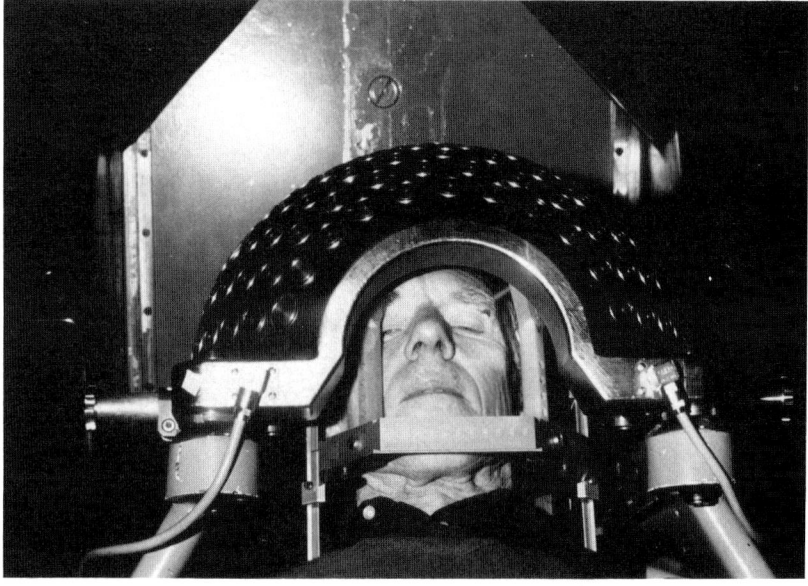

Figure 10.10. Patient with acoustic tumor has been fixed in collimator helmet. Patient is awake.

The introduction of CT revolutionized stereotactic localization and expanded the areas of interest for stereotactic surgery (8, 31). Localization is done by a simple manual technique (Fig. 10.7), or directly on the CT console by use of standard scanner software. With magnetic resonance (MR), localization is also done manually, with the added advantage of orthogonal imaging in three different, or even any arbitrary, planes (20). Recently, a dedicated stereotactic software program has been designed for use with some CT and MR scanners (Fig. 10.8) (34). Digital subtraction angiography and positron emission tomography (PET) scanning can also be used. The target coordinates are derived by the same means, manually or with computer assistance.

OPERATIVE PROCEDURE

When irradiation occurs by means of a cyclotron, the target is cross-irradiated by adjusting the position of the patient's head. With a linear accelerator, the position of the beam is also varied (Fig. 10.9). With the Gamma Unit, the head is fixed in the collimator helmet. The selected target is placed at the common point of intersection of the beams (Fig. 10.10), where it rests during the whole surgical procedure. This ensures a high degree of accuracy and simplifies the procedure, which is carried out by the surgeon and a physicist, without need for a large team of assisting personnel.

Only occasionally, with children or very agitated patients, will general anesthesia be required. The treatment is performed on an outpatient basis. There is no mortality and no risk of infections or other surgical complications.

CLINICAL APPLICATIONS

Functional

Intractable Pain

In the late 1960s, stereotactic surgery was still almost synonymous with functional neurosurgery. The first Gamma Unit was used in the treatment of a series of functional disorders (24, 27). Medial gammathalamotomy for intractable pain was an attractive means of achieving pain relief without sensory loss. A series of 50 gammathalamotomies gave a lot of information regarding the dose of radiation required. The results were somewhat inconsistent, but better for pain in the upper part of the body (45). Today, with better knowledge on functional neuroanatomy, this field will soon be explored further.

Psychiatric Disease

In psychosurgery, the advantages of radiosurgery seemed obvious (8) and a series of 30 gammacapsulotomies for severe anxiety and obsessive-compulsive states has given promising results. At a recent follow-up, five of seven patients treated by means of bilateral gammacapsulotomies were cured or significantly improved. Good correlation was seen between the surgical result and the placement of the lesion, as verified by postoperative MR scans (37). The opposition that exists has been countered by a very strict selection of cases.

Parkinsonism and Epilepsy

The functional visualization obtainable with magnetic resonance and PET scanning will become the basis for a considerable expansion in the field of functional radiosurgery. Stereotactically placed radiolesions of only a few millimeters in diameter in combination with improved localization techniques and computer-based brain atlas overlays, will make possible radiosurgical treatment of conditions such as parkinsonism.

MR makes possible immediate postoperative verification of the radiolesion (29), which may prove important in, for example, irradiation of some epileptic foci. The clinical result may be correlated to the radiosurgical parameters, a possibility that may be of help in answering some important questions, such as the optimal placement of the lesion as well as the best size of the lesion to be selected for different conditions.

Nonfunctional

With the advent of CT and the second generation Gamma Unit, the radiosurgical efforts were redirected toward the nonfunctional areas. Questions regarding the dose of radiation required in the various indications needed an answer.

In the beginning, each treatment was a "shot in the dark," and initial radiosurgical developments were therefore, by necessity, slow. Today, about 30% of the surgical procedures at the Karolinska Hospital in Stockholm are carried out with stereotactic techniques. Of these, about one-third are closed radiosurgical procedures. Most of the radiosurgical applications have been published, and a few of the more important indications will serve to illustrate the possibilities as well as some of the problems.

Acoustic Tumors

Ever since Sir Ballance made the first extirpation of an acoustic tumor in 1894 (7), the surgical treatment of these cerebellopontine angle lesions has represented a challenge and a very interesting, multifaceted problem. Since the early 20th century, many fine surgeons have contributed to the reduction of surgical mortality and postoperative morbidity (9, 11, 13, 16, 17, 40, 42). Their efforts were constantly aimed at finding ways to improve the surgical technique and instrumentation. The most important technical contribution came in the 1960s with the introduction of the surgical microscope (13, 16). With microsurgery, the removal of acoustic tumors has become a safe and elegant procedure, particularly in experienced hands. Nevertheless, in a global perspective, the results still need to be improved, particularly with respect to preservation of facial nerve function and hearing. Stereotactic radiosurgery appeared to be an alternative to the conventional techniques, particularly in small- and medium-sized tumors. The first trial was made in 1969 (25). It seemed possible to destroy the tumor with full preservation of facial nerve function (39). Today, 160 cases have been treated, and the longest observation time is 13 yr. Due to the absence of mortality in the radiosurgical series, it has been possible to obtain postmortem verification in only one case. The sharply focused high-dose radiation induces a central necrosis, and the tumor becomes acellular and rich in collagen. Very few vessels are observed. As a consequence, the tumors are not eradicated; they usually decrease in size and are gradually transformed into a mass of scar tissue. They therefore remain visible on CT for a long time, possibly forever.

In microsurgery, cure is defined as a total removal of the tumor. With radiosurgery cure is defined as a "dead" or inactive tumor. A recent review of 115 tumors (91 unilateral and 24 bilateral) showed that in the unilateral group, 49% of the tumors progressively decreased in size and 42% were arrested in their growth and remain stationary in size (Figs. 10.11 and 10.12).

Nine percent of the tumors are unaffected by the treatment, as seen on CT, and continue to grow. Of the patients with continued postoperative tumor growth, some have been reirradiated, while some have had their tumors surgically removed. Histopathologically, these tumors exhibit the same picture as described in the postmortem case above. However, in the removed tumors there are also areas unaffected by the radiation.

In the 24 bilateral tumors, the same percentages are 25, 42, and 33, respectively. The results are summarized in Tables 10.2 to 10.5. The reason why some tumors diminish in size while others just stop growing is largely unknown. It may well be a dose-related matter. It is not clear why 10% of the unilateral tumors continue to grow. There may be technical explanations for this, such as an error in localization or a suboptimal dose planning. In any event, observation times are sufficiently long, the radiosurgical indication is quite clear, and the method has proved to be safe and reliable. In the bilateral tumors, there is a larger percentage of continued postoperative growth (33%). These neurofibromatous tumors usually cannot be distinguished histologically from the unilateral ones. Nevertheless, they seem to react differently and less favorably to the irradiation. A correlation between dose of radiation delivered and the histology of the tumors remains to be done and may provide an explanation to this difference in results between uni- and bilateral tumors. As far as the facial nerve is concerned, there have been no permanent facial weaknesses among the 160 patients treated so far. Interestingly, 15% of the patients exhibit a tem-

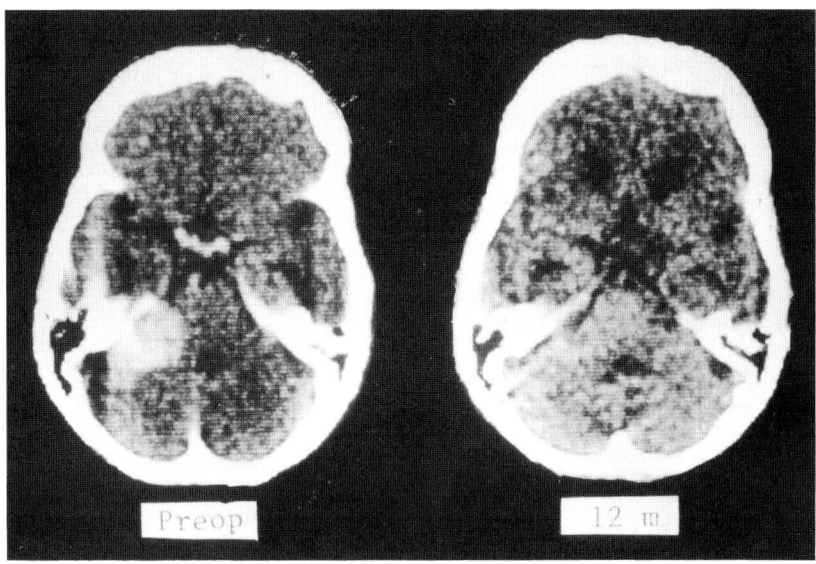

Figure 10.11. Acoustic tumor before and 12 months after stereotactic radiosurgery.

porary facial weakness which usually appears 6 months after the operation and disappears completely after another 6 months. Regarding hearing preservation, the results have been less encouraging. Twenty-five percent of cases retain their preoperative hearing levels, while 50% lose remaining hearing slowly over many years. Twenty-five percent of the patients experience a total loss of hearing within the first postoperative year. Of the 115 patients reviewed, five have had a permanent postoperative facial hypesthesia (Table 10.6). These results of stereotactic radiosurgery should be compared with those obtained by the best hands in the field. Still, even an experienced and skillful surgeon may have difficulty in reproducing the results obtained with radiosurgery; that is, no operative mortality, no permanent facial weak-

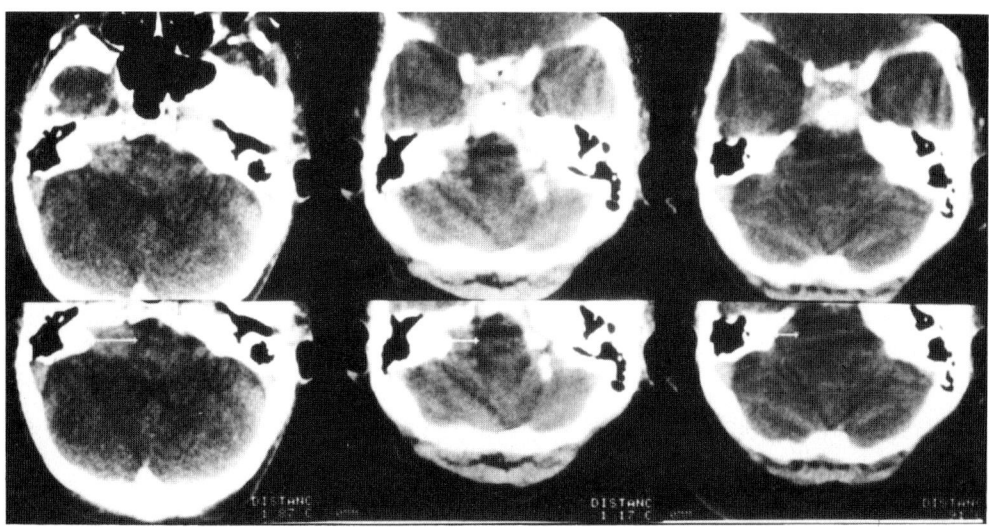

Figure 10.12. Acoustic tumor before, 18, and 48 months after stereotactic radiosurgery. Maximum tumor diameter is indicated in lower row.

TABLE 10.2
Stereotactic Radiosurgery in Acoustic Tumors*

Effect on Tumors	
Decreased	49%
Arrested growth	42%
Continued growth	9%

*n = 91.

TABLE 10.3
Stereotactic Radiosurgery in Von Recklinghausen's Disease*

Effect on Tumors	
Decreased	25%
Arrested growth	42%
Continued growth	33%

*n = 24.

TABLE 10.4
Stereotactic Radiosurgery in Acoustic Tumors*

Effect on Facial Nerve Function	
Temporary facial weakness	15%
Permanent facial weakness	0%
Facial paralysis	0%

*n = 115.

TABLE 10.5
Stereotactic Radiosurgery in Acoustic Tumors*

Effect on Auditory Function	
Preoperative hearing preserved	25%
Slow deterioration over several years	50%
Total deafness within 1 yr	25%

*n = 115.

TABLE 10.6
Stereotactic Radiosurgery in Acoustic Tumors*

Complications	
Temporary facial hypoesthesia	13%
Permanent facial hypoesthesia	4%

*n = 115.

nesses, preservation of hearing in 25% of cases, and no infections, CSF leaks, or other surgical complications. In those cases where the tumors continue to increase in size, the radiosurgical procedure can be repeated and conventional surgery is not precluded, if required later.

Stereotactic localization and dose planning for the acoustic tumors are expected to benefit from the use of MR (3), which may be of help in reducing the number of tumors that continue to grow after stereotactic radiosurgery.

MR is better than CT in outlining the intrameatal tumor boundaries that may be critical to save hearing. The tumor within the internal acoustic canal (IAC) is presently covered by the 4 mm collimator. The mechanical precision of the Gamma Unit makes possible the use of a 2-mm final collimator. Such a very small lesion in the IAC would probably also be of help with regard to hearing preservation.

The present policy in Stockholm is to treat radiosurgically all tumors with an extrameatal portion smaller than 25 to 30 mm.

Arteriovenous Malformations

The scope of microvascular surgery has expanded enormously since the 1960s, but there are still a number of vascular malformations that are considered inoperable or difficult to cope with because of their location.

In the first arteriovenous malformations (AVMs) treated radiosurgically, only the feeding arteries were irradiated (48). This attempt to occlude the feeders by means of a single heavy dose of ionizing radiation succeeded. The malformation was totally obliterated after 20 months. A renewed angiographical study of this patient after 56 months showed no signs of recanalization. At this time, the effect of the radiation on the vessels was largely unknown. A later study on the basilar artery of cats demonstrated how difficult it may be to obliterate normal vessels with irradiation alone (38). Because of difficulties in the localization of single vessels, this technique of selective gammaligature of feeding vessels was soon discontinued. Instead, the treatments have been based on irradiation of the whole malformation (43, 44, 47). At present, 550 AVMs have been treated by stereotactic radiosurgery and the results have been very rewarding. At the latest follow-up, on 104 cases after 2 yr, 86.5% of the malformations

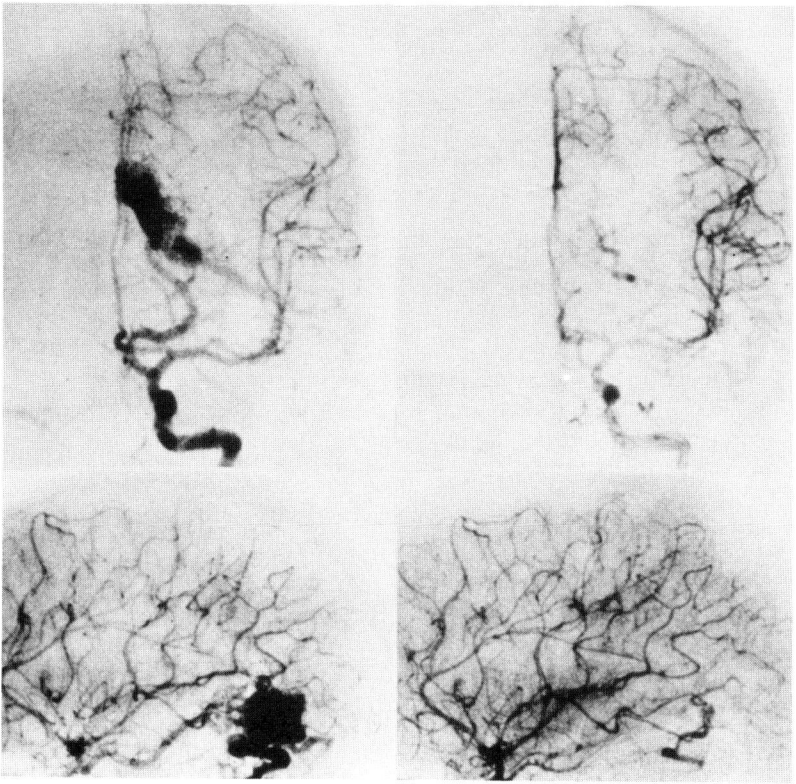

Figure 10.13. Intracerebral AVM before and 20 months after stereotactic radiosurgery.

were completely obliterated (Figs. 10.13 and 10.14); 11.5% were partially obliterated and 2% were unaffected by the procedure. There have been no recurrent hemorrhages after complete obliteration.

The long latency required for the AVMs to obliterate is a disadvantage, but the risks with radiosurgery, in small deep-seated and often inoperable AVMs, are minimal. In the whole series, 5% of the patients have bled during the postoperative latency period. Complications due to late radiation necrosis have occurred in 3% of the patients (46). The results are summarized in Table 10.7. Because of the risk for delayed radiation necrosis with very large fields of radiation, the AVMs in this series have had a maximum diameter of 30 mm or less. Larger AVMs may well be treated by irradiation of only their feeding arteries. New developments in neurovascular imaging are now expected to make the location of feeders easier, and the selective gammaligature of these will be taken up again.

The time required for total obliteration of the shunts has not been a problem. Nevertheless, a reduction of the latency is desirable, particularly in view of the possibility to also treat arterial aneurysms radiosurgically. New data regarding the effects of ionizing radiation, and various adjuvants on vessels are emerging (21). It is probable that the latency will soon be considerably reduced.

Craniopharyngiomas

Another indication that illustrates the potential benefits that may be achieved by maintaining a stereotactic attitude when looking for solutions to some difficult problems is represented by the craniopharyngiomas. Successful extirpation of these tumors requires long training. They are also relatively infrequent, which adds to the dif-

TABLE 10.7
Stereotactic Radiosurgery in AVMs*

Follow-Up 2 yr	
Total obliteration	86.5%
Partial obliteration	11.5%
No effect	2.0%
Late radiation necrosis	3.0%

*n = 104.

ficulty in obtaining such training. The problems to the patient are usually caused by the expanding cyst. The cystic portion is elegantly treated by stereotactic injection of a suitable isotope (5, 35). Backlund pioneered stereotactic radiosurgery in pituitary region tumors (4), and when a solid tumor is contributing to the symptomatology, it has been treated radiosurgically (Fig. 10.15). This has been necessary in only about 15% of cases, but the physical properties of the Gamma Unit, with the sharp limitation of the field of radiation, has been a prerequisite for this particular application (6).

Pituitary Tumors

Since 1975, more than 100 patients with Cushing's disease have been treated with the Gamma Unit (41). The sella was normal in size in the majority of these cases. The treatment has been based on the placement of one to four successive small radiolesions in the pituitary gland. The intervals between the procedures have ranged between 6 and 30 months. The first lesion has been placed in the center of the adenohypophysis. When this has failed to control the disease, additional lesions have been successively placed in the anterior and lateral parts of the sella.

A recent review of the results in 29 patients shows that 22 (76%) have obtained complete remission after a latency of between 1 and 3 yr. Two patients have im-

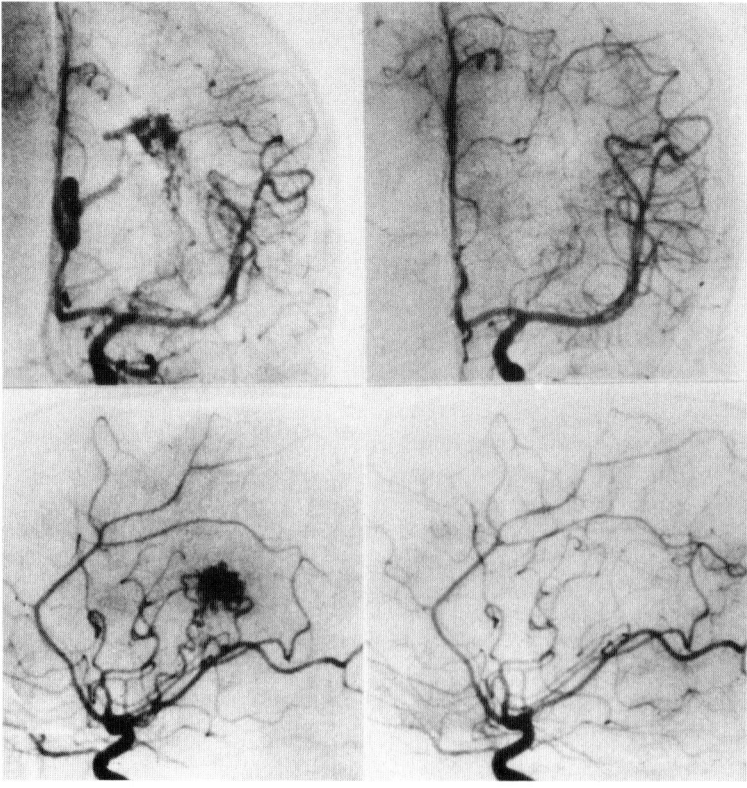

Figure 10.14. Intracerebral AVM before and 20 months after stereotactic radiosurgery.

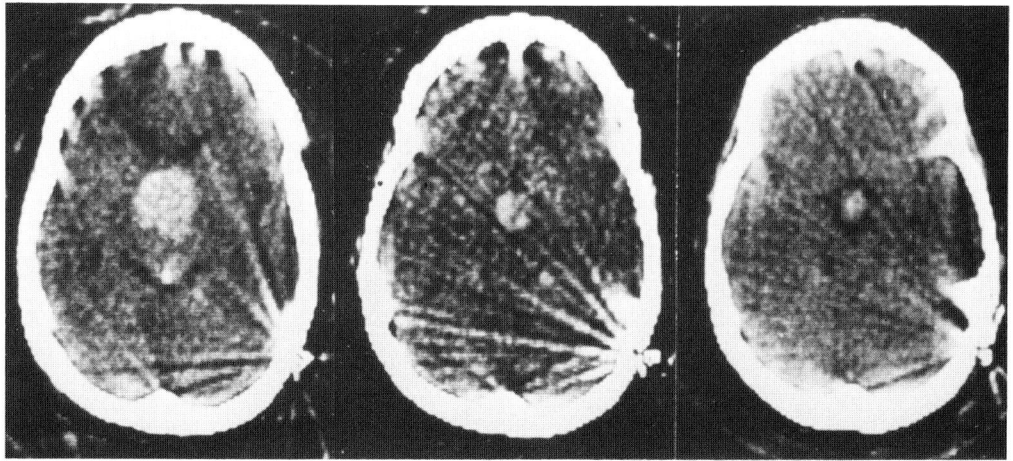

Figure 10.15. Solid craniopharyngioma before, 6, and 18 months after stereotactic radiosurgery.

proved and are not yet fully treated. Five patients had a symptomatology too severe to await full effect of the irradiation or to receive additional pituitary lesions. In these five cases, a bilateral adrenalectomy was performed. Twelve patients of the 22, in whom complete remission was achieved, developed pituitary insufficiency of varying severity. No local complications and no recurrences were observed (12).

It appears that in some instances with these microadenomas, the previously available radiological techniques have been partly inadequate to fully visualize some of the tumors. Again, with MR, a much finer intrasellar localization may be achieved. This will increase the precision, and the radiolesions can then be tailored to fit more exactly only onto the microadenomas.

CONCLUSION

New concepts are not always readily accepted by the medical community. New methods are often a source for controversy and skepticism. This has also been true with respect to some of the indications for stereotactic radiosurgery. Today, however, there are no objective reasons to dispute the validity of this surgical methodology. The results available today are based on 18 yr of experience. Successive reviews of the results have stimulated a continuous improvement of the technique as well as intense research in different areas of the field. The Gamma Unit has become an indispensable tool among other tools at the Department of Neurosurgery here in Stockholm. Stereotactic radiosurgery is not intended to replace conventional surgical techniques. Instead, it acts as an extremely valuable adjunct in the effort to provide each patient with the optimal treatment alternative for his or her particular disease. Over the years, there have been many cases in Stockholm that would have been difficult or impossible to treat without using the Gamma Unit. As already mentioned, much of what has been achieved so far has been based on the introduction of new imaging techniques. This will also be true for many future advances. Present indications will be perfected and new applications will result from the integration of stereotactic surgery and other related technologies. The depth of the brain is no longer inaccessible. Deep-seated and previously inoperable lesions are now amenable to surgical treatment.

Stereotactic radiosurgery should not be confused with other techniques in which various radiation delivery devices are used in connection with stereotactic positioning of the target. For example, the combined use of stereotactic surgery and linear accelerators (14, 15) is best called "stereotactic high-dose, single-radiation therapy" or, when fractionated, "stereotactic radiotherapy."

New Gamma Units have been installed in South America and in the United Kingdom. The Karolinska Hospital has ordered a third Gamma Unit, and new installations are underway in the United States and in Europe. This expanding "network" of radiosurgical Gamma Unit centers will jointly ensure a much faster development of the field than what has been possible so far in Stockholm alone. In the final analysis, our patients will become the beneficiaries of these joint efforts.

REFERENCES

1. Alberts W: Simple graphic stereotactic localization. *J Neurosurg* 18: 561–562, 1961.
2. Arndt J, Backlund E-O, Dahlin H, Ekstrm P: A computer controlled dose planning system for irradiation of small volumes of the brain with a multi-cobalt unit. Edinburgh, *Proc Third Cong Euro Soc Radiol*, 1975.
3. Arndt J, Hemmingsson A, Leksell D, Lindquist C, Tuomas K-H: Stereotactic radiosurgery in acoustic tumors with MRI based localization and dose-planning. *J Neurosurg* (in press).
4. Backlund E-O: Stereotaxic treatment of craniopharyngiomas. In Hamberger C-A, Wersall J (eds): *Nobel Symposium 10. Disorders of the Skull Base Region.* Stockholm, Almqvist & Wiksell, 1969, p 237.
5. Backlund E-O: Stereotaktisk behandling av kraniofaryngeom med intracystiskt Y-90 och extern Co-60 bestralning. (Thesis). Stockholm, *Acta Chir Scand* 1972.
6. Backlund E-O: Solid craniopharyngiomas treated by stereotactic radiosurgery. *INSERM* 12: 271–281, 1979.
7. Ballance CA: *Some Points in the Surgery of the Brain and its Membranes.* London, Macmillan, 1907, p 206.
8. Bergstrom M, Greitz T: Stereotaxic computed tomography. *Am J Roentgenol* 127: 167–170, 1976.
9. Cairns H: On conserving the facial nerve during removal of tumors of the cerebello-pontine angle. *Proc R Soc Med* 25: 1, 1931.
10. Carlsson CA, Leksell L: A diagram for determining space coordinates from two perpendicular roentgenograms (unpublished).
11. Cushing H: *Tumors of the nervus acusticus and the syndrome of the cerebellopontine angle.* Philadelphia, WB Saunders, 1917.
12. Degerblad M, Rahn T, Bergstrand G, Thoren M: Long-term results of stereotactic radiosurgery to the pituitary gland in Cushing's disease. *Acta Endocrinol* 112: 310–314, 1986.
13. Drake CG: Total removal of large acoustic neuromas. *J Neurosurg* 26: 554–561, 1967.
14. Hartmann GH, Schlegel W, Sturm V, Kober B, Pastyr O, Lorenz WJ: Cerebral radiation surgery using moving field irradiation at a linear accelerator facility. *Intl J Radiat Oncol Biol Physiol* 11: 1185–1192, 1985.
15. Heifetz MD, Wexler M, Thompson R: Single-beam radiotherapy knife. A practical theoretical model. *J Neurosurg* 60: 814–818, 1984.
16. House WF: Middle cranial fossa approach to the petrous pyramid. *Arch Otolaryngol* 78: 460–469, 1963.
17. House WF: Monograph II. Acoustic neurinoma. *Arch Otolaryngol* 88: 575–715, 1968.
18. Larsson B, Leksell L, Rexed B, Sourander P, Mair W, Andersson B: The high-energy proton beam as a neurosurgical tool. *Nature* 182: 1222–1223, 1958.
19. Larsson B, Liden K: Utlatande angaende apparatur for cerebral stralkirurgi med gammastralning fran Kobolt. *Uppsala/Lund,* 24: 6, 1963.
20. Leksell D: A simple manual method for multiplanar stereotactic MR localization (to be published).
21. Leksell D, Nilsson A, Wennerstrand J, Fredriksson G: Stereotactic gamma irradiation of the microcirculation using the rabbit ear chamber (to be published).
22. Leksell L: A stereotactic apparatus for intracerebral surgery. *Acta Chir Scand* 99: 229–233, 1949.
23. Leksell L: The stereotaxic method and radiosurgery of the brain. *Acta Chir Scand* 102: 316–319, 1951.
24. Leksell L: Cerebral radiosurgery I. Gammathalamotomy in two cases of intractable pain. *Acta Chir Scand* 134: 585–595, 1968.
25. Leksell L: A note on the treatment of acoustic tumors. *Acta Chir Scand* 137: 763–765, 1971.
26. Leksell L: Stereotaxis and radiosurgery. An operative system. Springfield, Charles C Thomas, 1971.
27. Leksell L: Stereotaxic radiosurgery in trigeminal neuralgia. *Acta Chir Scand* 137: 311–314, 1971.
28. Leksell L, Backlund E-O: Stereotaxic gammacapsulotomy. In Hitchcock ER, Ballantine HT, Meyerson BA (eds): *Modern Concepts in Psychiatric Surgery.* Amsterdam, Elsevier/North Holland, Biomedical Press, 1979, p 213.
29. Leksell L, Herner T, Leksell D, Persson B, Lindqvist C: Visualization of stereotactic radiolesions by nuclear magnetic resonance. *J Neurol Neurosurg Psychiatr* 48: 19–20, 1985.
30. Leksell L, Herner T, Liden K: Stereotaxic radiosurgery of the brain. Report of a case. *Kungl Fysiogr Sallsk Lund Forhandl* 25: 1–10, 1955.
31. Leksell L, Jernberg B: Stereotaxis and tomography. A technical note. *Acta Neurochir* 52: 1–7, 1980.
32. Leksell L, Larsson B, Andersson B, Rexed B, Sourander P, Mair W: Lesions in the depth of the brain produced by a beam of high-energy protons. *Acta Radiol* 54: 251–264, 1960.
33. Leksell L, Larsson B, Rexed B: The use of high-energy protons for cerebral surgery in man. *Acta Chir Scand* 125: 1–7, 1963.
34. Leksell L, Leksell D, Schwebel J: Stereotaxis and magnetic resonance. *J Neurol Neurosurg Psychiatr* 48: 14–18, 1985.

35. Leksell L, Liden K: A therapeutic trial with radioactive isotopes in cystic brain tumour. *Radioisotope Tech* 1: 1–4, 1951.
36. Liden K: Physikalische Grundlagen fur die Verwendung Ionisierender Strahlung bei gezielter Hirnchirurgie. In Olivecrona H, Tonnis W (eds): *Handbuch der Neurochirurgie, Band VI*. Heidelberg, Springer, 1957.
37. Mindus P, Bergstrom K, Lewander SE, Noren G, Hindmarsch T, Tuomas K: Magnetic resonance imaging and clinical outcome after psychosurgical intervention in severe anxiety disorder. *J Neurol Neurosurg Psychiatr* (submitted for publication).
38. Nilsson A, Wennerstrand J, Leksell D, Backlund E-O: Stereotactic gamma irradiation of basilar artery in cat. Preliminary experiences. *Acta Radiol Oncol* 17: 150–160, 1978.
39. Noren G: *Stereotactic radiosurgery in acoustic neurinomas. A new therapeutic approach.* (Thesis). Stockholm, Sundt Offset, 1982.
40. Olivecrona H: Acoustic tumors. *J Neurosurg* 26: 6–13, 1966.
41. Rahn T: *Stereotactic radiosurgery in Cushing's disease.* (Thesis). Stockholm, Sundt Offset, 1982.
42. Rand RW, Kurze T: Micro-neurosurgical resection of acoustic tumors by a transmeatal posterior fossa approach. *Bull LA Neurol Soc* 30: 17–20, 1965.
43. Steiner L: Radiosurgery in arteriovenous malformations in the brain. In Wilson C, Stein B (eds): *Intracranial Arteriovenous Malformations*. Baltimore, Williams & Wilkins, 1984.
44. Steiner L: Radiosurgery in arterio-venous malformations of the brain. In Flamm E, Fein J (eds): *Textbook of Cerebrovascular Surgery*. New York, Springer-Verlag, 1986.
45. Steiner L, Forster D, Leksell L, Meyerson BA, Boethius J: Gammathalamotomy in intractable pain. *Acta Neurochir* 52: 173–184, 1980.
46. Steiner L, Greitz T, Backlund E-O, Leksell L, Noren G, Rahn T: Radiosurgery in arteriovenous malformations of the brain. Undue effects. *INSERM* 12: 257–269, 1979.
47. Steiner L, Greitz T, Lindquist C, Arndt J: Radiosurgery in intracranial AV-malformations. XIII Symposium Neuroradiologicum, Stockholm, 23–28, 1986.
48. Steiner L, Leksell L, Greitz T, Forster D, Backlund E-O: Stereotaxic radiosurgery for cerebral arteriovenous malformations. Report of a case. *Acta Chir Scand* 138: 459–464, 1972.
49. Stereotaktisk gammaenhet-stralkniv-vid Karolinska sjukhuset. Ekonomisk kalkyl. Dept of Health, County of Stockholm, 12.9 1985 (unpublished).
50. Wennerstrand J, Ungerstedt U: Cerebral radiosurgery II. An anatomical study of gamma radiolesions. *Acta Chir Scand* 136: 133–137, 1970.

Chapter 11

Special Stereotactic Techniques: Single-Beam Photon Radiosurgery

J. L. BARCIA-SALORIO, M.D.

The term stereotactic irradiation is used to denote diverse procedures such as interstitial irradiation, curitherapy, or brachytherapy. In 1951, Leksell (9) first used "stereotactic radiosurgery" to describe closed surgery by use of external energy sources to avoid trephination and to thus eliminate the risk of infection or intracerebral bleeding. Originally, Leksell proposed using the necrotizing effect of ionizing radiations to produce very localized lesions of nuclei or fiber tracts, like thermo- or cryolesions. Thus appeared the terms "beam knife," "gamma knife," "gammathalamotomy," etc.

More recently, the term stereotactic radiosurgery has also referred to the use of ionizing radiations for their other biological effects, such as vessel thrombosis or cellular division interference. Because of its characteristic high dose that can be reached in a single application, stereotactic radiosurgery is now applied to treat arteriovenous malformations (AVMs) and benign tumors. As used in this chapter, the characteristics of radiosurgery are: (a) irradiation of a small intracerebral volume target, (b) localized by stereotactic techniques, (c) using external energy sources, and (d) a single application.

Thus, the definition of stereotactic radiosurgery is: The procedure of local irradiation, using external energy sources, destined for the destruction or treatment of small intracranial volumes, normal or pathological, of generally deep situation, localized by stereotactic methods and for therapeutic purposes.

PHYSICAL AND TECHNICAL FOUNDATIONS OF RADIOSURGERY

Ionizing radiations have been selected as the basis of radiosurgery because of their capacity to transport energy from external sources to the interior of the brain and their ability to produce long-term stabilized lesions of different size and form, according to the selected beam, without energy loss, through cerebral envelopes.

Different types of energy carriers have been used, all of which have advantages and disadvantages, from both theoretical and practical points of view. The larger cyclotrons are inaccessible to most neurosurgeons and need high technology and highly specialized staff. The Gamma Unit presents similar problems because of its high cost and its single application for neurosurgery. Nevertheless, the conventional radiotherapy units, such as telecobalt therapy or circular (Betatron) and linear accelerators, are common hospital equipment, so one can establish the possibility of performing radiosurgery with these machines, but with a minimum of accuracy and quality required. In this chapter, we shall describe the techniques of high-energy photons, as well as analyze and compare their results with the other stereotactic radiosurgical techniques used.

We must recognize that the heavily charged particles are ideal from the physical aspect. They include protons, which were used by Leksell and Larson in 1963, and Kjellberg from 1962, and alpha particles or helium nuclei used by Fabrikant since 1980. All these particles penetrate the cerebral tissue, more or less according to their weight and radiation energy. The greater the mass, the greater the energy necessary to produce a similar tract. The tract is 12 cm long with deuterons of 160 MeV energy of Harvard Cyclotron and 14.7 cm with helium nuclei of 230 MeV energy of Berkeley Synchrocyclotron.

All these particles create direct ionization by their positive electrical charges which change along the tract, since ionization is inversely proportional to the speed of the particles. At the beginning, the highly accelerated particles from the elevated energy apported by the cyclotron produce very little ionization and low dose, but on interacting with the matter and losing velocity, they gain ionization up to the point of stopping, where there is a burst of ionization in the interior of the brain. This ionization pattern is called the Bragg curve and the maximum, the Bragg peak. Another important quality of the ionization is that the particles travel in a direct line without scattering. Thus, the beams are very sharp in the lateral and final bands, and the ionization has a distinct end. The dose distribution is ideal for radiosurgery because with a single beam and entrance, a high dose can be delivered in a small target volume with a low dose in the rest of the brain. Nevertheless, the width of the peak also depends on the mass and energy utilized. With 196 MeV of Harvard Cyclotron, the width is about 1 cm, and it is inconvenient to produce a smaller lesion, and with 230 MeV of Berkeley Synchrocyclotron, the width is 0.7 cm, and it is inconvenient to produce a greater lesion.

On the contrary, photons are units that act as corpuscles of energy without mass, which have greater penetration with less energy. They are components of electromagnetic radiations, which are energy carrier waves that deliver their energy as a series of discrete quantities or amount of energy called "quanta" or photons. The energy is associated to the radiation frequency by $E = h\nu$ (E, photon energy; ν, radiation frequency; h, Planck's universal constant). X-rays, gamma rays, and light are examples of these radiations. Their different physical qualities depend on the frequency. Because they have no charge, the photons ionize indirectly on producing secondary electrons through the different interacting processes with the material. This interaction appears when an electromagnetic beam passes through the tissue. First, some of the radiation energy is ceded and is thus attenuated and absorbed by the irradiated material. Attenuation is due to the fundamental effects: photoelectric, Compton, and pair production.

The first is created at low-energy, less than 0.1 MeV, and is therefore of little importance in radiosurgery. Compton effect is the predominant process over medium-energy range of 1 to 40 MeV; therefore, it is the main effect of gamma radiation of cobalt and linear accelerators of 4 to 10 MeV, much used in radiosurgery. Pair production is created above 1.02 MeV, but its relative importance compared with Compton effect begins over 30 MeV.

Because of this attenuation phenomenon, there are two negative facts in the use of these radiations in radiosurgery. One is the diminishing of ionization and dose on deep penetration, which force the use of the so-called "cross-fire technique" with multiple beam entrances, and the other is the scattering of secondary radiation, which enlarges the beam out of the lateral bands of the selected beam, producing a "penumbra." But both disadvantages can be diminished by selecting the photon energy. Lateral scattering is mainly due to the Compton effect, that is, an interaction or collision of photons with free electrons. In each of these, the photon continues in a new direction, but the angle through which the photon is scattered depends on the energy of itself. At 1 MeV, the angle is 0 to 90° in 75%, and 40% is maintained with 45°, causing a forward dispersion but following the direction of primary radiation. At 10 MeV, forward dispersion is greater than at 1 MeV, and 60% of all Compton photons is maintained with 0 to 45°, and the broadening of the beam is less. At 35 MeV, the broadening is practically nothing.

Above 1.02 MeV, pair production begins. When a photon whose energy is greater passes close to the nucleus of an atom, the photon may disappear and in its place a positive and a negative electron appear, but without scattering effect. In contrast with the Compton effect, pair production increases with radiation energy, but its relative importance for brain tissue is small for beams less than 40 MeV. Above this energy, however, it is possible to find new disadvantages. The created positron soon links up with another negative electron producing the so-called "annihilation radiation," broadening the beam again.

The other negative fact, the diminishing of the dose on deep penetration, is also different according to the energy. With 1.25 MeV of cobalt gamma radiation, the slope is very pronounced. With 10 MeV, this slope is less pronounced, and with 30 to 45 MeV, the dose rises as the beam penetrates deeper, reaching its maximum at 7 cm depth, and the greater the energy, the less the number of entrances are needed to reach the same dose on the target. Lastly, the geometrical penumbra can also change the limits of the beam due to the size of the source and the relative distances among collimator, source, and target. The greater the source, the greater the penumbra. Cobalt standard sources are 1.5 cm in size while those of accelerators or betatrons are 0.2 to 0.3 cm. Relative distance among source, collimator, and target is limited by the range of the machine.

From all this we can conclude that, to date, the best high-energy photon sources for radiosurgery, from the physical, theoretical point of view, are the circular (betatron) or linear accelerators of 10 to 35 MeV. Nevertheless, in practice, there are not significant differences between accelerators and cobalt units. In Figure 11.1 we can compare the standard isodose curves computed for 10-mm collimator with seven entrances, each one separated 15°, in transversal plane at 8 cm depth, produced by a 4-MeV linear accelerator (A) with those computed for a patient's target, at 7 cm depth, using 10-mm collimator and 25 entrances, each one separated 15°, and those produced by a cobalt unit (B).

APPLICATION TECHNIQUES

Different techniques used by different authors may be classified as fixed-field therapy or rotation therapy. The former consists of the source being immobile during irradiation, the latter being the source rotating around a point called the isocenter.

In general, the advantages of rotating therapy are the reduction of irradiation time and the sharper deep isodose by infinite entrances, but it has less accuracy due to instability of energy emission, the vagueness of the mechanical isocenter ($\pm$ 2 to 6 mm), and the variability of the skin-target distance. The form and size of the collimator and energy intensity must be changing continuously. Modern linear and circular accelerators can vary the dose delivered per degree of rotation, guided by microprocessor, and change the form and size of a multileaf collimator during arc therapy, but are not actually available for small radiosurgical targets.

The fixed-field therapy has the advantage of greater accuracy because of the easy change of form and size of collimator in each entrance according to the form and size of the target and the facility to adapt the energy intensity of each beam according to skin-target distance. It has the disadvantage, however, of being much slower and having less uniform isodose.

For the small radiotherapy lesion, we prefer the fixed-field technique. Our method

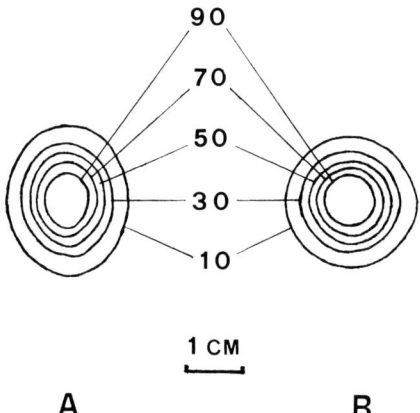

Figure 11.1. Isodose curves computed for 10-mm collimator with seven entrances, each one separated 15°, produced by a 4 MeV linear accelerator (*A*) and by a cobalt unit (*B*).

consists of the optical attachment of a radial stereotactical system to a cobalt unit or a circular or linear accelerator. The stereoguide is placed on the patient's head to localize and determine the stereotactic coordinates, the volume and form of the target, by means of x-ray-computed tomography (CT) or magnetic resonance imaging (MRI). Previous experimental study has been made to ascertain the isodose chart of beams and to determine the deep isodose, using films dosimetry and randophantom of human equivalent tissue. With computer assistance, the size, form, and geometry of the collimators are selected, which can vary in each entrance. The collimator is placed in the stereoguide to delimit the form and size of the beam, or the collimator can be situated on the source head of the counit or accelerator, and the stereoguide has only an optical device or telescopic sight to direct the beam.

The patient with the stereoguide is placed on the radiotherapy table, and the stereoguide is fixed in a special holder, moving the table up and down and right to left until the target coincides with the machine isocenter guided by laser or light-beam indicator. The patient can be in any position, right or left lateral, prone or supine, according to target situation, in order to be as close as possible to the source. The collimator-skin distance for each entrance is measured and thus the skin-target distance of each beam is calculated by the computer, and, in this way, a more accurate isodose can be calculated. The entrances are selected, changing the angles of the collimator or telescopic sight carrier. In this way, the entrances can be distributed over a spherical sector of 60° x 120°. The stereoguide was geometrically designed so that the beam passes through the target in any position of the collimator, or telescopic sight (Fig. 11.2). In this manner, the accuracy of the system depends on the stereoguide, which has a 0.1-mm error, but not on the accelerator mechanics, whose error is greater than 2 mm or 20 times more.

Berahas in Sao Paulo has coupled a 4-MeV accelerator to my stereoguide, following the same technique. Alternatively, Betti (3) in Buenos Aires has used rotatory therapy, in which the patient is placed in the sit-

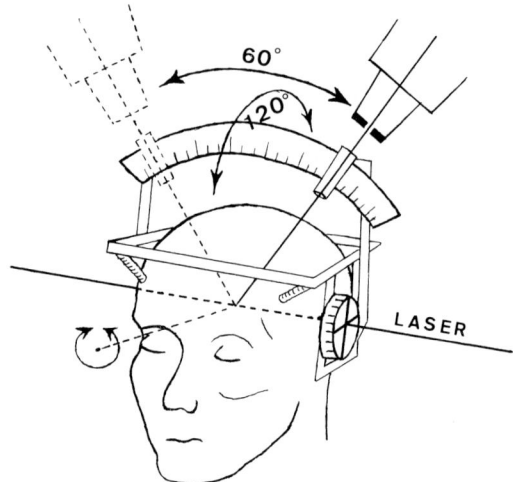

Figure 11.2. Optical attachment of stereoguide to external energy source. Beam-guide carrier allows for entrances over spherical sector of 60 x 120°.

ting position in a sliding chair on curved rails so that his head can be turned on a transverse axis that coincides with a 10-MeV accelerator isocenter. The patient and source head are combined so that infinite entrances from a spherical section are achieved. However, the accuracy of this system depends on the accelerator mechanics, having the forementioned disadvantages. In Italy, Collombo et al. (4) use a mixed technique, partly fixed and partly rotatory, with 5 to 10 arcs of 115° separated 15 to 30° each; however, they have used only relatively big collimators (25 mm diameter) in gliomas and AVMs, giving 2000 rads in two sessions separated 8 to 10 days. Heifetz et al. (6) have studied the feasibility of using a 10-MeV linear accelerator, applying rotatory therapy.

INDICATIONS AND RESULTS

In general, the indications and results of photon single-beam radiosurgery are the same as those of the Gamma Unit. The main indication, AVMs, is followed by deep tumors such as neurinomas, pinealomas, craniopharyngiomas, and, lastly, functional neurosurgery.

AVMs

We have calculated that more than 1900 AVMs have been treated in the world. Deep, small, and inaccessible AVMs are the most often selected.

In 1983, Kjellberg et al. (8) had 439 patients with AVMs treated by Bragg peak proton beam therapy, 244 of which had a follow-up over 2 yr, having a rate of total obliteration of 22% and a reduction in volume and density of AVMs in 87% of them. Fabrikant et al. (5) had 55 patients with deep intracranial AVMs treated by helium-ion Bragg peak beams, all of them with a follow-up of 18 months, and a significant decrease in size and blood flow through AVMs in seven cases.

Our personal experience with photon beam includes 65 patients with intracranial vascular disorders, 42 of them with AVMs and 15 with carotid-cavernous fistulae (CCF). Treatment was performed by means of stereotactic angiography and with 5 to 10-mm collimators, depending on the form and size of the malformation. In several cases, two targets were necessary in order to tailor the isodose curves inside the AVM limits. Total dose was 2500 to 4000 rads (25–40 Gy) depending on the irradiated volume. The results in the 18 first patients, 13 of which had a follow-up over 2 yr, were: complete obliteration in three cases (16%) within the first 6 months, in seven cases (41%) within the first year, and 11 cases (85%) after 2 yr.

CCF included 15 spontaneous, two dural AVMs and three traumatic, all being low-flow fistulae. Irradiation was performed with a 5-mm collimator (1), and a 10-mm collimator in the case of dural malformations, a total dose of 4000 rads (40 Gy) being delivered in all cases. Ninety-five percent of patients were symptom free from 2 to 7 months after treatment, and the angiographical control 1 yr later showed a total obliteration of the fistula and normal flow in the internal carotid.

In the great AVMs, more than 2 cm in diameter, we have performed stereotactic radiotherapy consisting of the use of a plastic helmet which allows the subsequent attachment of the stereoguide, day after day, a fractional dose being delivered during 4 weeks, until a total dose of 6000 rads (60 Gy) is reached. Irradiation is achieved through four to five entry portals and with collimator sizes, depending on the form and size of the lesion. The result of this accurate radiotherapy is not so effective as radiosurgery and, in our hands, the rate of nearly total obliteration was only 20%.

We have no morbidity due to radionecrosis, nor any neurological deficits after total thrombosis, so we can deduce—following Kjellberg et al. (8)—that AVM embryonic small vessels have a lower threshold for radiobiological effect than normal capillaries at the used dose. Histological observations in humans (8) and experimental fistulae produced in animals in our laboratory have shown that the main ionizing radiation effect upon small vessels is that of an endothelitis narrowing its lumen.

Deep Brain Tumors

Tumor necrosis is the main radiosurgical objective, but in special cases, it should be enough to obtain only growth arrest using a lower dose, taking advantage of its greater radiosensitivity. There is evidence that every kind of tumor has a different radiosensitivity, but one needs a greater number of clinical observations and experimental data to establish the single-dose sensitivity for each tumor.

In pituitary tumors, Kjellberg et al. (7) have the greatest experience with more than 1500 radiosurgical interventions with the Bragg peak heavy particles beam therapy, but there is no up-to-date experience using single-photon beam therapy. We have only a few cases of prolactinoma, hypophyseal adenoma, and craniopharyngioma, and through our results we can believe that these are similar to those of the heavy particles and the Gamma Unit. In acoustic neurinoma, the Gamma Unit has accumulated the greatest number of cases and the longest follow-up.

We have operated on 25 cases with our methods using a 5-mm collimator and a dose from 2500 to 9000 rads (25–90 Gy) according to the size of the tumor. About 6 months after irradiation, CT shows a ring image due to central necrosis; 1 yr later there is tumor shrinkage; and 7 yr later the image may have nearly disappeared. Our results in the first 16 cases are good in tumors smaller than 3 cm, and we have seen tumor shrinkage in 50% of cases. We have not had facial paresis nor facial hypoesthesia, and in some cases with previous audition, this can improve. With the same technique used in tumors greater than 30 mm, the results have been poor due to the periphery receiving a dose lower than 2000 rads. Biopsy and necropsy studies can demonstrate that 5000 rads are the necrosis dose, coinciding with Noren, who has also seen a necrosis sharp delimitation at 2000 rads. In conclusion, with adequated isodoses and technique, the results of radiosurgery can be similar to those of microsurgery, but are relatively risk free.

In deep and low-grade gliomas there is also little experience. They are radiosensitive tumors and can thus be treated by radiosurgery. Nevertheless, the main condition is for the tumor to be compact and sharply delimited and less than 2 cm in size. We have experience in brainstem and thalamic astrocytoma using 4000 to 9000 rads (40-90 Gy). In malignant gliomas, we have given a radiosurgical "boost" of 2 to 4000 rads in every tumor having a decrease in CT image after conventional radiotherapy but have achieved transient results. Colombo et al. (4) have recently reported their results in three thalamic, two pineal, and one parietal glioma using 400 rads in two sessions, with fields ranging from 2.5 to 5 cm and shrinkage or disappearance of tumor image in CT scans.

Functional Radiosurgery

Originally, Leksell sought to produce lesions like those of the stereotactical functional neurosurgery, but without trephination. This lesion was produced with 3 x 5 mm collimator and 15,000 to 25,000 rads. It was used in the treatment of pain, parkinsonism, and psychosurgery with habitual targets and same results, and with the advantage of being a bloodless and painless intervention. However, other qualities of low-dose irradiation have been favored.

We have, in the first place, the radiosurgery of trigeminal neuralgia. Leksell (10) reported two cases irradiated by 320 KeV x-ray with a dose between 1900 and 2100 rads. He then used the Gamma Unit in 63 cases. We have ourselves performed this intervention in 17 cases but with a different target. While Leksell irradiated the Gasserian ganglion, calling it "radiogangliothomy," we preferred the trigeminal root over the petrous ridge where Granit and Leksell supposed to be the site of the artificial synapses. Our dose was 4000 rads, and the results were very good initially, with all patients pain-free in the 24 hr after irradiation, with normal facial sensitivity, but later, 60% of them relapsed.

In the second place, radiosurgery is used in the treatment of epilepsy. After our experience in an experimental epileptic focus in the cat, we have applied this technique to man (2). Our series was 10 epileptic patients; eight of them presented with seizures and three with psychotic or behavioral disturbances. The focus was localized by means of chronic subarachnoidial and deep electrodes and irradiated with only 1000 rads with a 10-mm collimator. The follow-up was 9 months to 3 yr, and the overall results were excellent in three cases with complete clinical improvement and free of medical treatment. Four had good results; two, fair, and one, poor. The EEG was also normalized in patients with excellent results.

REFERENCES

1. Barcia-Salorio JL, Hernandez G, Broseta J, Gonzalez-Darder J, Ciudad J: Radiosurgical treatment of carotid-cavernous fistula. *Appl Neurophysiol* 45: 520-522, 1982.
2. Barcia-Salorio JL, Roldan P, Hernandez G, Lopez-Gomez L: Radiosurgical treatment of epilepsy. *Appl Neurophysiol* 48: 400-403, 1985.
3. Betti OO, Derechinsky VE: Hyperselective encephalic irradiation with linear accelerator. *Acta Neurochir Suppl* 33: 385-390, 1984.
4. Colombo F, Benedetti A, Pozza F, Avanzo RC, Marchetti C, Chierego G, Zenardo A: External stereotactic irradiation by linear accelerator. *Neurosurg* 16, 2: 154-160, 1985.
5. Fabrikant JK, Lyman JT, Hosobuchi Y: Stereotactic heavy ion Bragg peak radiosurgery for intracranial vascular disorders: method for treatment of deep arteriovenous malformations. *Br J Radiol* 57: 479-490, 1984.
6. Heifetz MD Wexler M, Thompson R: Single-beam radiotherapy knife. A practical theoretical model *J Neurosurg* 60: 814-8, 1984.
7. Kjellberg RN, Kliman B: Bragg-peak proton hypophysectomy for hyperpituitarism, induced hypopituitarism and neoplasm. *Prog Neurol Surg* 6: 295-325, 1975.
8. Kjellberg RN, Hanamura T, Davis KR, Lyons SL, Adams, RD: Bragg peak proton beam therapy for arteriovenous malformations of the brain. *N Engl J Med* 5: 269-274, 1983.

9. Leksell L: The stereotaxic method and radiosurgery of the brain. *Acta Chir Scand* 102: 316–319, 1951.

10. Leksell L: Stereotaxic radiosurgery for trigeminal neuralgia. *Acta Chir Scand* 137: 311–324, 1971.

Chapter 12

Special Stereotactic Techniques: Robotic Methods Applied to Stereotactic Surgery

YIK SAN KWOH, Ph.D.

INTRODUCTION AND HISTORICAL DEVELOPMENTS THAT LED TO THE ROBOT

Stereotactic brain surgery is a technique for guiding the tip of a probe or other delicate surgical instrument into the brain through a small burr hole drilled in the skull without direct visualization of the surgical site.

Minimizing brain damage as the probe travels from the skull to the surgical target deep in the brain requires a straight-line trajectory that avoids such vital parts of the brain as major vessels and the motor strip. If the probe trajectory is selected by an experienced surgeon, and if the probe is inserted along a straight trajectory, there will be no identifiable neurological damage due to probe insertion. Straight-line trajectory probe insertion is most easily accomplished by inserting the probe through a probe guide, which is itself supported by a sturdy mechanical structure. This overall design for very stable trajectory control is referred to as the *stereotactic frame*. This device usually takes the form of some apparatus, affixed to the patient's skull, that allows the probe guide to be positioned along any preassigned trajectory by means of a system of angular settings, scales, and verniers.

The second problem inherent to stereotactic procedures is that the surgeon has no visual contact with the surgical site. Therefore, some three-dimensional (3-D) localization of the target area is required. In other words, the surgeon must know through what angle and what depth he has to insert the probe in order to reach the target. This 3-D localization is usually accomplished by coupling the frame with some x-ray device or by making use of the standard atlas of the brain.

The basic process of stereotactic neurosurgery has been used both clinically and as a research tool for nearly 80 yr, following the pioneering work of Sir Victor Horsley and Robert Clarke (5), Queen's Square Hospital, London, England, in the first decade of this century. Horsley and Clarke developed the first 3-D stereotactic apparatus. The Clarke apparatus (6) was an adjustable mechanical structure to be affixed to the cranium of an animal and is specially devised for accurate positioning of an electrode in a precise cerebellar nucleus with minimum injury to the surrounding brain structures. This apparatus exploited the nearly constant proportionality relationship between external landmarks on the cranium and the head encephalic content. The variability in location of brain structures with reference to anatomical landmarks on the skull was observed to be small among animals of such species as Macacus rhesus and cats.

The stereotactic apparatus for human neurosurgery was developed by Drs. Spiegel and Wycis. Since the human brain is anatomically much more complex than animals' brain, a more accurate 3-D localization system was required for humans. Spiegel and Wycis solved this 3-D localization problem by interfacing the stereotactic frame with a conventional x-ray device.

Since these pioneering efforts, many stereotactic devices have been developed (9). In the early stereotactic procedures, the road to the target was provided by conventional x-ray pictures, which were often enhanced by contrast material techniques. Another aid is the standard atlas of the brain. This accurate chart shows the position of such an important surgical target as the thalamus with respect to the brain ventricular system, a landmark easily identifiable via x-ray pneumoencephalography. Sometimes, because of unpredictable variability of brain structures with respect to landmarks, clinical confirmation of the site is necessary. For example, this confirmation of site could be done by stimulating or cooling the cells of the target area and observing the neurophysiological response.

In the late 1970s stereotactic surgery received new impetus with the advent of computer tomographic (CT) scanning. This technique provides two-dimensional (2-D), high resolution pictures, which show the details of the soft tissue anatomy in precise transverse sections of the craniovault and the spinal canal. This strongly contrasts with conventional x-ray pictures that show projections of the anatomy along lines radiating from the x-ray tube. It was soon realized that the unsurpassed density resolution of the CT images could significantly enhance the accuracy of stereotactic target localization. In the late 1970s, Memorial Medical Center of Long Beach developed its own CT-guided stereotactic apparatus (1). This device is shown in Figure 12.1. The apparatus is mounted on the CT scanner couch. The patient lies on the CT scanner couch with his/her skull affixed to the frame by four screws inserted by the surgeon under local anesthesia. Three N-shaped locators localize the scan plane with respect to the frame. Any target—say, a tumor—identified on the CT picture can be easily localized in three dimensions in the frame coordinate system. Once the (x, y, z) coordinates of the tumors in the apparatus reference frame are computed, some trigonometric calculations allow one to determine the four angular settings of the frame—base ring, arch pitch, carriage, and probe—such that the probe guide is pointing toward the target. The probe depth, i.e., the distance between the distal end of the bushing and the tumor, is also computed. The surgeon burrs a hole in the skull, inserts the probe in the brain through the probe guide at the appropriate depth, and the tip of the probe is exactly at the target previously identified on the CT

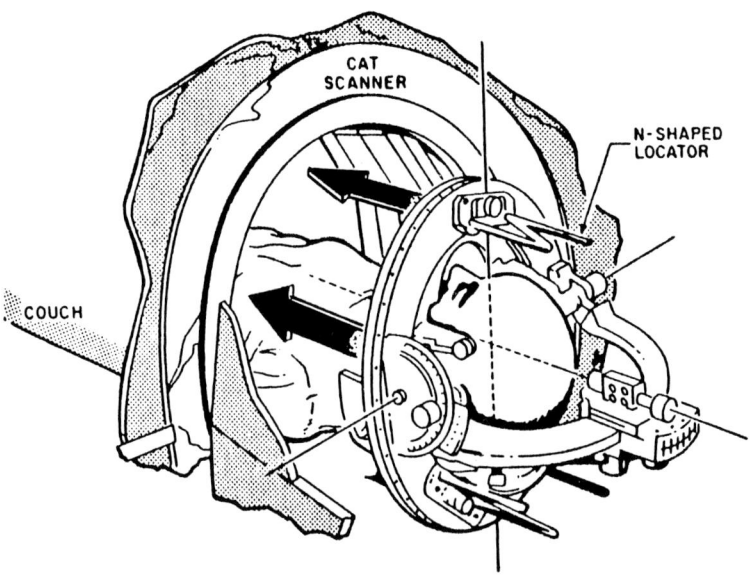

Figure 12.1. Memorial Hospital stereotactic head frame.

picture. At this point, the surgeon is ready for tissue biopsy, abscess drainage, cryogenic or electrolytic ablation, or any other hollow-needle procedure.

In the course of many stereotactic procedures conducted at Memorial Medical Center from 1980 to 1984, it soon became evident that reading the scales on the frame and adjusting the frame according to the computer output was a tedious and time-consuming procedure, especially in the case of tumors that had to be approached from several different directions. Adjustments after the first trajectory setting were almost impossible because the frame had already been draped under sterile conditions. The multiple, time-consuming, and manual adjustments of the frame motivated the search for a new procedure, a procedure that was going to be faster, more automated, more flexible, more reliable, and more accurate; a procedure that could be used for both the body and the head. The solution appeared to be the radical replacement of the stereotactic frame—a device more than 80 yr of age—by a high-precision, versatile, computer-controlled, latest generation robot, fully interfaced with the CT scanner and with the probe guide at its "end effector."

THE ROBOT

The very first phase of this project was a careful evaluation of the industrial robot available on the market in order to determine whether a robot with enough dexterity, accuracy, and reliability to operate in the surgical environment was available. After a long screening procedure, although the ideal robot was not available on the market, we have nevertheless found that the robot best suited to our purposes is the Unimation Puma 200 robot. This decision involved, among other things, the following considerations: The Unimation Puma 200 is a programmable, computer-controlled, versatile robot. The Unimation Puma 200 robot has been especially designed for accurate, delicate work, yet it is sturdy enough to provide very stable trajectory. The Unimation Puma 200 robot motions are similar to those of the human body and can be described in human terms: waist, shoulder, elbow, wrist, flange rotation, and wrist bend. The Unimation Puma 200 robot is designed to work with humans and at human tempos so that it will mesh with existing surgical procedures. The Puma 200 robot has a relative accuracy of 0.05 mm. The Puma 200 robot has been devised to be very versatile; its computer is compatible with a variety of imaging computers currently used in the biomedical field. The Unimation Puma 200 robot is safe. The waist, shoulder, and elbow joints are equipped with spring-applied, solenoid-released brakes which are automatically clamped should any mechanical or electrical defect occur. The wrist of the robot—or the end effector in the more technical jargon—is designed and manufactored so that it can receive a variety of tools and instruments, in particular, a bushing for probe guidance would not constitute a major problem to be adapted.

Mathematically, the Puma robot is a series of *links* interconnected by *six revolute joints*. Each link is characterized by its *joint angle theta*. The *joint angle vector* is defined as q = (θ1, θ2, θ3, θ4, θ5, θ6).

The numbering of the angles goes from the waist (#1) to the wrist (#6). In the nominal mode of operation of the robot, the operator enters the θs from the robot computer keyboard, and the robot automatically moves to the configuration specified by the joint angles. The position of the end effector in space—which is of paramount importance in stereotactic surgery, since this is the entrance point—requires six parameters: three parameters, i.e., the x, y, and z coordinates, to specify the position of the wrist, and three more parameters, i.e., three Euler angles, to specify the orientation of the wrist. These six parameters are concatenated into an array of numbers, referred to as the homogenous transformation T in the mathematical jargon (8). The mapping from the *joint angle vector q* to the (translational and rotational) position T of the end effector is referred to as *forward kinematic:*

$$T = f(q).$$

However, in most robotic problems, the position of the end effector T is specified, and the problem is to determine the joint angles that place the end effector at the pre-specific position: this is the *reverse kinematic* problem:

$$q = \text{inverse} (f) (T).$$

The reverse kinematic problem is not easy, because it is nonlinear and has a nonunique solution. However, several methods of solutions are known.

Also observe that both the forward and the reverse kinematic problems, i.e., the *f* and inverse (*f*) functions, depend on such geometric parameters as the lengths of the links, i.e., the length of the upper arm, the length of the lower arm, and many other subtle parameters, the details of which are not expanded upon here. We will just mention that, mathematically, the set of all of these parameters is usually referred to as Hartenberg-Denavit parameters. The manufacturer only specifies the nominal values of the parameters of the robot family; this is to say that a particular robot within the family will have its parameters slightly off the nominal values, because of small errors occuring during manufacturing and assembly of the robot (2).

ORGANIZATION OF SURGICAL FIELD, CALIBRATION, TESTING, AND FIRST BRAIN OPERATION

After choosing the Unimation Puma 200 robot, it was decided to use the former stereotactic frame, with the arch removed, to affix the patient's head to the CT scanner couch. This setup is shown in Figure 12.2. The main reason for using part of the manually adjustable stereotactic equipment to organize the robotic surgical field is reliability: in the unlikely event of a problem with the robot, it would be possible to put the arch back on the base ring and proceed with the operation using the manually adjustable frame.

As before, the base ring is mounted on the CT scanner couch. The patient lies on the CT scanner couch, and the surgeon surgically affixes the patient's head to the frame base ring. The N-shaped locators are mounted on the base ring, and CT pictures of the brain are taken. The target is localized on the CT picture, and the (x, y, z) coordinates of the target are computed in the base ring reference frame. After CT scan, the patient is moved out of the scanner to an area convenient to the surgeon. The robot, which is bolted on a pedestal, is brought in operation by hooking up the robot's pedestal to the base ring. The target coordinates are located in the robot's reference frame. After solving the *inverse kinematic problem,* the robot is programmed to swing smoothly and to point the probe guide exactly toward the target. The surgeon has the option to manipulate the trajectory in a variety of different ways, yet the robot always points toward the same target, as shown in Figure 12.3. After deciding which trajectory is best, the surgeon perforates the skull and inserts the probe.

After envisioning this robotic stereotactic procedure, several simulation experiments and tests were conducted. The first phase consisted of some calibration tests. The robot was mounted on a "chessboard" with equally spaced holes on which several cylindrical objects (with vertices pointing upward) were mounted, shown in Figure 12.4. The purpose of that test was to evaluate the software and also to calibrate the robot so that it could reach the vertex of an object placed anywhere on the chessboard. Afterward, a great number of experiments were conducted. A watermelon embedded with a small lead BB simulating a lesion in the human brain was CT-scanned; the robot swung to the desired position, guiding a small needle so that it met the BB. A great number of watermelon experiments were conducted before applying the procedure to a human (7).

Finally, on April 11, 1985, a 52-yr-old man, who wants to remain anonymous, was admitted to the hospital with a suspicious brain lesion. The surgeon wanted to obtain a tissue sample for positive diagnosis. The surgeon, assisted by two electrical engineers, decided to use the robot. The 52-yr-old man was put on the CT scanner couch, CT pictures of the brain were taken, the target was

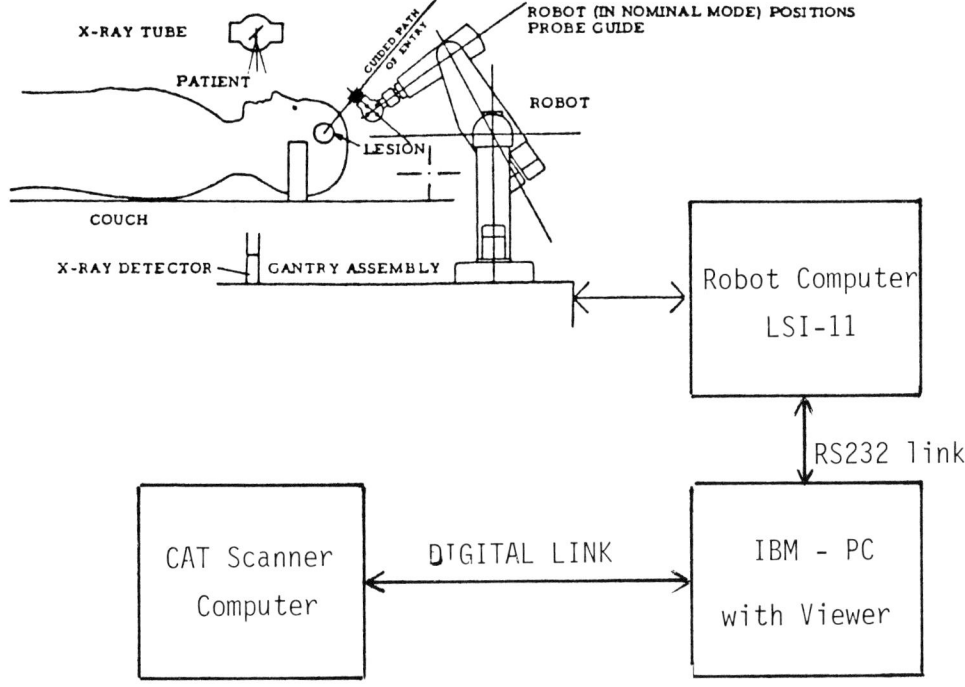

Figure 12.2. Overall robot-automated stereotactic procedure.

identified on the CT pictures, the robot was brought in operation, and quickly the robot oriented the bushing toward the suspected area in the brain. The biopsy needle was inserted through the bushing, and a sample of tissue was sucked with a syringe. The tissue sample was sent to the pathology lab, where a positive biopsy was confirmed on the first sample. As of September 1986, 22 patients have undergone the same procedure.

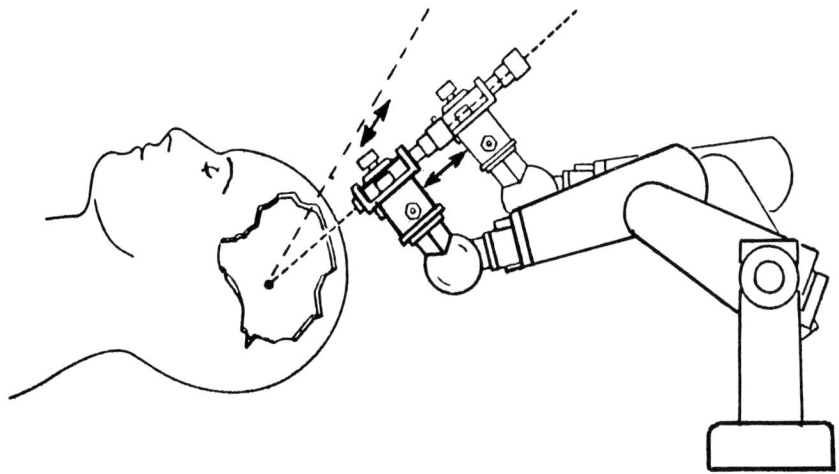

Figure 12.3. Flexible arm movement.

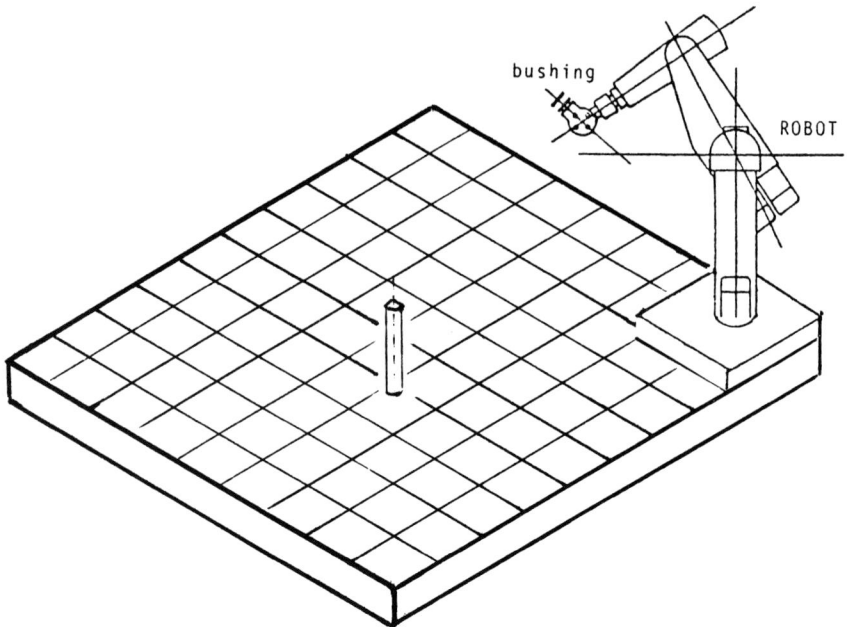

Figure 12.4. Calibration is done on a precision chessboard.

IMPROVING THE ABSOLUTE POSITIONING ACCURACY OF THE ROBOT

While the commercially available Unimation Puma 200 robot proved accurate enough for operations on big tumors (0.5 cm) located in noncritical areas of the brain (e.g., corpus callosum), it soon became evident that operating on smaller size lesions located deep in the brain was going to require some sort of improvement of the accuracy.

Unimation specifies that the Puma 200 robot has a *relative accuracy* of 0.05 mm. *Relative accuracy* is also referred to as *repeatability*. Repeatability is a measurement of the deviation between a position previously held by the end effector and the position to which it returns in a *repetitive* motion.

However, in such an application as CT-guided surgery, in which the robot is guided by some external sensory device, the notion of accuracy should refer to some external reference frame. The *accuracy* (or *absolute accuracy*) of a robot arm is defined to be the mismatch between, on the one hand, the actual position of the end effector and, on the other hand, the end effector position as it has been specified by its coordinates in some external reference frame.

The repeatability tolerance is finer than the accuracy tolerance. The difference between accuracy and repeatability stems from the fact that all the robot arms within the same family are not exactly similar. Because of finite precision manufacturing, the link parameters of a particular robot within a family do not exactly have the nominal values of the robot family. Repeatability is a characteristic of a robot arm family; accuracy is a characteristic of a particular robot within the family. This is the reason why manufacturers specify repeatability rather than accuracy. However, the accuracy tolerance can be brought to about the same level as the repeatability tolerance, provided one can compensate for the imperfections of the robot. This process is referred to as *calibration* of the robot or *improvement of its absolute positioning accuracy* (3).

In our setup, it is required that the tip of the needle mounted at the robot's end effector be positioned at the precise point in the brain defined by the cursor position on the CT image of the brain. The cursor position, together with the signature of the base ring N-shaped locators, yields the (x, y, z) coordinates of the target in the base ring reference frame. This, in turn, can be converted into (x, y, z) coordinates in the robot's reference frame. Therefore, the problem is: to solve the inverse kinematic problem in such a way that if the precision coordinates (i.e., joint angles) are entered from the robot computer keyboard, the needle tip will be exactly at the (x, y, z) point. If this is done without compensation for the inherent geometric errors of the particular robot being used, the needle tip could be as much as a few millimeters off the specified target. However, for some delicate neurosurgical applications, the consensus among neurosurgeons is that submillimeter accuracy is required. The purpose of our calibration is to compensate for the robot error in order to reach submillimeter accuracy.

The essential factor limiting the absolute accuracy of a particular robot within a family is the imprecise knowledge of the robot's geometry. In a certain way, one must compensate for the offset between nominal and actual kinematics.

The idea is, through some kinematic experiments with the robot, to estimate, i.e., to identify, the geometric parameters of our particular robot. The geometric parameters of our robot will not be exactly the same as the "nominal" parameters specified by the manufacturer.

Practically, this is done as follows: The robot is mounted on the high precision chessboard. On the chessboard is mounted a high precision object with a receptacle that can receive a special tool mounted on the robot end effector. The receptacle can receive the tool mounted on the wrist only when the latter is in a very precise position together with a very precise orientation. This provides a very accurate measure of the (translation and rotation) position T of the end effector. In this configuration, the precision joint angles vector $q = (\theta 1, \ldots, \theta 6)$ is measured. This operation is repeated for many different locations of the object on the chessboard, and the data $[T, q]$ are accumulated. From this data, and through some least squares techniques, the robot geometric (Hartenberg-Denavit) parameters are computed. The computation software is implemented on an IBM PC.

A second package, also implemented on an IBM PC, makes use of the precise estimates of the Hartenberg-Denavit parameters to solve, in a very accurate fashion, the inverse kinematic problem (4).

Experiments have confirmed the targeted submillimeter accuracy of our system.

APPLICATIONS

So far, the stereotactic robot has been used only for brain tumor biopsy.

However, it is anticipated that soon the robot will be used for radioactive implantation directly inside malignant tumors. If the biopsy confirms glioma, i.e., malignant brain lesion, the standard treatment is destruction of the malignant cells by radiation. However, an external beam radiation, even when focused on the lesion, is likely to create radionecrosis of surrounding tissues. A more sensible approach is endocurietherapy, i.e., the deposition of a radioactive seed directly inside the malignant tumor. This allows for higher doses of radiation to be delivered to the malignant lesion, yet the risk of destroying the surrounding tissues is significantly reduced. This could be accomplished with the robot as follows: The probe would be inserted in the lumen of the afterloading catheter; both the probe and the catheter would be inserted in the brain through the bushing held in position by the robot; the probe would be removed, leaving the catheter in position. Then the patient would be moved to a lead-shielded room, where a seed of Iridium 192 (^{192}-Ir) would be inserted in the catheter down to the lesion area.

Another neurosurgical application where the high accuracy of the robot would be needed is deep brain stimulation to help patients suffering from chronic pain due to industrial accidents, nerve injuries, metabolic disorders, acute dental problems, etc. The aqueduct of Sylvius, which goes from the third to fourth ventricle of the human brain, is surrounded by a thin layer of cells called the periventricular gray. When these cells are electrically stimulated, they release in the spinal canal β-endorphines, a morphine-like compound, that create a profound analgesia relieving the patient from pain. However, deep cerebral stimulation requires the accurate stereotactic positioning of an electrode in the periventricular gray. This could be accomplished with the robot, provided that a new design for the effector is completed.

REFERENCES

1. Brown RA: A stereotactic head frame for use with CT body scanners. *Invest Radiol* 15: 308–312, 1980.
2. Hayati S: Robot arm geometric link parameter estimation. *Trans Biomed Engin* 22: 1477–1483, 1983.
3. Hayati S, Mirmirani M: Improving the absolute positioning accuracy of robot manipulators. *Robotic Syst* 2: 307–413, 1985.
4. Hayati S, Roston G: Inverse kinematic solutions for near-simple robots and its application to robot calibration. Proceeding of International Symposium on Robot Manipulators: Modeling, Control and Education. Albuquerque, New Mexico, Nov 11–16, 1986
5. Horsley V, Clarke RH: On the intrinsic fibers of the cerebellum, its nuclei and its efferent tracts. *Brain* 28: 12–29, 1905.
6. Horsley V, Clarke RH: The structure and functions of the cerebellum examined by a new method. *Brain* 31: 45–124, 1908.
7. Kwoh YS, Reed IS, Chen, Shao H, Truong TK, Jonckheere EA: A new computerized tomographic aided robotic stereotactic system. *Robotics Age* pp 17–21, 1985.
8. Paul R: *Robot Manipulators: Mathematics, Programming and Control.* Cambridge, MIT Press, 1984.
9. Second Annual Symposium on Parkinson's Disease. *J Neurosurg* 24: 430–481, 1966.

Chapter 13

Special Stereotactic Techniques: Hyperthermia Techniques

MICHAEL SAPOZINK, M.D, Ph.D.

The success rate for the control of malignant gliomas with conventional modalities, surgery, ionizing radiation, and cytotoxic chemotherapy has been disappointing. More aggressive use of these modalities is limited by the necessities of preventing neurological injury and serious systemic toxicity. Therefore, innovative additional local treatment modalities are being actively sought. Hyperthermia is a local modality that has recently undergone a renaissance of extensive investigation and, theoretically, should be very applicable to brain tumor therapy (5). The mechanisms of thermal cytotoxicity are quite complex, but well documented (3). Temperatures greater than 42.5°C are associated with exponentially decreased survival of proliferating cell populations in vitro and in vivo as a function of temperature or the duration of exposure to elevated temperature. This direct thermal cytotoxicity is most pronounced for cells in S-phase and for hypoxic, acidotic, nutritionally deprived cells, such as might be found near poorly vascularized necrotic regions in glioblastomas. Hyperthermia will also synergistically potentiate cellular injury by ionizing radiation, primarily by inhibiting repair of sublethal molecular damage. Thermal radiosensitization can be inferred from laboratory models at temperatures less than 42.5°C. Although the relationship is also exponential with respect to temperature and time of exposure, the rate constant differs at lower temperatures (3). Cytotoxicity of some chemotherapeutic agents may be synergistically potentiated by heat as well. The mechanisms of these interactions are complex, agent dependent, and not well elucidated; however, for one group of drugs, which includes alkylating agents, nitrosoureas, *cis*-platinum, and Mitomycin C, thermal chemosensitization is an exponential function of temperature even at small increments above base line. Local heating of brain tumors therefore has the potential for direct cytotoxicity as well as synergistic enhancement of the cell kill by active conventional modalities.

TECHNIQUES

Local heating of brain tumors, temperature documentation, and temperature control are formidable technical challenges that have only recently become approachable with refinements in stereotactic neurosurgery. Tissue temperature elevation is most easily induced by electrical or mechanical excitation or molecular vibratory and rotational energy states in the target site. Externally applied hyperthermia devices are poorly suited to the treatment of brain tumors because of poor penetration through skull (ultrasound), unfavorable patterns of energy deposition (magnetic induction), or rapid attenuation of the incoming signal (radiative rf and microwave devices). Although tumor-to-normal brain temperature gradients might occur with such devices because of relatively decreased conductive cooling secondary to poorer tumor perfusion, the overall effect of using external heating devices would be unpredictable, and temperature elevation would be poorly localized.

The same CT-stereotactic neurosurgical techniques that permit temporary implantation of a precisely defined array of encapsulated radioisotope sources within a brain tumor (2), also permit temporary placement of microwave dipole antennas in a precise spatial array. Such antennas are designed to be linear in shape in order to fit within a conventional radioisotope afterloading catheter, so that interstitial irradiation and interstitial hyperthermia can be performed sequentially without truly increasing the invasiveness of the procedure. The lengths of the radiating antenna segments and coaxial insulation can be designed such that an essentially cylindrically divergent wave form will be optimally radiated. Two-dimensional computer simulations have been used to predict isothermal distributions about individual antennas and parallel arrays in regions of differing blood flow (Fig. 13.1), using the bioheat transfer equation (8). In this model temperature is dependent on energy deposition (a function of the electrical properties of the antennae and the absorbing tissues and the operating frequency), on thermal convection (primarily a function of the thermal gradient between the target area and surrounding tissues), and on thermal conduction by the local vasculature (a function of basal perfusion rates). Although this model is simplistic in that three-dimensional relationships and dynamic time-temperature dependent changes in vascular perfusion rates are ignored, its predictions have been reasonably accurate when tested by static phantom measurements and controlled animal experiments (9). Interstitial microwave antenna arrays (IMAA) are thus physically capable of producing highly localized elevation of temperatures in brain tumors. The magnitude of the thermal gradient which may be established between the target volume and surrounding normal brain will be dependent upon tissue electrical properties and local perfusion. The effective treatment volume will be dependent on antenna design, number, spacing, and operating frequency. Tissue attenuation of the primary wave front is directly proportional to frequency. Optimal spacing between adjacent antennae balances attenuation of the primary wavefront by permitting maximal constructive interference of convergent waves in the intervening space. At the frequencies commonly employed with IMAA systems, 633 to 2450 MHz, optimal spacing is in the 1- to 2-cm range for parallel arrays. This, fortunately, is similar to catheter spacing for interstitial ^{125}I and ^{192}Ir irradiation, allowing both modalities to be delivered sequentially through the same set of CT stereotactically placed catheters.

Predicted temperature distributions should not be entirely relied upon in clinical situations, since the latter differ greatly with respect to tissue inhomogeneities and dynamic perfusion rates. Since noninvasive thermometry does not exist, invasive temperature measurement is mandatory. Commercially available microwave antennas almost always are designed with a single thermistor located at the hottest point on the antenna. Usually, more catheters are required to achieve a satisfactory interstitial radiation dose distribution over the target volume than are required for IMAA heating, and catheters without antennas can be used for thermometry. Techniques are available for "mapping" temperatures at various spatial loci along a given catheter, either by mechanically translating a thermistor (1), or by using multiple sensor thermometry. Thus, the amount of information can be maximized from a given catheter without increasing invasiveness.

The surgical techniques for CT-stereotactic catheter placement are identical to the methodologies discussed in Chapter 4 for temporary radioisotope placement, with a few important exceptions. The distal end of the outer afterloading catheter must be exteriorized through the scalp, necessitating meticulous postoperative wound care to avoid cerebrospinal fluid (CSF) leakage and infection. The inner catheters containing the radioactive seeds are not placed during the initial operation. However, a Silastic ventricular catheter may be stereotactically

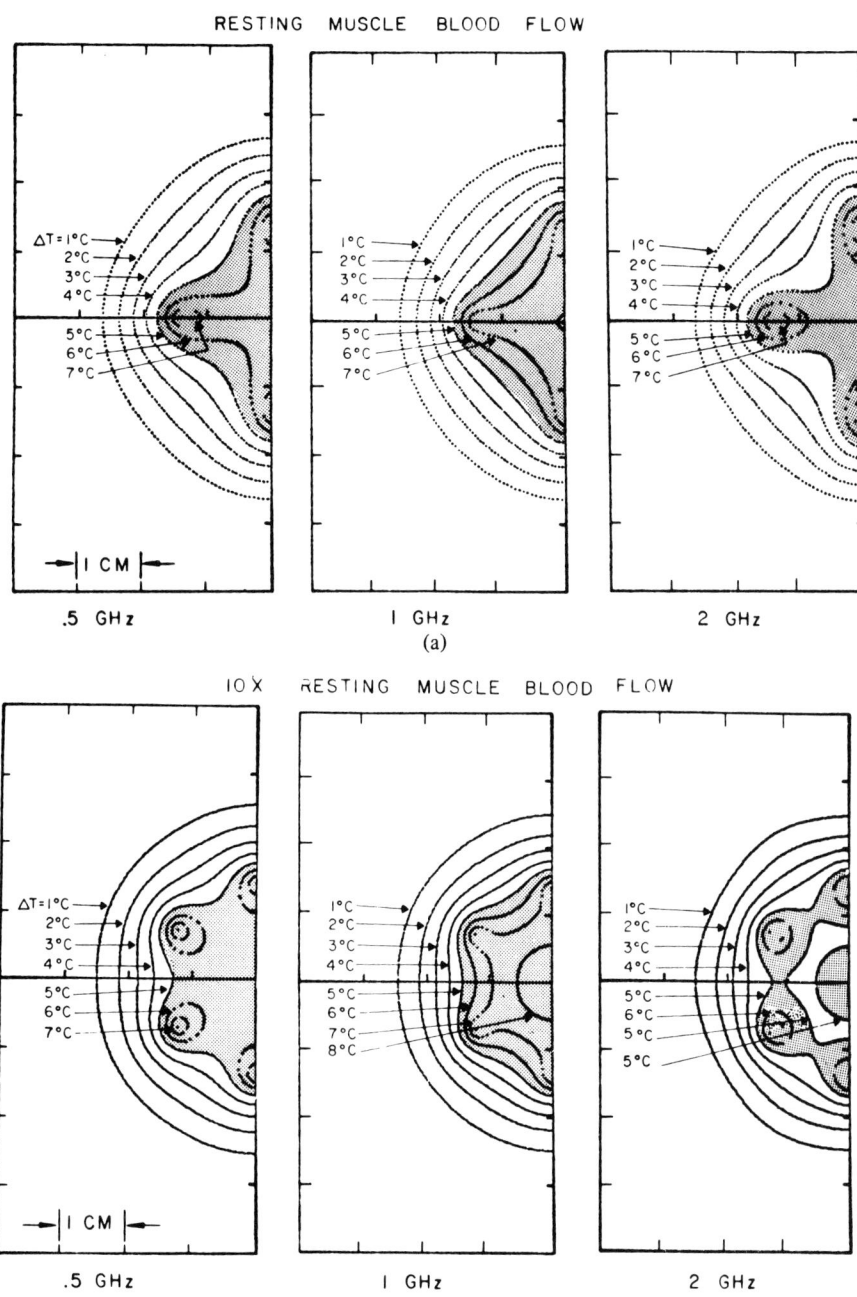

Figure 13.1. Effects of frequency on temperature distributions: $R_o = 1.414$ cm. Specific parameters: $f = 0.5$ GHz, $e = 52.7$, $o = 1.2$ mhos/m, $h = 1.93$ cm; $f = 1$ GHz, $e = 50$, o 1.3 mhos/m, $h = 1.03$ cm; $f = 2$ GHz, $e = 48$, $o = 1.94$ mhos/m, $h = 0.53$ cm. (a) Blood flow = 2.7 ml/(100 g min) (resting muscle), four antennas, $t = 15$ min. (b) Blood flow = 27 ml (100 g min) (10 x resting muscle), six antennas, $t = 5$ min. (Reprinted with permission from Strohbein JW, Trembly BS, Douple EB. Blood flow effects on the temperature distributions from an invasive microwave antenna array used in cancer therapy. IEEE Trans Biomed Engin 29: #1 649–661, 1982.)

placed through a separate drill hole for subsequent monitoring of intracranial pressure (ICP).

When the patient achieves postoperative stabilization and is alert, usually within 24 hr, the microwave antennas are inserted in the outer catheters and the target volume is heated with the general objective of maintaining minimum target temperatures of 42 to 43°C for 30 to 60 min, as measured within catheters not containing antennas, which have attained thermal equilibrium with the target tissues. Thermometry information from thermistors located on the antennas will always be artifactually higher than would be found in adjacent tissue because of attenuation of radiated waves across the catheter. Such information, however, can be useful if each individual antenna or antenna pairs are driven by independently controlled power sources. Since electromagnetic energy may be coupled more or less effectively by different antennas within an array, different antenna power levels may be required to heat the target tissues with optimal uniformity. Temperature information from the antenna thermistors can help to determine individual power levels, which are generally in the 1- to 10-W range for each antenna. Since the patient is alert, frequent neurological examinations and ICP measurement can be used for routine clinical monitoring, although electroencephalography and visually evoked potentials have been used as well.

At the conclusion of the hyperthermia session, the antennas and thermometry devices are replaced with sterile inner catheters containing the encapsulated radioisotopes, spaced to achieve optimal isodose distributions over the target volume, and glued in place. When the prescribed minimum tumor dose has been achieved, the inner catheters are carefully removed, and a second hyperthermia treatment is performed. The outer afterloading catheters are then removed, although the intraventricular catheter may be left in place if further ICP monitoring is desired. When clinical stability is evident, the patient is discharged on oral antiepileptic, antibiotic, and tapering corticosteroid regimens, and followed at frequent intervals.

CLINICAL RESULTS

Interstitial hyperthermia of human brain tumors is a new technique, and only a few series have been reported in the literature. Salcman and Samaras (6) reported the initial clinical experience with interstital microwave (2450 MHz) hyperthermia in six patients with recurrent malignant gliomas. A single antenna was used to deliver two 60-min hyperthermia treatments on alert patients after a 60-min intraoperative treatment that followed limited surgical debulking. Sophisticated CT-stereotactic placement was not employed, and detailed measurement of spatial temperature distributions was only performed in two of six patients. Complications were not severe, and consisted of one transient deterioration of existing neurological deficits, and two CSF leaks, which required surgical repair. Objective decrease in tumor volume was documented by CT in three out of six patients; however, the contributions of surgical debulking alone and subsequent or concurrent chemotherapy (three of six patients) to response rate were likely to have been significant. Nevertheless, survivals of 6, 7, 18+, 18+, 18+, and 27+ months postimplant were observed, which is rather encouraging.

Winter *et al.* (10) reported 12 patients with a variety of recurrent brain tumors who were treated with a range of 1- to 12-microwave (2450 MHz) interstitial hyperthermia treatments, using a range of one to six antennas. Only 2 of 12 of these pateints underwent CT-stereotactic catheter placement, and no thermometry data were reported. No acute or chronic toxicity was observed, and relief of headaches was noted in 5 of 12 patients, as well as objective neurological improvement in 5 of 12 patients. Postmortem findings in two patients were presented, which demonstrated regions of local necrosis, however, the lack of thermometry and CT-stereotactic confirmation of antenna location does not really permit any scientific conclusion to be drawn from this information.

Roberts *et al.* (4) have presented the most complete report to date of a Phase I clinical trial of interstitial thermoradiotherapy that

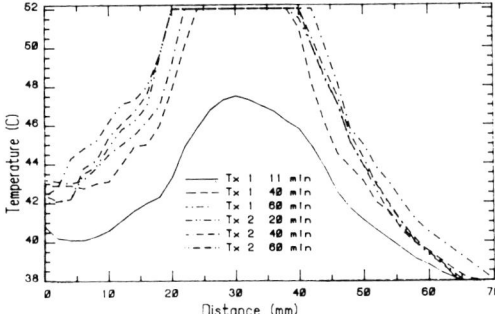

Figure 13.2. Temperature distribution during hyperthermia treatment (Tx) in case 3. Medial margin of tumor (distance = 0) was maintained at 42° to 43° C after the warm-up period. Left lateral tumor margin was estimated to be at 55 mm. (Reprinted with permission from Roberts DW, Coughlin CT, Wong TZ, Fratkin MD, Douple EP, Strohbein JW: Interstitial hyperthermia and iridium brachytherapy in treatment of malignant glioma: A phase I clincical trial. *J Neurosurg* 64: 581–587, 1986.)

employed CT-stereotactic localization, extensive preplanning of both temperature and isotope distributions, rigorous documentation of temperatures on the antennas as well as at multiple points within the treatment volume, and clinical monitoring of ICP and electroencephalography. A minimum of four microwave (915 MHz) antennas were used to treat each of three patients with untreated and three patients with recurrent malignant gliomas. Minimum "boundary" radioisotopes (^{192}Ir) doses ranged from 17.5 to 65.8 Gy. Minimum boundary temperatures of 39 to 43°C were reported and maximal temperatures of 46 to 52°C were observed, usually in the center of the IMAA. Figure 13.2 illustrates an example of the temperature distributions which were documented in one case. One patient could not be adequately heated because of significant temperature-dependent transient arm paresis. Three other patients experienced transient deterioration of existing neurological deficits, and one other patient developed a cutaneous CSF leak and bacterial meningitis which responded to antibiotic therapy. One patient developed temperature-dependent ICP elevation to 30 cm of water above baseline during the first treatment, and 17 cm above baseline during the subsequent treatment. ICP measurements during and after interstitial hyperthermia were not significantly different from baseline in the other five patients. Follow-up CT scans generally demonstrated decreased contrast enhancement and increased "edema." Survivals of 5, 10+, 12, 13, and 16 months postimplant were observed, with one patient dying of unrelated causes at 1.5 months.

These studies are all quite preliminary, but do demonstrate that interstitial brain tumor hyperthermia is technically feasible, and many of the clinical responses have been encouraging. No fatal complications have been reported in the 24 cases discussed above, although the incidences of transient neurological deterioration and CSF leak are not insignificant. Major questions that remain unanswered involve optimal achievement of desired thermal distributions, optimal prescribed "thermal dose" (7), and optimal radiation dose when delivered with thermal enhancement. Precisely quantitated CT-stereotactic information and correlation with rigorous thermometric measurement are critical to the scientific determination of the solutions to these dilemma. Precise definition of "tumor volume" is, of course, a continuing challenge, as with any other local brain tumor treatment technique. When the quality assurance and dose questions have been satisfactorily answered, CT-stereotactic interstitial microwave hyperthermia should be able to be tested in controlled prospective clinical trials.

REFERENCES

1. Gibbs FA Jr: Thermal mapping in experimental cancer treatment with hyperthermia: description and use of a semiautomatic system. *Int J Radiol Oncl Biol Physiol* 9: 1057–1063, 1983.
2. Gutin PH, Phillips TL, Hosobuchi Y, Wara WM Leibel SA, Levin VA, Weaver KA, Lamb S: Removable high activity ^{125}-Iodine implants for the brachytherapy of recurrent malignant brain tumors. *J Neurosurg* 60: 61–68, 1984.
3. Hahn GM: *Hyperthermia and Cancer.* New York, Plenum, 1982.
4. Roberts DW, Coughlin CT, Wong TZ, Fratkin MD, Douple EB, Strohbein JW: Interstitial hyperthermia and iridium brachytherapy in

treatment of malignant glioma: A phase I clinical trial. *J Neurosurg* 64: 581–587, 1986.
5. Salcman M, Samaras GM: Hyperthermia for brain tumors: Biophysical rationale. *Neurosurgery* 9: 327–335, 1981.
6. Salcman M, Samaras GM: Interstitial microwave hyperthermia for brain tumors. Results of a phase-I clinical trial. *J Neurooncol* 1: 225–236, 1983.
7. Sapozink MD, Gibbs FA Jr, Sandhu TS Practical thermal dosimetry. *Int J Radiol Oncol Biol Physiol* 11: 555–560, 1985.
8. Strohbein JW, Trembly BS, Douple EB: Blood flow effects on the temperature distributions from an invasive microwave antenna array used in cancer therapy. *IEEE Trans Biomed Englin* 29: 649–661, 1982.
9. Strohbehn JW: Temperature distributions from interstitial RF electrode hyperthermia systems: theoretical predictions. *Intl J Radiol Oncol Biol Physiol* 9: 1655–1667, 1983.
10. Winter A, Laing J, Paglione R, Sterzer F: Microwave hyperthermia for brain tumors. *Neurosurgery* 17: 387–399, 1985.

Chapter 14

Special Stereotactic Techniques: Stereotactic Laser Resection of Deep-Seated Tumors

P.J. KELLY, M.D., B.A. KALL, M.S., and S.J. GOERSS, B.S.

INTRODUCTION

Computer reconstruction of planar tumor boundaries defined by stereotactic computed tomography (CT) scanning and magnetic resonance imaging (MRI) allow the representation of a tumor volume in stereotactic space. This volume may then be resected by a stereotactically directed CO_2 laser since its beam can be mechanically directed and computer monitored in three-dimensional (3-D) space. The CO_2 laser is particularly applicable to the stereotactic method because of its precision in cutting and vaporization, especially when applied to the resection of intraaxial neoplasms from neurologically important areas.

We began stereotactic CO_2 laser resections of deep-seated intracranial lesions in January 1980. As clinical experience was acquired, technical innovations were incorporated into the procedures, which increased the facility and accuracy with which these operations were performed. Our first procedures were based on coronal and sagittal reconstructions of CT data superimposed on stereotactic x-ray pictures (5, 6). Preoperative treatment planning for these early operations was cumbersome and tedious, and intraoperative monitoring was done by time consuming anteroposterior (AP) and lateral teleradiographs. In order to facilitate preoperative treatment planning and streamline intraoperative calculations and graphic displays, we incorporated an operating room computer system into the procedure. The computer has proven itself invaluable for the transposition of volumetric information derived from axial stereotactic CT scans into 3-D space (1, 4, 7–9). In addition, the position of a stereotactically directed CO_2 laser is monitored by computer and displayed on an operating room computer graphics terminal in relation to computer-generated reconstructions of the tumor sliced orthogonal to the surgical approach. Later, we developed a servomotor-controlled stereotactic frame which allows rapid stereotactic access to multiple regions within a tumor volume for computer-monitored laser vaporization. Thus, it was theoretically possible to remove all CT-detectable neoplasm through a transcortical approach opening smaller than the tumor itself.

The following report will describe our current methodology for computer-assisted stereotactic laser microsurgical extirpation of deep-seated lesions. In addition we will report on the clinical results in the first 191 patients treated by this method.

MATERIAL AND METHODS

Data Base Acquisition

Patients undergo stereotactic CT scanning and MRI with their heads fixed in CT-

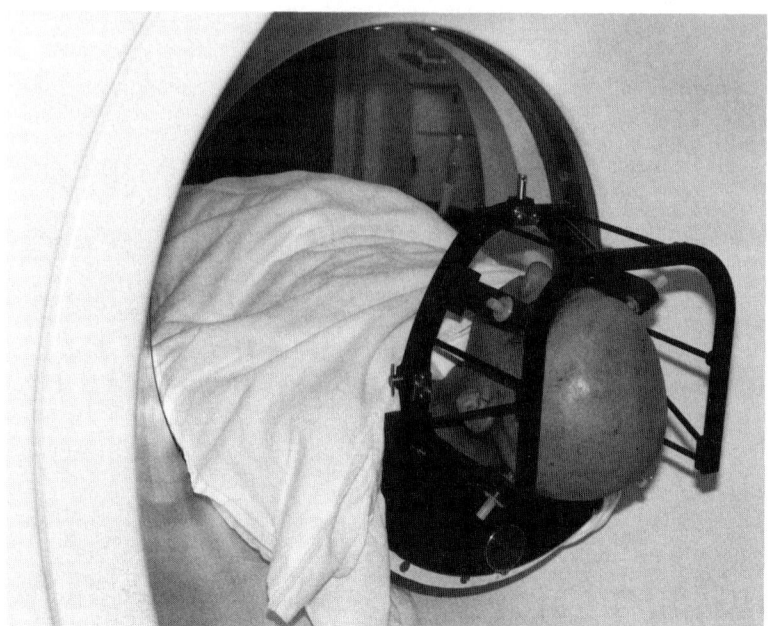

Figure 14.1. CT-compatible stereotactic head holder mounted in a CT table adaptation plate on a GE 8800 CT scanner.

and MRI-compatible stereotactic head holders. CT- and MRI-localizing devices attach to the head holders, and create a series of nine reference artifacts on each CT and MRI slice (Fig. 14.1). The archived CT data tapes are input to the operating room computer system (Independent Physicians Display Console for General Electric 8800 CT Scanner—Data General Eclipse S140 with 192 megabyte disc and Ramtek Raster Display Terminal). The surgeon digitizes each CT/MRI slice which demonstrates the tumor as follows: First, the localizing artifacts on each CT and MRI slice are digitized automatically by the computer-utilizing cursor and trackball subsystem of the Ramtek display terminal (Fig. 14.2). A tumor volume is created in stereotactic space by an interpolation program which may be sliced orthogonal to any specified surgical approach angle. Furthermore, the computer calculates the volume of the lesion and the x, y, and z mechanical adjustments of the stereotactic frame, which bring a selected point within the tumor volume into the focal point of an arc-quadrant stereotactic frame.

The stereotactic surgical instrument consists of an arc-quadrant frame in which the patient's head is moved with three degrees of freedom to place an intracranial target point into the center of the sphere described by arc and quadrant. Movement of the head in three dimensions is controlled by servomotors and displayed by a digital calibration system (Acu-Rite, Bausch and Lomb). The surgical laser is directed from a carriage which runs perpendicular to the tangent of a 400-mm arc. The center of the arc is at the focal point of the stereotactic frame. An operating microscope is also fixed to the carriage (Acu-Rite, Bausch and Lomb). The laser beam is controlled by x, y galvanometers operated by a remote joystick. The position of the laser beam is relayed to the computer system by optical encoders activated by the joystick (Fig. 14.3).

The surgical procedure is performed under general anesthesia through a linear scalp incision. Prior to the actual craniotomy, the tumor is first traversed by a stereotactic biopsy cannula directed through a twist drill hole and a series of tiny stainless steel balls at 5-mm intervals along the surgical viewline are deposited (Fig.

LASER RESECTION OF DEEP-SEATED TUMORS 235

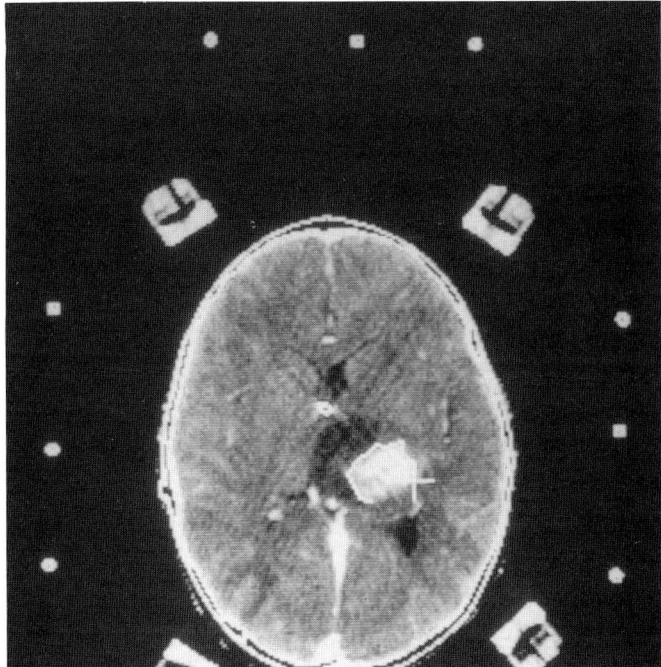

Figure 14.2. Each CT slice demonstrates nine reference marks. Height of slice is related to distance of middle reference marks from others on each localizing set. Reference marks are digitized by an intensity detection program. Surgeon outlines boundaries of tumor on each CT slice, utilizing cursor and trackball.

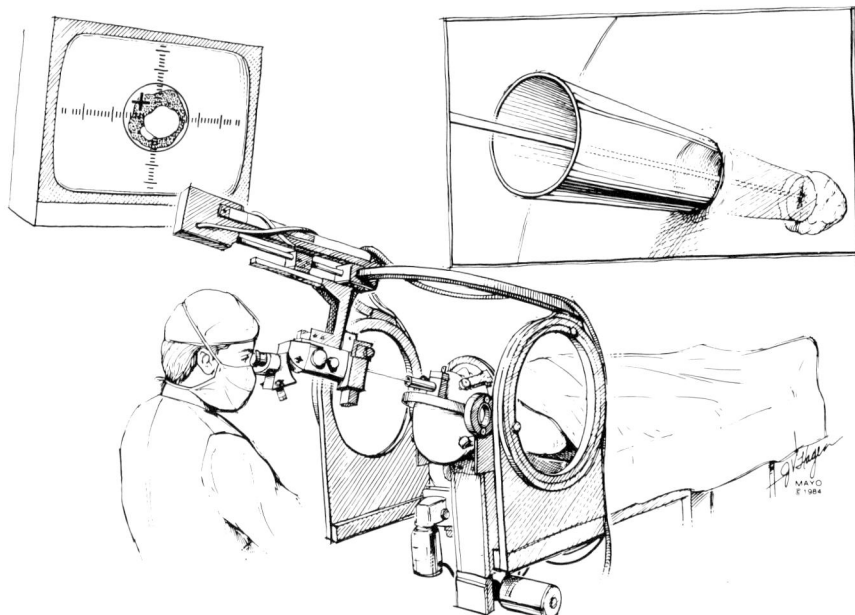

Figure 14.3. Custom arc-quadrant stereotactic frame mounted on operating table. Three-dimensional mechanical slide moves head to place an intracranial target point in focal point of a 135-mm and a 400-mm arc-quadrant. Microscope and laser manipulator mechanism run on a carriage which travels perpendicular to a tangent of 400-mm arc. Tumors are vaporized by stereotactically directed laser aimed through stereotactically held retractor. Computer display monitor shows position of laser (cursor), retractor (circle), and slice from CT- (and/or MRI-) defined tumor volume. Tumor volume sliced perpendicular to surgical viewline at level of depth to which retractor has been inserted.

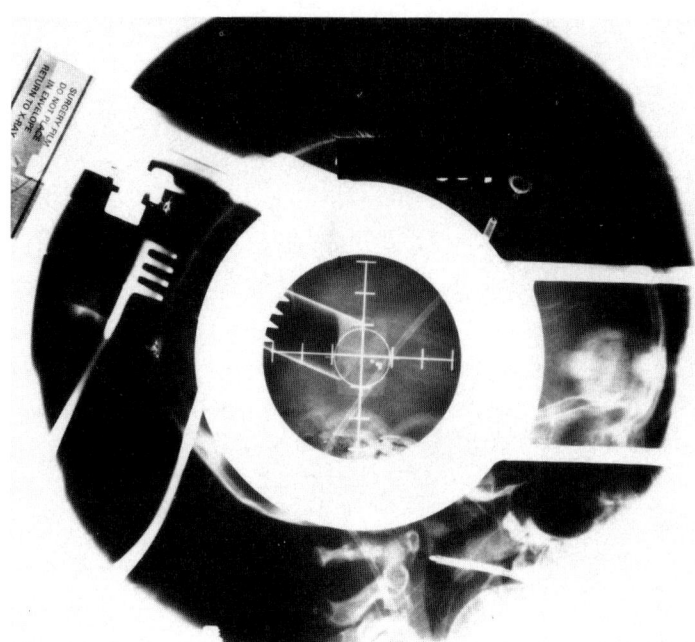

Figure 14.4. Lateral stereotactic teleradiograph showing stereotactic retractor. Also demonstrating position of steel reference balls which were inserted along surgical viewline.

14.4). AP and lateral radiographs are obtained and used as reference for movements of the tumor within the intracranial space following removal of a circular trephine plug and opening of the dura. An incision in the brain is made with the CO_2 laser and deepened as the microscope and laser directed toward the focal point of the frame are advanced by the carriage. At the outer border of the tumor, a stereotactic retractor is placed which creates a shaft through the brain to the tumor. The tumor is vaporized slice by slice progressing from the most superficial layer to the deepest. The surgeon monitors the position of the laser (represented by the cursor) in relationship to reformatted planar tumor boundaries on an operating room graphics monitor (Fig. 14.5). Ultimately, a cavity is produced and is documented by AP and lateral teleradiographs. These may be compared with coronal and sagittal reconstructions of CT data through the tumor.

RESULTS

One hundred ninety-seven (197) computer-assisted stereotactic craniotomies have been performed on 191 patients since 1980. Five patients underwent repeat procedures for residual (3 patients) and recurrent (2 patients) tumors, and one of these patients underwent a third procedure for recurrent tumor. Patients ranged in age from 2 to 78 yr, with an average of 46.8 yr. Lesion locations are illustrated in Fig. 14.6, and histologies are listed in Table 14.1. Postoperative contrast-enhanced CT scans failed to demonstrate residual contrast-enhancing tumor in 38 of 42 patients with grade 4 astrocytomas, 11 of 14 patients with grade 3 astrocytomas, and all of the 12 patients having grade 2 pilocytic astrocytomas. The remainder of the grade 2 astrocytomas were low density on CT. Postoperative CT scanning revealed that a significant internal decompression (greater than 80% of the original tumor volume) was achieved in all of the oligodendrogliomas. Complete resection of all metastatic tumors, vascular, and miscellaneous lesions was confirmed by postoperative CT scanning. Figure 14.7 demonstrates examples of pre- and postoperative CT scans obtained in this group of patients. Neurological ex-

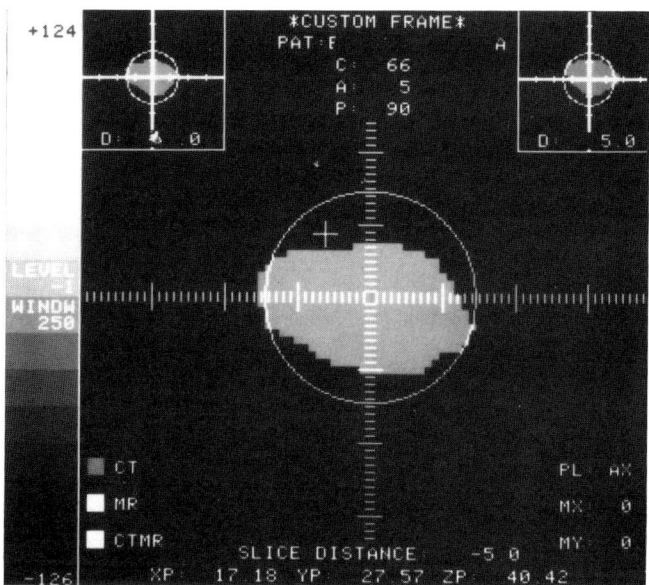

Figure 14.5. Computer-generated display showing section of tumor sliced along surgical viewline, outline of stereotactic retractor, and position of surgical laser in reference to tumor represented by a cursor. "Look ahead" sequence shows deeper slices of tumor.

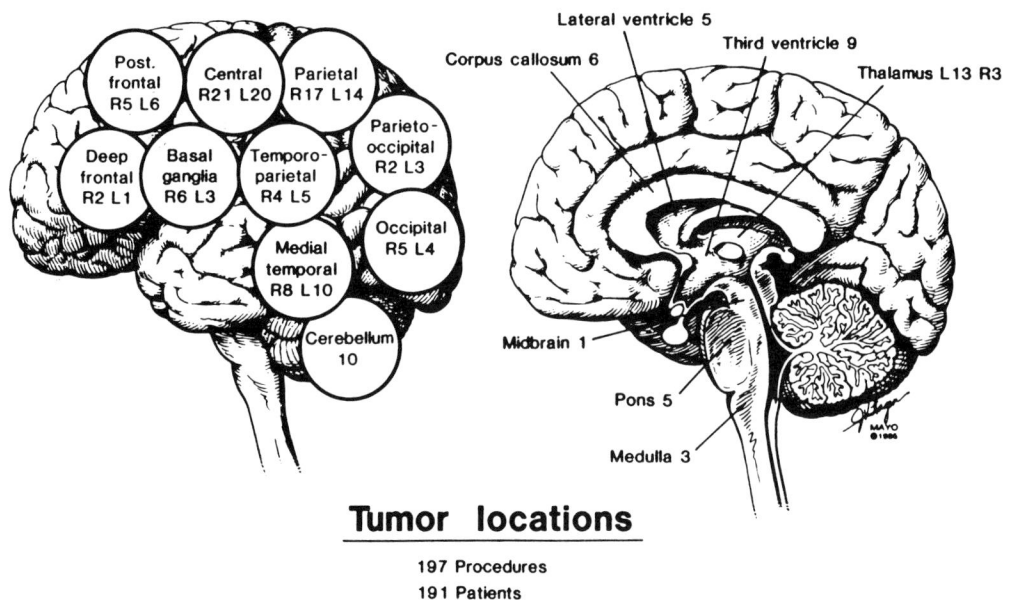

Tumor locations

197 Procedures
191 Patients

Figure 14.6. Location of lesion in 140 patients undergoing 146 procedures.

TABLE 14.1
Tumor Histology in 191 Patients Undergoing Computer-Assisted Stereotactic Resections

Astrocytoma grade 4	42
Astrocytoma grade 3	14
Astrocytoma grade 2	32
Metastatic	48
Oligodendroglioma	10
Vascular	22
Miscellaneous	23
Lymphoma	2
Tub, sclerosis	4
Meningioma	4
Abscess	3
Choroid plexis papilloma	1
Colloid cyst	2
Ganglioglioma	3
Radiation necrosis	2
Others	2
Total	191

aminations performed 1 week following the 197 procedures revealed that 101 patients had improved from preoperative levels, 77 patients were neurologically unchanged postoperatively (52 had been normal preoperatively and remained normal postoperatively, 25 patients had preoperative neurological deficits which did not improve postoperatively).

Nineteen (19) patients were neurologically worse: seven patients developed superior quadrant visual field deficits following posterior temporal approaches to medial temporal or thalamic lesions, one patient had a complete homonymous hemianopsia following an occipital approach to a posterior thalamic lesion, and 11 patients experienced worsening of neurological deficits noted preoperatively. Three (3) deaths occurred within 1 month following surgery:

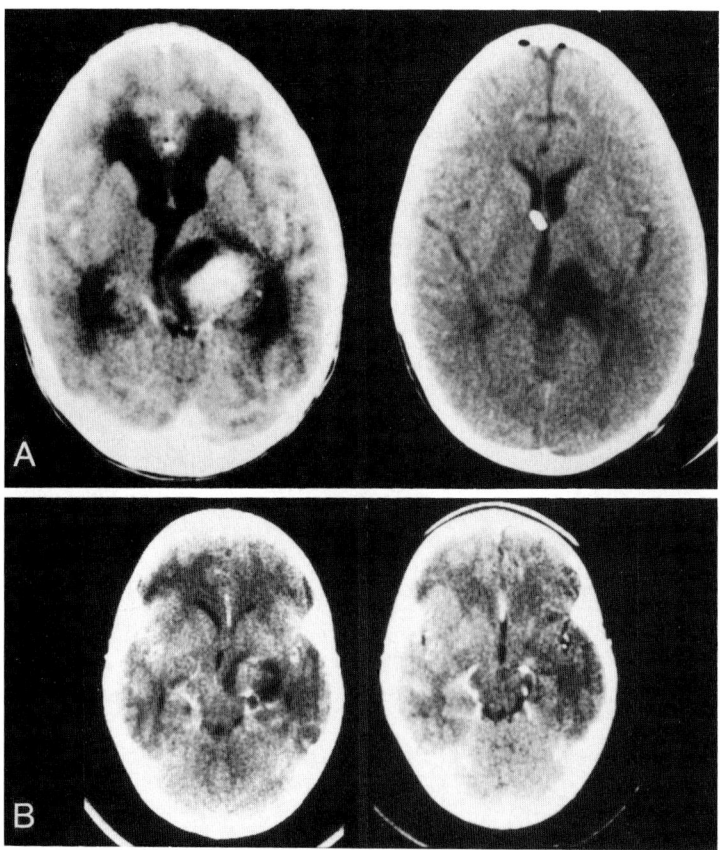

Figure 14.7. Representative pre- and postoperative CT scan in two patients having thalamic pilocytic astrocytomas.

one from massive brainstem edema following removal of a ventral thalamic astrocytoma with brainstem infiltration apparent on MRI, one from a ventricular infection after resection of a previously irradiated teratoma from the third ventricle, and one from massive pulmonary embolis 2 weeks following resection of a thalamic cavernous hemangioma.

DISCUSSION

Stereotactic laser microsurgical resection of deep-seated intracranial lesions allows maintenance of 3-D surgical orientation in subcortical procedures. Tumors in important subcortical areas may be approached through nonessential brain tissue and the resection of the lesion is precise and monitored not only by the visualization of the surgeon but also computer graphics and teleradiography. Thus, aggressive and safe resection of deep-seated neoplasms is possible (Fig. 14.7) (8).

With the stereotactic method described, it is possible to resect all tumor detected by CT scanning. Nevertheless, correlation studies of histology from stereotactic serial biopsies and CT-defined tumor boundaries indicated that the CT scan may not accurately represent the histological limits of primary intracranial neoplasms (2). Our experience indicates that the histological boundaries of primary glial neoplasms extend beyond the boundaries indicated by CT scanning. Thus, some form of adjuvent therapy must be directed at the cells of the neoplasm remaining in the hypodense zone surrounding the area of contrast enhancement, which is resected by the stereotactic procedure. Nevertheless, a significant reduction of tumor cell burden may favorably influence survival and response to external radiation and chemotherapy. In addition, photoradiation therapy is considered to supplement standard radiation therapy and chemotherapy (3). We believe that this will further reduce the tumor cell population that remains following CT-based stereotactic laser resection of the lesion.

SUMMARY

The CO_2 laser has been incorporated into a computer-assisted stereotactic system for precision resection of deep-seated intraaxial neoplasms. Stereotactic CT scanning provides a precise 3-D tumor volumetric data base in relationship to a custom arc-quadrant stereotactic frame. A CO_2 laser beam is directed by the stereotactic instrument. It is monitored by an interactive computer graphic system in relation to boundaries of the tumor volume, which has been sliced orthogonal to the surgical viewline. Theoretically, the procedure allows removal of all tumor identified by CT scanning. One hundred ninety-seven of these procedures have been performed on 191 patients having a variety of neoplasms in various deep-seated locations. Postoperative results have been satisfactory in regards to the postoperative condition of the patient in consideration of the completeness of tumor removal achieved.

REFERENCES

1. Alker GJ, Kelly PJ, Kall BA, Goerss SJ: Stereotactic laser ablation of intracranial lesions. *Am J Neuroradiol* 4: 727–730, 1983.
2. Daumas-Duport C, Monsaingeon V, Szenthe L, Szikla G: A double histological code of gliomas according to malignancy and 3-D configuration, as an aid to therapeutic decision and assessment of results. *Appl Neurophysiol* 45: 431–437, 1982.
3. Dougherty TJ, Kaufman JE, Goldfarb A, Weishaupt KR, Boyle D, Mittleman A; Photoradiation therapy for the treatment of malignant tumors. *Canc Res* 38: 2628–2635, 1978.
4. Goerss S, Kelly PJ, Kall B, Alker GJ Jr: A computed tomographic stereotactic adaption system. *Neurosurg* 10: 375–379, 1982.
5. Kelly PJ, Alker GJ Jr: A stereotactic approach to deep seated CNS neoplasms using the carbon dioxide laser. *Surg Neurol* 15: 331–334, 1981.
6. Kelly PJ, Alker GJ Jr: A microstereotactic approach to deep-seated arteriovenous malformation: case report and technical note. *Surg Neurol* 17: 206–262, 1982.
7. Kelly PJ, Alker GJ Jr, Goerss SJ: Computer assisted stereotactic laser microsurgery for the treatment of intracranial neoplasms. *Neurosurg* 10: 324–331, 1982.
8. Kelly PJ, Alker GJ Jr, Kall B, Goerss S: Precision resection of intra-axial CNS lesions by CT-based stereotactic craniotomy and computer monitored CO_2 laser. *Acta Neurochir* 68: 1–9, 1983.
9. Kelly PJ, Kall B, Goerss S, Earnest F: Computer-assisted stereotaxic resection of intra-axial brain neoplasms. *J Neurosurg* 64: 427–439, 1986.

Chapter 15

Special Stereotactic Techniques: Stereotactic Interstitial Brachytherapy

PHILIP H. GUTIN, M.D., NICHOLAS M. BARBARO, M.D., and STEVEN A. LEIBEL, M.D.

INTRODUCTION

Interstitial brachytherapy has been used extensively for the treatment of prostate, breast, head and neck, and gynecological tumors (3). Because most malignant gliomas recur locally without causing the difficult oncological problem of widespread metastatic deposits seen in many systemic cancers, and because radiation therapy is the most effective therapy for malignant gliomas, there has been an increased interest recently in the use of brachytherapy for brain tumors (4). The principal advantage of brachytherapy, the ability to deliver a high, focal dose of radiation with relative sparing of normal tissue (9), is the same for brachytherapy at any site. Yet, because of the relative inaccessibility of intracranial lesions, brain tumor brachytherapy is more difficult to perform than brachytherapy at other sites. The recent availability of computed tomography (CT)-directed stereotactic systems makes it possible to implant radioactive sources into targets within brain tumors with great precision. Over the past 6 years, we have used these techniques to perform more than 250 implantations into primary and metastatic malignant brain tumors. The approach has been used both to administer a second dose of radiation to recurrent tumor and to "boost" the focal dose to tumor immediately after conventional teletherapy. In this chapter, we discuss our promising results and the special problems of and constraints upon this method.

ADVANTAGES OF INTERSTITIAL BRACHYTHERAPY

Radiation from implanted sources is delivered continuously at the low dose of approximately 1 cGy/min compared with the 200 cGy/min delivered from conventional cobalt sources or linear accelerators. The lower, continuous dose rates used in brachytherapy and physical principles allow the total dose to the lesion to be delivered over a few days rather than over the several months needed to deliver a course of conventional teletherapy at high dose rates. The radiophysical advantages of brachytherapy are obvious. An implanted isotope delivers a maximum radiation by dose to the tumor, while the dose to surrounding tissue is dramatically reduced. This is the result of attenuation of radiation by interposed tissues and by the constraints of the inverse square law, which states that the intensity of radiation from any point source is inversely proportional to the square of the distance from the source. Moreover, as the dose rate is lowered, the biological effect of radiation is reduced, principally because tissue exposed to the low-dose rate radiation can repair sublethal damage during the time of exposure. Normal tissues may repair sublethal damage more efficiently than tumor tissue does, which may explain the efficacy of brachytherapy against a variety of tumors and the relative sparing of exposed surrounding normal tissue.

CHOICE OF ISOTOPE

After the early experience with implantation of radium sources for treatment of gliomas, gold 198 and iridium 192 (^{192}Ir) were used most extensively for the interstitial irradation of brain tumors. ^{192}Ir is still receiving considerable attention for this purpose, but iodine-125 (^{125}I), which emits characteristic x-rays of a far lower energy (27–35 keV) than the gamma rays emitted by ^{192}Ir (300–610 keV), is preferred by several groups. The lower energy of photons emitted from ^{125}I simplifies the problems inherent in protecting medical personnel (12). ^{125}I is provided as a standard low activity source (0.5mCi) that has proven useful for permanent implantation into lower grade gliomas. The large number of these low activity sources necessary to treat the faster-growing, more malignant gliomas, however, makes them less practical. Higher activity ^{125}I sources (30–50 mCi) are available by special order (Medical Product Division, 3M Company, St. Paul, MN); implantation with a few sources provides higher, more suitable dose rates. High-activity sources cannot be left implanted permanently because of the unacceptable high dose that would be guaranteed by this strategy. For this reason, we implant high-activity ^{125}I sources housed in catheters that can be removed after the appropriate dose has been delivered. A number of centers now have experience with removable, high-activity sources for malignant brain tumors (1, 2, 5, 8, 14, 15).

PATIENT SELECTION

Tumors are selected for treatment based on a high quality, contrast-enhanced CT scan and, in general, are supratentorial, small, well circumscribed lesions that do not extend to or across the midline. Although we have no limit on the maximum size of a lesion that may be treated, tumors less than 3.5 cm in diameter are best suited for treatment. Tumors in the corpus callosum tend to invade the deep white matter bilaterally and diffusely, and the total volume of these lesions is difficult to predict from CT scans; therefore, accurate treatment planning for brachytherapy is impossible because isodose contours cannot be determined. Tumors with subependymal spread, multifocal tumors, and posterior fossa tumors are not treated with brachytherapy.

IMPLANTATION TECHNIQUE AND RADIATION DOSIMETRY

By using a CT-stereotactic system, targets for implantation can be selected based on the tumor geometry seen on a CT scan, and sources may be implanted precisely within the tumor, using stereotactic guidance. When the stereotactic system is integrated with a brachytherapy treatment-planning computer program (see below), stereotactic targets may be determined after various arrays and the corresponding radiation isodose lines are simulated and displayed on the computer screen. A multiplanar appreciation of the tumor is more important in interstitial brachytherapy than in tumor biopsy procedures. Reformatting of dosimetry simulations in sagittal and coronal planes provides information necessary to perform the implantation.

We now use the Brown-Roberts-Wells (BRW) stereotactic system (10) (Trent Wells Inc., South Gate, CA) for implantation of ^{125}I sources. The entire procedure is performed under local anesthesia in adults and under general anesthesia in children. The patient is scanned with the localizing system fixed to the skull. We take 3mm cuts that begin well above and end well below the lesion. The computer tape from the CT scanner is taken to the Department of Radiation Oncology and read into the planning computer.

Our treatment-planning computer program includes a VAX computer-based package that has evolved from extensive modifications of software provided by Drs. Sturm and Schlegel of the German Cancer Research Center in Heidelberg (16). Hardware includes a VAX-11/780 computer, an FPS array processor, and a Lexidata 3700 color display system. The CT-data tape is read directly by the computer. Because we implant high-activity sources housed in

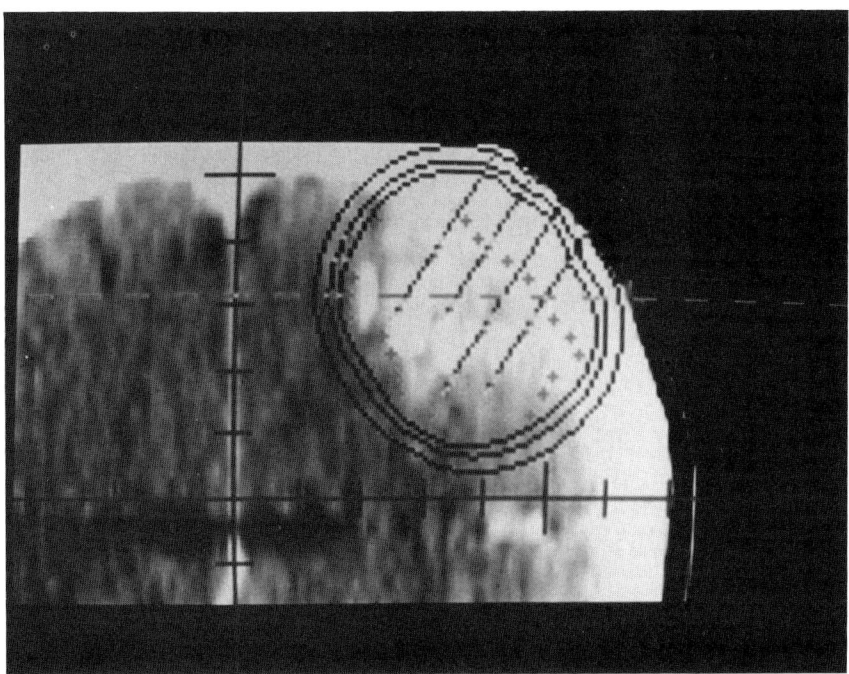

Figure 15.1. Treatment-planning computer simulation for a four catheter implantation into a left parietal glioblastoma. Isodose curves are for 50 cGy/hr (inner), 40 cGy/hr (middle), and 30 cGy/hr (outer). The computer program generates the target coordinates and the BRW angles for each catheter simulated.

catheters, the program provides us the opportunity to plan catheter arrays (number of catheters, catheter location, number of sources, source strengths, source spacing) prospectively on CT images projected onto the computer display, which allows visualization of the isodose curves created by the arrays on axial or reformatted images (Fig. 15.1). Source strengths from our bank of ^{125}I sources and their distribution are chosen to deliver a minimum tumor dose rate of 40 to 60 cGY/hr to a distance of 0.5 cm beyond the periphery of the tumor. When the lesion is seen to be well covered by the appropriate isodose curves of one of the simulated arrays, the stereotactic coordinates of the catheter targets are generated rapidly and trajectories planned based on either skull entry points selected from the display screen or on a desired azimuth and declination; these correspond to the BRW and BRWT programs in the traditional BRW stereotactic system. Integration of the necessary calculations of the BRW stereotactic system into our treatment-planning software has expedited this process. For a "typical" tumor, 4 to 6 catheters, each containing several sources and spacers, are implanted (Fig. 15.2).

A coaxial afterloaded silicone catheter system consisting of an outer catheter placed initially and an inner catheter that contains sources is used to hold them within the often soft necrotic tumor center and to allow removal of sources after the desired dose has been delivered (7). After the number of sources to be used and their spacing have been determined, they are loaded into the inner catheter, and the entire assembly is autoclaved.

Using stereotactic guidance, the outer catheter is inserted into the tumor with the aid of a removable metal stylet through either burr or twistdrill holes. The choice between the burr hole and twistdrill technique depends on the possible presence of major vascular structures beneath the site of implantation. Burr holes are recommended for implantation over the temporal lobe near the Sylvian fissure and the parasagittal region where large bridging veins are present, and twistdrill holes can be used at

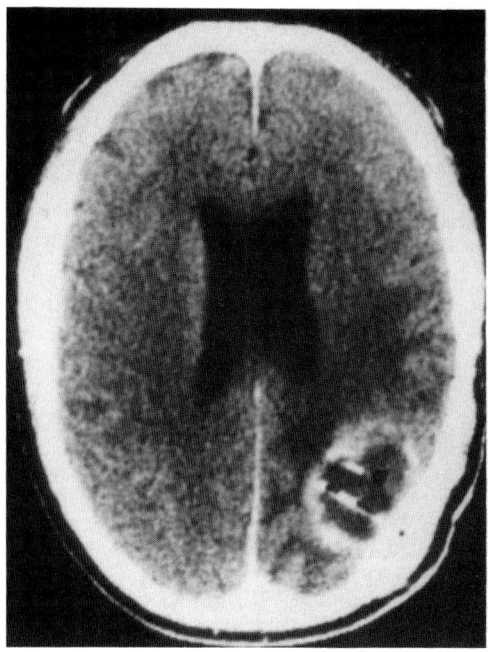 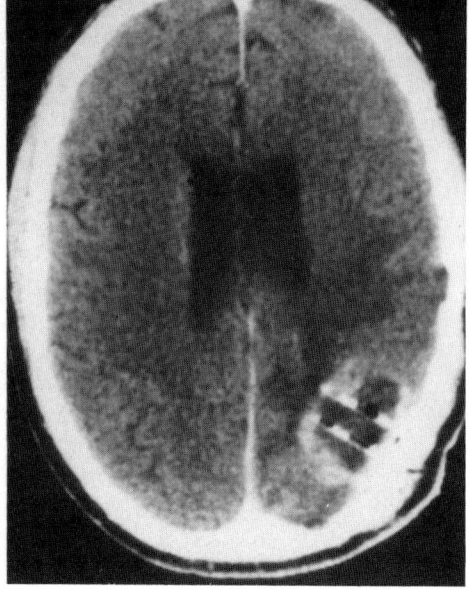

Figure 15.2. CT scan that localizes the position of the ^{125}I source in four catheters implanted into a left parietal glioblastoma. Two catheters each containing three sources can be seen at an inferior (left) and two at a more superior (right) position within the tumor.

other sites. Before radioactive sources are loaded, the outer catheters are implanted and glued to the Silastic ring through which they pass. The ring is then either cemented to the skull if a burr hole is used or sutured to the skull if a twistdrill technique is used. After all outer catheters are fixed in position, the inner catheters holding sources are carefully placed and cemented to the outer catheter. Care must be taken to ensure that the inner catheter slides to the bottom of the outer catheter. Any stricture in the outer catheter that may be created by bone or dura will prevent the inner catheter from being properly positioned, which will adversely affect dosimetry.

The patient is isolated in a private room that is surveyed by a radiation physicist who determines the safe exposure time to nurses and visitors. A helmet lined with lead foil is worn by the patient when visitors or medical personnel enter the room. Anticonvulsant medications must be monitored carefully because manipulation of tumor during implantation may lead to an increase in the number of seizures in the early postoperative period.

After implantation, a CT scan is obtained to confirm that sources have been placed accurately, and orthogonal radiographs are obtained to index source relationships. These data are converted by a computer program into dose rate contours in any plane through the tumor volume. The implantation time necessary to deliver the desired dose is calculated, and the catheters are removed either in the operating room if a burr hole was used or in the patient's room if a twistdrill technique was used. Patients are usually discharged the day after sources are removed.

RESULTS

Between 1980 and 1986, 77 patients with recurrent malignant gliomas—42 with anaplastic astrocytoma and 35 with glioblastoma multiforme—were treated with temporarily implanted, high-activity ^{125}I sources. At the time of analysis, 45% of patients with anaplastic astrocytoma and 34% of patients with glioblastoma were alive (median follow up of 13 and 9 months, respectively). The median survival after brachytherapy for recurrence was 22 months for patients with anaplastic astrocytoma and 14.5 months for those with glioblastoma multiforme.

Twenty-seven of 77 patients (35%) required reoperation after brachtherapy because their neurological condition deteriorated and because there was evidence of an increase in the size of their lesions on CT scans, consistent with either focal radiation necrosis or tumor progression. Time to reoperation ranged from 9 to 80 weeks (median of 34 weeks). At reoperation, lesions were generally firm and avascular. Patients generally improved after reoperation. In most instances, histopathological evaluation of resected material showed a combination of radiation-induced necrotic tissue and recurrent tumor. There was no correlation between the histopathology of resected material and outcome, however. Compared with patients harboring the same tumor type who did not have subsequent surgery, reoperated patients generally had a significant improvement in survival. In addition, despite the presence of apparently viable tumor in resected specimens in most patients, in many instances, tumor cells present did not grow in culture, which suggests that while radiation did not kill these cells, many of them apparently lost the growth characteristics that led to rapid tumor recurrence.

Complications in 77 patients treated with brachytherapy included infection in six patients, wound breakdown in two, acute cerebral edema in two, and intracranial hemorrhage in one. Preliminary evidence suggests that the incidence of infection may be reduced by the routine use of perioperative antibiotics.

Based on the promising results for our treatment of recurrent gliomas with removable ^{125}I sources, we have begun a study through the Northern California Oncology Group in which aggressive brachytherapy is used near the beginning of treatment rather than at the time of recurrence. Patients are irradiated using conventional teletherapy with 60 Gy of radiation to the tumor volume, administered concomitantly with hydroxyurea as a radiosensitizer. This was followed within 2 weeks by brachytherapy to deliver an additional minimum tumor dose of 60 Gy. A 12-month course of cyclical chemotherapy with procarbazine (CCNU), and vincristine is then administered. This therapeutic approach is based on our previous best-treatment protocol that combines external irradiation, hydroxyurea, and the cyclic chemotherapy regimen.

The risk of focal radiation necrosis in patients receiving the aggressive treatment described above is unknown as is the extent of neurological deficit that might be induced or exacerbated by such treatment. Unfortunately, the usual criteria for evaluating patients for tumor recurrence do not distinguish between recurrent disease and focal radiation necrosis. Positron emission tomography (PET) scanning may help distinguish between these two lesions. Our experience suggests that surgery will be helpful in ameliorating these complications.

More than 80 patients have been placed on the protocol, but the length of follow-up is insufficient for analysis at this time. When analysis is possible, it must show brachytherapy to be dramatically superior in patients with well circumscribed tumors, or the risk of increased deficit and expense of this treatment will not be considered worthwhile.

CONCLUSIONS AND FUTURE DIRECTIONS

CT stereotactic neurosurgery permits the accurate placement of radioactive sources into malignant gliomas, and this treatment appears to cause tumor regression and prolonged survival in patients with recurrent malignant gliomas. Results for patients with glioblastoma are inferior to those for patients with anaplastic astrocytoma, either because the dose of radiation is too low or, more probably, because the tumor volumes are being underestimated from the CT scans. Kelly's work with stereotactic biopsies based on CT scans has shown that cells with an abnormal appearance can be harvested from regions at relatively great distances from the contrast-enhancing zone in both anaplastic astrocytoma and glioblastomas (11). It is not clear that MRI scanning will help define tumor margins better than those seen on CT scans. Certainly, malignant brain tumors are not the only malignant tumors that do not have well-defined margins, and brachytherapy is surely helpful for the treatment of malignant tumors at other sites; the diffuse nature of glioblastoma is not a cause for nihilism about local therapy. From the results of an autopsy study of patients with glioblastoma, Burger and his coworkers have shown that tumor margins are far better defined immediately after external beam irradiation, the infiltrative, presumably well-oxygenated tumor cells being killed by this treatment (6). These results provide a further rationale for performing brachytherapy in an adjuvant setting than holding treatment until tumors have recurred, at which time Burger found very diffuse margins (6). Brachytherapy radiation "boosts" in the adjuvant setting after external beam irradiation are routine for breast carcinomas, head and neck tumor, and gynecological tumors (3).

There are many issues to be addressed in an attempt to optimize brain tumor brachytherapy. These include which isotope is most ideally suited for this treatment, determination of the minimum tumor dose necessary for local control of these tumors, and which tumor geometries and which locations are best suited to treatment. In addition, the use of brachytherapy in combination with chemotherapy, radiation sensitizers, or hyperthermia must be studied because these modalities may offer the opportunity to reduce the brachytherapy dose and thereby reduce or ameliorate the problem of focal radiation necrosis. Combination treatment with hyperthermia is particularly promising because heat is a potent radiosensitizer and can be delivered locally to the tumor with antennae for hyperthermia inserted through the same catheters used for the implantation of sources. This treatment is being tested extensively in our laboratory and by others, and has received limited clinical testing (13).

REFERENCES

1. Abrath FG, Henderson SD, Simpson JR, et al: Dosimetry of CT-guided volumetric Ir-192 brain implant. *Int J Radiat Oncol Biol Physiol* 12: 359–363, 1986.
2. Apuzzo MLJ, Jepson JH, Luxton G, et al: Ionizing and nonionizing radiation treatment of malignant cerebral gliomas. *Clin Neurosurg* 31: 470–496, 1983.
3. Aristizabal S, Oleson JR: Combined interstitial irradiation and localized current field hyperthermia: results and conclustions from clinical studies. *Canc Res* 44(Suppl): 4757s–4760, 1984.
4. Bernstein M, Gutin PH: Interstitial irradiation of brain tumors: A review. *Neurosurgery* 9: 741–750, 1981.
5. Bouzaglou A, Dyck P, Solt-Bohman LG, et al: Stereotactic interstitial implantation of brain tumors. *Endocurie Hyperthermia Oncol* 1: 99–112, 1985.
6. Burger PC, Dubois PJ, Schold CS Jr, et al: Computerized tomographic and pathologic studies of the untreated, quiescent, and recurrent glioblastoma multiforme. *J Neurosurg* 58: 159–169, 1983.
7. Gutin PH, Dormandy, RH Jr: A coaxial catheter system for afterloading radioactive sources for the interstitial irradiation of brain tumors. Technical note. *J Neursurg* 56: 34–735, 1982.
8. Gutin PH, Phillips TL, Wara WM, et al: Brachytherapy of recurrent malignant brain tumors with removable high-activity iodine-125 sources. *J Neurosurg* 60: 61–68, 1984.
9. Hall EJ: The biological basis of endocurietherapy. The Henschke Memorial Lecture 1984. *Endocurie Hyperthermia Oncol* 1: 141–152, 1985.
10. Heilbrun MP, Roberts TS, Apuzzo MLJ, et al: Preliminary experience with the Brown-Roberts-Wells (BRW) computerized tomographic stereotaxic guidance system. *J Neurosurg* 59: 217–222, 1983.
11. Kelly PJ: Computer-assisted stereotaxis: New approaches for the management of intracranial intra-axial tumors. *Neurology* 36: 535–541, 1986.
12. Liu J, Edwards FM: Radiation exposure to medical personnel during iodine-125 seed implantation of the prostate. *Radiology* 132: 748–749, 1979.
13. Roberts DW, Coughlin CT, Wong TZ, et al: Interstitial hyperthermia and iridium brachytherapy in treatment of malignant glioma. *J Neurosurg* 64: 581–587, 1986.
14. Rossman KJ, Shelter AJ, Speiser BL: Stereotactic afterloading iridium implants in the treatment of high grade gliomas. *Endocurie Hyperthermia Oncol.* 1: 49–58, 1985.
15. Salcman M, Sewchand W, Amin PP, et al: Technique and preliminary results of interstitial irradiation for primary brain tumors. *J Neuro-Oncol* 4: 141–149, 1986.
16. Schlegel W, Scharfenberg H, Doll J, et al: CT-images as the basis of operation planning in stereotactical neurosurgery. Proceedings of the 1st International Symposium on Medical Imaging and Image Interpretation, Berlin, October 1982, ISMII 82. New York: IEEE 1982, pp 172–177.

Chapter 16

Future Developments in Stereotactic Neurosurgery

EDWARD GANZ, M.D.

INTRODUCTION

This chapter will present an overview of both the anticipated and potential future developments in the discipline of stereotactic neurosurgery. Some current developments are noteworthy because they make available the precision of stereotactic localization to the majority of practicing neurosurgeons. Others demand recognition because they are specialized techniques and procedures that, while not generally available, make possible neurosurgical intervention of a type not previously possible or considered. Earlier chapters in this volume have detailed specific stereotactic procedures and technology. This section will attempt to integrate these findings, emphasizing the rapid growth and exciting future possibilities for image-guided stereotactic procedures.

IMAGING

Prior to the advent of the CT scan, stereotactic technique was quite limited in that it was confined to targets whose location could be defined in relation to a coordinate system tied to ventricular and periventricular anatomy. Standardized atlases defined the most probable position of functional targets with respect to a coordinate system related to the brain, using intraoperative ventriculography. With the advent of CT scanning, the situation changed dramatically. To generate such a scan, as with all computed tomographic techniques, a digital image is synthesized from a series of projections taken about the object of interest; in this case, the brain.

The tomographic data are reconstructed and projected into a rectangular array consisting of individual picture elements, each of which occupies a fixed and identifiable locus in space. In principle, any small group of such picture elements may then serve as the region of interest that constitutes the target for a stereotactic approach. The specific task to be performed in the target region may vary from focal thermal ablation, to biopsy, to implantation of a radionuclide, to extracellular microelectrode recording.

The fundamental feature of computed tomographic imaging, whether that imaging technique be x-ray transmission tomography, magnetic resonance imaging, or positron emission tomography, is that the scanning device is able to provide the neurosurgeon with the three-dimensional spatial data required to access targets defined by that particular scanning modality. It is the function of the stereotactic frame and its localizing system to relate the spatial data contained within the image to the operating platform fixed to the calvarium. In a typical system, the orientation of the tomographic plane is determined in the coordinate system of the stereotactic apparatus affixed to the head. It is then possible to determine the location of each of the discrete points comprising the image in stereotactic space.

Each imaging modality provides unique data to the stereotactic neurosurgeon. Conventional x-ray transmission computed tomography produces images that are essentially maps of x-ray attenuation. Iodinated intravascular agents are frequently used to enhance regional contrast. As is well familiar, such techniques are useful for the delineation of neoplasm, focal infection, cerebrospinal fluid containing spaces, as well as normal parenchymal structures differentiable from one another by the contrast between gray and white matter. Currently, magnetic resonance imaging (MRI) is superior to the CT scan for delineating gray/white differences. This is true because the relaxation parameters of anatomical components differ from one another much more strikingly than do their x-ray attenuation coefficients. For this reason, MRI has been superb in depicting normal cerebral structure. It is also true that many abnormalities, such as most forms of neoplasia, as well as such entities as focal inflammation or demyelinating/degenerative disease, are seen with a high degree of image contrast. The arrival of a generation of stereotactic instruments able to utilize MRI spatial data has been most exciting. After resolution of initial problems with incompatibility of stereotactic instrumentation and the MR imaging environment, the ability to access regions of interest as defined by MR scanning has evolved quickly. Although positron emission tomography (PET) is not widely available, those neurosurgeons with access to this imaging modality will be able to utilize conventional image-guided stereotactic technique because the PET scan is also a computed tomographic image. In this case, rather than maps of x-ray attenuation coefficients, or magnetic relaxation parameters, an image represents the quantitative distribution of a physiologically or metabolically significant radionuclide. While the spatial resolution of this modality is poor compared with CT and MR, the fact that it is a functional map rather than an anatomical one is of great significance. A neurosurgeon seeking, for instance, to biopsy the most metabolically active portion of a neoplasm could direct a probe to that region of the tumor having the highest cerebral metabolic rate for glucose or oxygen, or alternatively, the highest focal uptake of a particular amino acid.

While in the preceding discussion the various imaging modalities have been considered separate from and in comparison with one another, there is great appeal to a stereotactic system that works with a variety of computed tomographic images, where the same regions of interest on different types of image can be related to one another. Thus, with current and future "universal" stereotactic devices that are compatible with CT, MR and PET, important information will be available based upon the ability to relate the images to one another stereotactically. This maneuver may be accomplished through normalization of the images to one another with subsequent histological correlation of lesions characterized both anatomically and physiologically.

Various techniques exist for integrating yet another imaging modality, in this case, that is not tomographic, into the milieu of stereotactic localization. If cerebral angiography (either cut film or DSA) is performed while the patient is positioned in a stereotactic localizer, it is now feasible to derive an entire angiographic spatial data set that can be used either independently, primarily for vascular lesions such as arteriovenous malformations, or integrated into the CT and MR images, thus superimposing those structures of vascular significance. It is anticipated that this technique will be of increasing importance for both selecting safe trajectories that avoid vulnerable vascular structures during CT or MR image-guided stereotactic procedures, as well as enabling the stereotactic surgeon to identify intrinsically vascular structures, including the afferent vessels supplying arteriovenous malformations.

In summary, the future possibilities for stereotactic neurosurgery, based on the extensive spatial data available from the computers that synthesize tomographic images, are virtually unlimited. The stereotactic surgeon will be able to define targets virtually anywhere within the brain based on a spectrum of anatomical and/or physiological attributes. Stereotactic frames are compatible with these various modalities and are also capable of relating one to another. The current marked increase in the popularity and availability of stereotactic procedures has largely resulted from the application of stereotactic techniques to the newer imaging modalities, and it is likely to improve and to expand greatly in the future.

COMPUTER TECHNOLOGY

In addition to the growth of new imaging modalities for stereotactic neurosurgery, there have been spectacular advances in sophisticated computer hardware and software increasingly available to the neurosurgeon. Computation for image-guided stereotactic procedures is now most frequently carried out either on the console of the scanner itself or in small stand-alone microcomputers. A number of individuals and centers have explored the more comprehensive application of larger scale computers to stereotactic neurosurgery. By utilizing the principles of computer graphics, it has been possible, for instance, to store the relevent data from complete sets of CT or MRI scans, and then to perform a variety of relevant spatial transformations. Such techniques make it possible to rotate the image of the brain to any degree of obliquity so as to delineate an electrode track or path for biopsy instrument, as though the surgeon were looking directly down the axis of the probe. Surface-rendered features of subcortical targets have been demonstrated in convincing three-dimensional perspective by slowly moving rotation or multiple projection. Application of computer-aided design/computer-aided manufacture, (CAD/CAM) techniques makes it possible to realize such goals as radiation treatment planning for both highly collimated swept external beams as well as for arrays of implanted radionuclides. Computers are now able to do the type of normalization from one scanning modality to another, which is required for the most sophisticated approach to a difficult lesion. As the availability of powerful supermicro- and minicomputers becomes more universal and their prices become lower, it is very likely that the techniques now in prototype development at relatively few centers, will one day be available to the vast majority of neurosurgeons performing stereotactic surgery.

STEREOTACTIC TECHNIQUES FOR CRANIOTOMY

While the majority of stereotactic surgery is performed with narrow probes introduced through small calvarial openings, such as burr or twist-drill holes, a growing application is to be anticipated in the area of craniotomy aided by stereotactic guidance. Utilizing this technique, the patient preparing to undergo craniotomy for tumor or arteriovenous malformation, for example, is first placed in a stereotactic frame, and the scan data are collected. These will be used to intraoperatively relate specific points in the operative field to identifiable points in the tomographic image. For example, a small tumor in a subcortical location cannot only be unequivocally localized, but its borders with surrounding brain and potential impingement on eloquent structures can be identified and flagged with markers introduced stereotactically during the operation. A subcortical lesion residing beneath an eloquent area need not be approached by the shortest possible path. Rather, a "quiet" area of cortex may be chosen for entrance and the stereotactic apparatus employed to guide the operator from the surface to the target at some degree of obliquity. In a similar fashion, the feeding vessels of an arteriovenous malformation can all be identified using both stereotactic angiography and contrast-enhanced CT. By locating these vessels stereotactically prior to direct approach of the vascular malformation itself, it should be possible to significantly diminish hazard. While combining stereotactic technique with craniotomy has just been described, it is also the case that certain lesions traditionally treated by formal craniotomy may well be attacked using purely stereotactic means. For example, significant success has been reported in the aspiration of colloid cysts of the third ventricle using only stereotactic technique. Individuals so treated are able to have this lesion managed effectively without the need for conventional operation by either the interhemispheric or transventricular approach.

In a number of institutions, stereotactic guidance has been combined with the laser and operating microscope to make possible resection of neoplasms whose position is defined stereotactically and which are able to be resected through rather narrow specula introduced from the surface of the brain. An exciting further development of this basic approach could provide the operator with a maplike overlay derived from one or a combination of imaging modalities, which would then be continuously visible or able to be instantly called up during craniotomy.

FUNCTIONAL NEUROSURGERY AND EPILEPSY

Recent advances have also stimulated renewed interest in functional stereotactic neurosurgery. Sophisticated microelectrode recording techniques have increased the precision with which discrete lesions may be placed for the purpose of controlling such disorders as the tremor of parkinsonism. Thalamotomy performed using the best image-guided stereotactic localization, in addition to electrophysiological mapping, is able to be considerably more precise and effective than had previously been possible. Intraoperative graphics displays generated by computer have made it feasible for the surgeon to visualize the advance of the operating probe through anatomical structures defined by normalized atlases, as well as to identify physiologically characterized cell populations within those structures. The prospect is excellent for this sophisticated approach to develop further and also to become much more widely available than in the specialized centers where it is currently practiced. The implantation of stimulating systems for the control of chronic intractable pain has not been widely practiced, but the same sort of technological advances that have made movement disorders more accessible should also aid those exploring stimulation-produced analgesia.

The primary rationale for the application of stereotactic technique to epilepsy is the more accurate delineation of the epileptogenic focus. While some centers rely heavily upon recording from the cortical surface with electrode arrays, others have and continue to depend upon multiple depth electrodes. These electrodes may be introduced to a variety of targets using image-guided stereotactic technique. Both anatomical criteria in the temporal lobe, as well as preliminary functional and metabolic criteria using positron emission tomography, have been employed. In practice, the unequivocal identification of the epileptogenic focus is essential before any consideration of extirpation may take place. Stereotactic placement of electrodes has been successfully employed for this purpose in a significant number of centers. Because there is growing recognition that a considerable number of individuals with anticonvulsant refractory epilepsy may well be candidates for surgery, it is expected that this particular application of stereotactic surgery will increase significantly. In a specific subgroup of patients, it is possible to achieve a salutary effect upon seizure frequency and severity by the placement of destructive lesions in the amygdala-hippocampal complex. A variation of the thermal ablative lesion is the stereotactically guided resection of the same target site.

STEREOTACTIC RADIOSURGERY

Radiosurgery may be defined as the use of a highly collimated external beam of ionizing radiation for the purpose of causing focal ablation of an intracranial structure. A variety of radiation sources exists. The gamma knife, developed by Leksell, uses an array of individual ^{60}Co sources distributed over a fairly large solid angle and brought to focus at a single point. Targets such as arteriovenous malformations are placed at the focus of the sources and are irradiated intensely for short periods of time. Another approach has been to use a charged particle beam comprised of protons or helium ions to achieve a similar end. Both of these techniques have been demonstrated to be effective, but both are very specialized pieces of apparatus whose availability has been limited to a few sites in the neurosurgical community. The prospect for future expansion of stereotactic radiosurgical techniques is based upon the combination of a conventional linear accelerator, using a highly collimated beam, with a stereotactic apparatus. Using this technique, the lesion is stereotactically positioned at the isocenter of rotation of the linear accelerator, and a series of arcs swept out such that the adjacent brain through which the beam passes receives only modest amounts of radiation, whereas the volume at the isocenter receives a large dose with rapid fall-off at the margins.

Because such linear accelerators are widely available and are able to be effectively mated to stereotactic localizing systems, the prospect is good for a significant increase in the use of this modality. As is true in a number of the other applications described, heavy reliance is placed upon the computer hardware and software necessary to both localize the lesion to be treated, as well as to determine accurately the radiation dosimetry. Preliminary work is underway to characterize the spectrum of biological effects produced by these nonfractionated, high-flux bursts of photon irradiation.

BRACHYTHERAPY

Another approach to the focal irradiation of intracranial targets is through the use of stereotactically implanted radionuclides. In practice, the volume to be treated—typically, a malignant glial tumor—is defined using the spatial information derived from a series of CT and/or MR scans. The studies are performed with the patient's head in a localizer and the position of the lesion volume determined in stereotactic space. Radiation dosimetry is then performed and a series of isodose profiles generated for an appropriate geometric distribution of implants. Most frequently, the implanted sources are in the form of afterloaded catheters that are first positioned stereotactically and are then subsequently filled with emitting sources. The more popular radionuclides used for this purpose have been the isotopes iodine-125 (^{125}I) and iridium-192 (^{192}Ir). It is possible to deliver very high doses to the tumor volume by using a combination of the implants supplemented by conventional external beam therapy.

Lately, much interest has been shown in treating both recurrent and first-occurence malignant glial tumors in this fashion, and it is likely to grow in popularity as the requisite stereotactic expertise, as well as the treatment planning capability, develops in more centers. Early problems with radiation necrosis due to the use of relatively few sources of extremely high activity have been ameliorated by distributing the radionuclide to a greater number of sources, thus achieving greater homogeneity of activity. While data are preliminary, it appears that, at least in some patient populations, a significantly greater degree of tumor control has resulted from interstitial irradiation than would have been anticipated from external beam therapy alone. A variation of the use of stereotactically positioned afterloaded catheters is the direct injection of radioactive colloidal material into cystic tumors.

BIOPSY

The greatest numbers of patients operated upon using image-guided stereotactic techniques have been those undergoing biopsy of some parenchymal lesion. The mass lesions being approached are most frequently neoplastic or infectious. Biopsy of these masses has done much to stimulate the recent remarkable growth in stereotactic neurosurgery. There is little to suggest that this form of operative intervention will do anything but increase in importance and in numbers. Stereotactic technique has made the definitive tissue diagnosis of deep-seated lesions both safe and accurate. There is now little reason to initiate any form of treatment without histological diagnosis. Such definitive diagnosis makes it possible to plan the optimal form of adjunctive therapy and does away with uncertain etiology or the hazards associated with craniotomy, particularly in the sick and fragile individual. From an investigational standpoint, recent work has demonstrated the significant extension of neoplastic cellular elements beyond the boundaries normally associated with tumor on conventional scans. Indeed, this ability of stereotactic technique to correlate a specific region of an image or lesion with a precise histological characterization makes it valuable for the derivation of new information regarding tumor growth and metabolism. Very likely many neurosurgeons will initially be trained in, or will bring stereotactic techniques to their practice for the purpose of biopsy. In many instances, however, this application will serve as a first step in their growing familiarity with the technique and may well lead to more general applications of stereotactic procedures in their practice.

TISSUE TRANSPLANTATION

Much recent work has explored the possibility that groups of cells of either neuronal or endocrine origin can be transplanted to, and will survive in, the adult central nervous system. A tremendous increase in the volume of research delineating the survivability and functional parameters of these transplanted cell populations has recently taken place. Preliminary clinical application has focused on the use of cells that produce neurotransmitters which may be useful in a deficiency state, such as the autologous transplantation of adrenal medulla to the brain of an individual with Parkinson's disease. Both open and stereotactic placement of implants have been employed, and a promising technique is one wherein the adrenal medullary explant is placed such that it is partially within the substance of the caudate nucleus and partially within the ventricular cerebral spinal fluid. Transplanted tissue so placed produces neurotransmitter and is able to survive in situ.

This preliminary work opens entire areas of potential applicability of transplanted tissue to the central nervous system. Several broad categories of such transplantation exist. Cell populations that release neurotransmitter globally may well function in a much more efficient fashion than if exogenous transmitter were systemically administered. In this fashion, they are analogous to biological "chemodes." Recent work on reinnervation of specific neural pathways, perhaps aided by factors uniquely elaborated by populations of fetal cells, further gives rise to the potential for functional reinnervation of pathways that have been damaged or lost. In the second case, very specific points of delivery of the transplanted cells will clearly be of import. While transplantation as a therapeutic modality is still very much in its infancy, it is clear that extraordinary potential exists for a prospect considered fantastic only a few years ago—the restoration of central nervous function through the successful regeneration of interrupted pathways, or the specific repopulation of cellular elements able to produce a deficient neurotransmitter.

SUMMARY

Earlier chapters in this volume have detailed some specific techniques and approaches to particular problems in stereotactic neurosurgery. It has been the goal of this section to briefly survey those areas that are either currently well established or are the object of active development, to indicate how each fills a unique niche within the practice of neurosurgery, and to extrapolate the potential directions for future growth. It is clear that a number of these areas hold promise for either quite universal application in neurosurgical practice, or for the fruitful accumulation of new information about the brain and diseases that affect it.

What has become quite evident is that the introduction and maturation of image-guided stereotactic neurosurgery has transformed a valuable neurosurgical technique from one originally practiced almost exclusively by a small group of specialists, to one that is widely available in the neurosurgical community. The extent to which a neurosurgeon will incorporate stereotactic procedures into his or her practice will vary greatly. Much of the technical development at the forefront of investigation will continue to be performed by individuals whose principal interest is stereotactic technique. "Friendly" computer software and sophisticated hardware have broadened the availability of stereotactic technique dramatically. As the stereotactic specialists evaluate, refine, and ultimately simplify the techniques currently being investigated, it is anticipated that those techniques will also find their way to the practice of surgeons both willing to learn and use them effectively. Stereotactic neurosurgery promises to result in a significant transformation of the way neurosurgery is practiced, in that the spatial information which is its province will become increasingly available to all neurosurgeons in conducting more precise, rational, and safe operative intervention.

SUGGESTED READINGS

Anderson RE, Thomas DGT, du Boulay GH: Radiological aspects of CT-guided stereotactic neurosurgical procedures. *Neuroradiol* 24:163-166, 1983.

Andrew J, Fowler CJ, Harrison MJG: Stereotaxic

thalamotomy in 55 cases of dystonia. *Brain* 106:981-1000, 1983.

Asakura T, Uetsuhara K, Kanemaru R, Hirahara K: An applicability study on a CT-guided stereotactic technique for functional neurosurgery. *Appl Neurophysiol* 48:73-76, 1985.

Barcia Salorio JL, Vanaclocha V, Cerda M, Roldan P: Focal irradiation in epilepsy. Experimental study in the cat. *Appl Neurophysiol* 48:152, 1985.

Bergstrom M, Greitz T, Ribbe T: A method of stereotaxic localization adopted for conventional and digital radiography. *Neuroradiology* 28:100-104, 1986.

Betti OO, Derechinsky VE: Hyperselective encephalic irradiation with linear accelerator. *Acta Neuochir* 33:385-390, 1984.

Birg W, Mundinger F, Mohadjer M, Weigel K: Fuermaier R: X-ray and magnetic resonance stereotaxy for functional and nonfunctional neurosurgery. *Appl Neurophysiol* 48:22-29, 1985.

Boethius J, Bergstrand G, Collins VP, Edner G, Tribukait B: DNA distribution in various parts of malignant gliomas assayed on stereotactic biopsies. *Appl Neurophysiol* 43:216-221, 1980.

Bohm G, Greitz T, Kingsley D, Berggren BM, Olsson L: Adjustable computerized stereotaxic brain atlas for transmission and emission tomography. *AJNR* 4:731-733, May/June 1983.

Bosch DA: Indications for stereotactic biopsy in brain tumours. *Acta Neurochir* 54:167-179, 1980.

Bowyer KW, Starmer F, DuBois P: Error sensitivity of computerized tomography guided stereotaxis. *Comput Biomed Res* 15:272-280, 1982.

Broggi G, Franzini A: Value of serial stereotactic biopsies and impedance monitoring in the treatment of deep brain tumours. *J Neurol Neurosurg Psychiatr* 44:397-401, 1981.

Broggi G, Franzini A, Costa A, Melcarne A, Allegranza A: Cell kinetics of neuroepithelial tumors in serial stereotactic biopsies. A new combined approach. *Appl Neurophysiol* 48:472-476, 1985.

Broggi G, Franzini A, Peluchitti D, Servello D: Treatment of deep brain abscesses by stereotactic implantation of an intracavitary device for evacuation and local application of antibiotics. *Acta Neurochir* 76:94-98, 1985.

Brown RA, Roberts TS, Osborn AG: Stereotaxic frame and computer software for CT-directed neurosurgical localization. *Invest Radio* 15(4):308-312, 1985.

Brown RA, Roberts T, Osborn AG: Simplified CT-guided stereotaxic biopsy. *AJNR* 2:131-184, March/April 1981.

Bullard DE: Role of stereotaxic biopsy in the management of patients with intracranial lesions. *Neurologic Clinics* 3(4):817-830, November 1985.

Bullard DE, Makachinas TT, Nashold BS Jr: Use of intraoperative stimulation in the selection of target sites for CT-guided stereotactic biopsies. *Appl Neurophysiol* 48:454-459, 1985.

Bullard DE, Nashold BS: Stereotaxic thalamotomy for treatment of posttraumatic movement disorders. *J Neurosurg* 61:316-321, 1984.

Bullard DE, Nashold BS Jr, Osborne D, Burger PC, Dubois P: CT-guided stereotactic biopsies using a modified frame and Gildenberg technique. *J Neurol Neurosurg Psychiatry* 47:590-595, 1984.

Bullard DE, Osborne D, Burger PC, Nashold BS Jr: Further experience utilizing the Gildenberg technique for computed tomography-guided stereotactic biopsies. *Neurosurgery* 19(3):386-391, 1986.

Burger PC: Pathologic anatomy and CT correlations in the glioblastoma multiforme. *Appl Neurophysiol* 46:180-187, 1983.

Carol M: A true advanced imaging assisted skull-mounted stereotactic system. *Appl Neurophysiol* 48:69-72, 1985.

Coffey RJ, Lunsford LD: Stereotactic surgery for mass lesions of the midbrain and pons. *Neurosurgery* 17(1):12-18, 1985

Colombo F, Benedetti A, Pozza F, Avanzo RC, Marchetti C, Chierego G, Zanardo A: External stereotactic irradiation by linear accelerator. *Neurosurgery* 16(2):154-160, 1985.

Colombo F, Benedetti A, Pozza F, Zanardo A, Avanzo RC, Chierego G, Marchetti C: Stereotactic radiosurgery utilizing a linear accelerater. *Appl Neurophysiol* 48:133-145, 1985.

Daumas-Duport C, Blond S, Vedrenne C, Szikla G: Radiolesion versus recurrence: bioptic data in 39 gliomas after interstitial, or combined interstitial and external radiation treatment. *Acta Neurochir* 33:291-299, 1985.

Daumas-Duport C, Mann M, Manari C, Blonde S, Musolino A, Monsaingeon V, Chodkiewicz JP: Cryptic vascular malformations diagnosed by stereotactic biopsies—a preliminary study. *Appl Neurophysiol* 48:440-443, 1985.

Daumas-Duport C, Monsaingeon V, N'Guyen JP, Missir O, Scikla G: Some correlations between histological and CT aspects of cerebral gliomas contributing to the choice of significant trajectories for stereotactic biopsies. *Acta Neurochir* 33:185-194, 1984.

Daumas-Duport C, Monsaingon V, Szenthe L, Szikla G: Serial sterotactic biopsies: a double histological code of gliomas according to malignancy and 3-D configuration, as an aid to therapeutic decision and assessment of results. *Appl Neurophysiol* 45:431-437, 1982.

de Divitiis E, Sqaziante R, Cappabianca P, Caputi F, Pettinato G, Del Basso De Caro M: Reliability of stereotactic biopsy. A model to test the value of diagnoses obtained from small fragments of nervous system tumors. *Appl Neurophysiol* 46:295-303, 1983.

Degerblad M, Rahn T, Bergstrand, Thoren M: Long-term results of stereotactic radiosurgery to the pituitary gland in Cushing's disease. *Acta Endocrinolog* 112:310-314, 1986.

Dubois PJ, Nashold BS, Perry J, Burger P, Bowyer K, Heinz ER, Drayer BP, Bigner S, Higgins AC: CT-guided stereotaxis using a modified conventional stereotaxic frame. *AJNR* 3:345-351, May/June 1983.

Dyck P, Bouzaglou A, Solti-Bohman LG, Gruskin P: CT-compatible system for stereotactic biopsy and brachytherapy of infratentorial tumors. *Appl Neurophysiol* 49: 53-61, 1986.

Eddy MS, Selker RG, Anderson LL: On a method of dosimetry planning and implantation of Iodine-125 for interstitial irradiation of malignant gliomas. *J Neurooncol* 4:131-139, 1986.

Engle DJ, Lunsford LD, Panichelli T: Rigid head fixation for intraoperative computed tomography. *Neurosurgery* 19(2):258-262, 1986.

Fabrikant JI, Lyman JT, Frankel KA: Heavy charged-particle bragg peak radiosurgery for intracranial vascular disorders. *Radiat Res* 104:S-244-S-258, 1985.

Fabrikant JI, Lyman JT, Hosobuchi V: Stereotactic heavy-ion bragg peak radiosurgery for intra-cranial vascular disorders: method for treatment of deep arteriovenous malformations. *Br J Radiol* 57:479-490, June 1984.

Fox PT, Perlmutter JS, Raichle ME: A stereotactic method of anatomical localization for positron emission tomography. *Comput Assist Tomogr* 9(1): 141-153, January/February 1985.

Frank F, Fabrizi AP, Frank-Ricci R, Sturaile C, Nuzzo G: Treatment of low malignancy brain neoplasms by means of stereotactic interstitial radiotherapy. *Appl Neurophysiol* 48:121-126, 1985.

Frank F, Gaist G, Piazza G. Ricci RF, Sturiale C, Galassi E: Stereotaxic biopsy and radioactive implantation for interstitial therapy of tumors of the pineal region. *Surg Neurol* 23:275-280, 1985.

Franzini A, Broggi G, Allegranza A, Melcarne A, Ventura L, Costa A: Cell kinetics of gliomas by serial stereotactic biopsy. *Bas Appl Histochem* 30:203-207, 1986.

Fratkin JD, Ward MM, Roberts DW, Sullivan MM: CT-guided stereotactic biopsy of intracranial lesions: correlation between core biopsy and aspiration smear. *Diag Cytopathol* 2(2):126-132, 1986.

Froder M, Seitzer D, Buren G, Dieckmann G: Digital radiography for target point evaluation in stereotactic neurosurgery. *Appl Neurophysiol* 46:206-210, 1983.

Gahbauer H, Sturm V, Schlegel W, Pastyr O, Scharfenberg H, Zabel HJ, van Kaick G, Netzeband G, Scheer KE, Schabbert S: Combined use of stereotaxic CT and angiography for brain biopsies and stereotaxic irradiation. *AJNR* 4:715-718, May/June 1983.

Garcia de Sola R, Cabezudo J, Areitio E, Bravo G: Combined approach (stereotactic-microsurgical) to a paraventricular arteriovenous malformation. *Acta Neurochir* 33:413-416, 1980.

Gildenberg PL: Stereotactic neurosurgery and computerized tomographic scanning. *Appl Neurophysiol* 46: 170-179, 1983.

Gildenberg PL: Combining CT scanning with stereotactic surgery. *Comput Radiol* 9:91-100, 1985.

Gildenberg PL, Franklin P: Survey of CT-guided stereotactic surgery. *Appl Neurophysiol* 48:477-480, 1985.

Gildenberg PL, Kaufman HH: Direct calculation of stereotactic coordinates from CT scans. *Appl Neurophysiol* 45:347-351, 1982.

Giorgi C, Gartibotto G, Garozzo S, Micca G, Piretta G: Three-dimensional precession of a stereotactic brain atlas. *Appl Neurophysiol* 45:419-425, 1982.

Goethius J, Bergstrom M, Greitz T, Ribbe T: CT localization in stereotactic surgery. *Appl Neurophysiol* 43:164-169, 1980.

Gouda KI, Freidberg SR, Larsen CR, Baker RA, Silverman ML: Modification of the Gouda frame to allow stereotactic biopsy of the brain using the GE 8800 computed tomographic scanner. *Neurosurgery* 13(2):176-181, 1983.

Greitz T, Lax I, Bergstrom M, Arndt J, Benggren BM, Blomgren H, Boethius J, Lindqvist M, Ribe T, Steiner L: Stereotactic radiation therapy of intracranial lesions. *Acta Radiol* 25:81-89, 1986.

Gutin PH, Leibel SA: Stereotaxic interstitial irradiation of malignant brain tumors. *Neurol Clin* 3:883-893, November 1985.

Hadley MN, Shetter AG, Amos MR: Use of the Brown-Roberts-Wells stereotactic frame for functional neurosurgery. *Appl Neurophysiol* 48:61-68, 1985.

Haynor DR, Borning AW, Griffin BA, Jacky JP, Kalet IJ, Shuman WP: Radiotherapy planning: direct tumor location on simulation and port films using CT. *Radiol* 158:537-540, 1986.

Heilbrun MP: Computed tomography-guided stereotactic systems. *Clin Neurosurg* 31:564-581, 1983.

Heilbrun MP, Brown RA, McDonald PR: Real-time three-dimensional graphic reconstructions using Brown-Roberts-Wells frame coordinates in a microcomputer environment. *Appl Neurophysiol* 48:7-10, 1985.

Heilbrun MP, Roberts TS, Apuzzo MLJ, Wells TH, Sabshin JK: Preliminary experience with Brown-Roberts-Wells (BRW) computerized tomography stereotaxic guidance system. *J Neurosurg* 59:217-222, 1983.

Higgins AC, Nashold BS Jr: Stereotactic evacuation of large intracerebral hematoma. *Appl Neurophysiol* 43:96-103, 1980.

Higgins, AC, Nashold, BS, and Cosman E: Stereotactic evacuation of primary intracerebral hematomas: new instrumentation, *Appl Neurophysiol* 45:438-442, 1982.

Hood TW, Gebarski SS, McKeever PE, Venes JL: Stereotaxic biopsy of intrinsic lesions of the brain stem. *J Neurosurg* 65:172-176, 1986.

Houdek PV, Fayos JV, VanBuren JM, Ginsberg MS: Stereotaxic radiotherapy technique for small intracranial lesions. *Med Phys* 12(4):469-472, July/August 1985.

Huk WJ, Mahlstedt J: Intracystic radiotherapy (^{90}Y) of craniopharyngiomas: CT-guided stereotaxic implantation of indwelling drainage system. *AJNR* 4:803-806, May/June 1983.

Iacono RP, Osborne DR, Nashold BS Jr: CT analysis of stereotactic thalamotomy. *Adv Neurol* 40:453-458, 1984.

Johnston LE Jr, Behrents RG: A system for graphic representation during stereotaxic procedures. *Brain Res Bull* 12:335-337, 1984.

Kall BA, Kelly PJ, Goerss SJ: Interactive stereotactic surgical system for the removal of intracranial tumors utilizing the CO_2 laser and CT-derived database. *IEEE* Vol. BME-32 No. 2:112-116, February 1985.

Kandel EI, Peresedov VV: Stereotaxic evacuation of spontaneous intracerebral hematomas. *J Neurosurg* 62:206-213, 1985.

Kelly PJ: Applications and methodology for contemporary stereotactic surgery. *Neurol Res* 8:2-12, March 1986.

Kelley PJ: Computer-assisted stereotaxis: new approaches for the management of intracranial intraaxial tumors. *Neurology* 36:535-541, 1986.

Kelley PJ, Alker GJ, Kall BA, Goerss S: Method of computed tomography-based stereotactic biopsy with arteriographic control. *Neurosurgery* 14(2):172-177, 1984.

Kelly PJ, Goerss S, Kall BA, Kispert, DB: Computed tomography-based stereotactic third ventriculostomy: technical note. *Neurosurgery* 18(6):791-794, 1986.

Kelly PJ, Kall B, Georss S: Preoperative computer determination of interstitial irridium-192 source placement into CNS tumor volumes. *Acta Neurochir* 33:377-383, 1984.

Kelly PJ, Kall BA, Goerss S: Transposition of volumetric information derived from computed tomography scanning into stereotactic space. *Surgical Neurology* 21:465-471, 1984.

Kelly PJ, Kall B, Goerss S, Alker GJ Jr: Precision resection of intra-axial CNS lesions by CT-based stereotactic craniotomy and computer monitored CO_2 laser. *Acta Neurochir* 68:1-9, 1983.

Kelly PJ, Kall BA, Goerss S, Cascino TL: Results of computer-assisted stereotactic laser resection of deep-seated intracranial lesions. *Mayo Clin Proc* 61:20-27, 1986.

Kelly PJ, Kall BA, Goerss D: Computer simulation for the stereotactic placement of interstitial radionuclide sources into computed tomography-defined tumor volumes. *Neurosurgery* 14(4):442-448, 1984.

Kelly, PJ, Kall B, and Goerss S, Earnest F: Present and future developments of stereotactic technology. *Appl Neurophysiol* 46:193-199, 1983.

Kelly PJ, Kall BA, Goerss S, Earnest F: Present and future developments of stereotactic technology. *Appl Neurophysiol* 48:1-6, 1985.

Kiessling M, Kleihues P, Gessaga E, Mundinger F, Ostertag CB, Weigel K: Morphology of intracranial tumours and adjacent brain structures following interstitial iodine-125 radiotherapy. *Acta Neurochirur* 33:281-289, 1984.

Kim GM: A three-dimensional graphics system for the stereotactic placement of heavy-ion beams. *Computer Methods Programs Biomed* 23:73-81, 1986.

Kleihues P, Volk B, Anagnostopoulos J, Miessling M: Morphologic evaluation of stereotactic brain tumour biopsies. *Acta Neurochir* 33:171-181, 1984.

Laitinen LV: Brain targets in surgery for Parkinson's disease. *J Neurosurg* 62:349-351, 1985.

Laitinen LV: CT-guided ablative stereotaxis without ventriculography. *Appl Neurophysiol* 48:18-21, 1985.

Laitinen LV, Liliequist B, Fagerlund M, Eriksson AT: An adapter for computed tomography-guided stereotaxis. *Surg Neurol* 23:559-566, 1985.

Latchaw RE, Lunsford LD, Kennedy WH: Reformatted imaging to define the intercommissural line for CT-guided stereotaxic functional neurosurgery. *AJNR* 6:429-433, May/June 1985.

Le Bas JF, Leviel JL, Decorps M, Benabid AL: NMR relaxation times from serial stereotactic biopsies in human brain tumors. *J Comput Assist Tomog* 8(6): 1048-1057, December 1984.

Leksell L: Stereotactic radiosurgery. *J Neuro Neurosurg Psychiatr* 46:797-803, 1983.

Leksell L, Herner T, Leksell D, Persson B, Lindquist C: Visualization of stereotactic radiolesions by nuclear magnetic resonance. *J Neurol Neurosurg Psychiatr* 48:19-20, 1985.

Leksell L, Leksell D, Schwebel J: Stereotaxis and nuclear magnetic resonance. *J Neurol Neurosurg Psychiatr* 48:14-18, 1985.

Lunsford LD, Deutsch M, Yoder V: Stereotactic interstitial brachytherapy—current concepts and concerns in twenty patients. *Appl Neurophysiol* 48:117-120, 1985.

Lunsford LD, Gummerman L, Levine G: Stereotactic intracavitary irradiation of cyctic neoplasms of the brain. *Appl Neurophysiol* 48:146-150, 1985.

Lunsford LD, Latchaw RE, Vries JK: Stereotactic implantation of deep brain electrodes using computed tomography. *Neurosurgery* 13(3):280-286, 1983.

Lunsford LD, Martinez AJ, Latchaw RE: Stereotaxic surgery with a magnetic resonance- and computerized tomography-compatible system. *J Neurosurg* 64:872-878, 1986.

Lunsford LD, Rosenbaum AE, Perry J: Stereotactic surgery using the "therapeutic" CT scanner. *Surg Neurol* 18(2):116-122, 1982.

MacKay AR, Gutin PH, Hosobuchi V, Norman D: Computed tomography-directed stereotaxy for biopsy and interstitial irradiation of brain tumors: technical note. *Neurosurgery* 11(1):38-42, 1982.

Mansaingeon V, Daumas-Duport C, Mann M, Miyahara S, Sxikla G: Stereotactic sampling biopsies in a series of 268 consecutive cases—validity and technical aspects. *Acta Neurochir* 33:195-200, 1984.

Maruyama Y, Chin HW, Young AB, Wang PC, Tibbs P, Beach JL, Goldstein S: Implantation of brain tumors with Cf-252. *Radiol* 152:177-181, 1984.

Montagno E de A, Nashold BS Jr: A new stereotactic instrument for use with computed tomography and magnetic resonance imaging. *Appl Neurophysiol* 48: 34-38, 1985.

Munari C, Musolino A, Daumas-Duport C, Missir O, Brunet P, Giallonardo AT, Chodkiewica JP, Bancaud J: Correlation between stereo-EEG, CT-scan and stereotactic biopsy data in epileptic patients with low-grade gliomas. *Appl Neurophysiol* 48:448-453, 1985.

Mundinger F, Ostertag CB, Birg W, Weigel K: Stereotactic treatment of brain lesions. Biopsy, interstitial radiotherapy (Iridium-192 and Iodine-125) and drainage procedures. *Appl Neurophysiol* 43:198-204, 1980.

Mundinger F, Weigel K: Indication and results of stereotactic curietherapy with Iridium-192 and Iodine-125 for non-resectable tumours of the hypothalamic region. *Acta Neurochirur* 33:323-330, 1984.

Mundinger F, Weigel K: Long-term results of stereotactic interstitial curietherapy. *Acta Neurochirur* 33:367-371, 1984.

Naquet R: Neurophysiological remarks. *Acta Neurochirurg* 30:83-89, 1980.

Netzeband G, Sturm V, Georgi P, Sinn H, Schnabel K, Schlegel W, Schabbert S, Marin-grez M, Gahbauer H: Results of stereotactic intracavitary irradiation of cycstic craniopharyngiomas. Comparison of the effects of Yttrium-90 and Rhenium-186. *Acta Neurochir* 33:341-344, 1984.

Olivier A, Bertrand G, Peters T: Stereotactic systems and precedures for depth electrode placement: technical aspects. *Appl Neurophysiol* 46:37-40, 1983.

Olivier A, Gloor P, Andermann F, Quesney LF: The place of stereotactic depth electrode recording in epilepsy. *Appl Neurophysiol* 48:395-399, 1985.

Olivier A, Peters T, Bertrand G: Stereotactic system and apparatus for use with magnetic resonance imaging, computerized tomography, and digital subtraction imaging *Appl Neurophysiol* 48:94-96, 1985.

Osborne DRS, Iacono R, Nashold BS, Dubois PJ, Drayer BP, Heinz ER: Computed tomography in the planning and evaluation of therapeutic stereotaxic surgical procedures of the brain. *AJNR* 4:807-809, May/June 1983.

Ostertag CB, Groothius D, Kleihues P: Experimental data on early and late morphologic effects of permanently implanted gamma and beta sources (Iridium-192, Iodine-125 and Yttrium-90) in the brain. *Acta Neurochir* 33:271-280, 1984.

Ostertag CB, Mennel HD, Kiessling M: Stereotactic biopsy of brain tumors. *Surg Neurol* 14:975-283, 1980.

Perry JH, Rosenbaum AE, Lunsford LD, Swink CA, Zorub DS: Computed tomography-guided stereotactic surgery: conception and development of a new stereotactic methodology. *Neurosurgery* 7(4):376-381, 1980.

Peters TM, Clark JA, Olivier A, Marchand EP, Mawko G, Dieumegarde M, Muresan LV, Ethier R: Integrated stereotaxic imaging with CT, MR imaging and digital subtraction angiography. *Radiol* 161:821-826, 1986.

Ransohoff J, Kelly P, Laws E: The role of intracranial surgery for the treatment of malignant gliomas. *Semin Oncol* 13(1):27-37, 1986.

Rhodes ML, Glenn WV, Azzawi YM, Slater R: Stereotactic neurosurgery using 3-D image data from computed tomography. *J Med Syst* 6:(1):105-119, 1982.

Rivas JJ, Lobato RD: CT-assisted stereotaxic aspiration of colloid cysts of the third ventricle. *J Neurosurg* 62:238-242, 1985.

Roberts DW, Coughlin CT, Wong TZ, Fratkin JD, Douple EB, Strohbehn JW: Interstitial hyperthermia and irridium brachytherapy in treatment of malignant glioma. *J Neurosurg* 64:581-587, 1986.

Roberts DW, Strohbehn JW, Hatch JF, Murray W, Kettenberger H: A frameless stereotaxic integration of computerized tomographic imaging and the operation microscope. *J Neurosurg* 65:545-549, 1986.

Rougier A, Pigneax J, Cohadon F: Combined interstitial and external irradiation of gliomas. *Acta Neurochir* 33:345-353, 1984.

Salcman M, Sewchand W, Amin PP, Bellis EH: Technique and preliminary results of interstitial irradiation for primary brain tumors. *J Neurooncol* 4:141-149, 1986.

Shao HM, Truong TK, Reed IS, Slater RA: A new CT-aided stereotactic neurosurgery technique. *IEEE BME-32* 540-544, July 1985.

Sigfried J, Comte P, Meier R: Intracerebral electrode implantation system. *J Neurosurg* 59:356-359, 1983.

Suetens P, Gybels J, Jansen P, Oosterlinck A, Haegemans A, Dierckx P: A global 3-d image of the blood vessels, tumor and simulated electrode. *Acta Neurochir* 33:225-232, 1984.

Szikla G: Progress and problems in tumour stereotaxis. *Acta Neurochir* 33:391-394, 1984.

Thomas DGT, Davis CH, Ingram S, Olney JS, Bydder GM, Young IR: Stereotaxic biopsy of the brain under MR imaging control. *AJNR* 7:161-163, January/February 1986.

Thomson GSM, Kingsley DPE, Afshar F, Wylie IG: Stereotactic brain biopsy using a narrow aperture computed tomography scanner. *Clin Radiol* 34:209-214, 1984.

Thoren M, Rahn T, Hallengren B, Kaad PH, Nilsson KO, Ravn H, Ritzen M, Ptersen KE, Aarskog D: Treatment of Cushing's disease in childhood and adolescence by stereotactic pituitary irradiation. *Acta Padiatr Scand* 75:388-395, 1986.

Index

Page numbers in *italics* denote figures; those followed by "*f*" denote footnotes.

A

A-delta fibers, 190
  in pain, 149
Abscess
  brain
    CT-monitored aspiration of, 37
    diagnostic aspiration of, 37
    therapeutic aspiration of, 37
Absorption bands
  of porphyrins, 123–124
Accelerator
  circular (betatron), 213
  linear, 213, 241, 250
  source, 213
Acetylcholine
  from grafted source, 39
Acoustic neuroma
  Gamma Unit for, 44, 215
  radiosurgery for, 44, 126
Acquired immunodeficiency syndrome (AIDS), 96
  CT-stereotactic surgery in, 11
Acromegaly
  hypophysectomy for, 45
Acrylic cement
  used to hasten thrombosis, 33–34
  used to prevent CSF leakage
    after hypophysectomy, 30
Acta Neurochirurgica, 8
Activities of daily living (ADL) assessment, 145, 145*f*
Adenocarcinomas
  bone metastases in
    pain of, 22
  pain of, 22
  renal, 96
Adenoma
  hypophyseal
    single-photon beam therapy for, 215
  pituitary, 97
    radiosurgery for, 44, 46, 124, 126
  radiosurgery for, 126
  recurrent
    proton beam therapy for, 45
Adrenal medullary tissue
  human
    transplantation of, 39
Adrenalectomy, 207
Affective reactions, fearful
  after DBS operations, 28

Afshar atlas, 4
AIDS. *see* Acquired immunodeficiency syndrome
Air cystography, 43
Alcohol injection, 6
α-fetoprotein, 97, 98
α-HCG, 98
α-Human chorionic gonadotrophin (α-HCG), 97
α-particle, 211
Alzheimer's disease
  CNS transplantation in, 40
Amphetamine
  administration into rat nigrostriatal pathway, 39
Amygdala
  in epilepsy, 31, 161, 162, 164, 168
Amygdalotomy
  for aggressive behavior, 31
  for behavior disorders, in children, 31
  for drug addiction, 31
  for hemiplegia, in children, 31
  in mental retardation, 31
  for pain, 32–33
  for psychomotor seizures, 31
  for seizures, in children, 31
  stereotactic
    complications of, 31
Analgesia
  from central cord lesion, 189*f*
  hemibody
    after tractotomy, 25
  stimulation produced, 250
Andrew-Watkins atlas, 4, 136
Anesthesia dolorosa, 22
  after surgery for trigeminal neuralgia, 22
  facial
    thalamic stimulation for, 28
    VPM stimulation for, 27
  nucleotomy for, 189
  pain of, 7–8
Aneurysm
  angiography for, 33
  anterior communicating artery, 33
  arterial, 205
  coagulation of lumen of, 7
  radiosurgery for, 124, 126
  surgery for
    complications of, 34
    to induce thrombosis, 33
Angina
  cingulotomy for, 32

Angiography, 170
  cerebral, 33
    CT integrated, 248
    MRI integrated, 248
  in foreign body surgery, 36
  intraoperative, 34
  stereotactic, 215, 249
    in radiosurgery, 44
  for target localization, 199
Anorexia nervosa
  cingulotomy for, 32
Ansa lenticularis
  epileptic discharge in, 31
  lesions in, 6, 133–134
Ansotomy, 6
Anterior choroidal artery
  ligation of, 6
Antibiotics
  after hyperthermia, 230
  application to catheter, 114f
  application to catheter complex, 112f
Anticholinergic drugs
  for tremor, 134
Anticonvulsants
  in brachytherapy, 244
Antiepileptics
  after hyperthermia, 230
Anxiety
  cingulotomy for, 32
  radiosurgery for, 201
Anxiety neurosis
  electrical discharge in, 162
Aphasia
  after thalamotomy, 137
  in epilepsy, 165
Apomorphine
  administration into rat nigrostriatal pathway, 39
Applied Neurophysiology, 8–9
Arc principle, 195
  target in, 197f
Arc-radius system, 57f, 50, 105–106
  adjustment of, 81f
  catheter settings, 109f
Arteriography
  stereotactic stereoscopic, 168
Arteriovenous malformation (AVM), 126, 199
  angiograms of, 33
  Gamma Unit treatment for, 44
  intracerebral, 205f
  radiosurgery for, 45–46, 126, 204–205, 206f, 211, 214–215
  stereotactic treatment of, 34
Artery
  carotid
    cervical
      in subarachnoid hemorrhage, 33
Aspiration devices, 82f
Astrocytoma, 41, 236
  anaplastic, 94
    brachytherapy for, 245
    diagnosis of, 94
    differential diagnosis, 94–95
    multifocal, 96
  brainstem
    radiosurgery for, 216

cell population of, 94
grading system for, 94
malignant
  response to treatment, 115
smear of, 94
thalamic
  radiosurgery for, 216
thalamic pilocytic
  CT scan of, 238f
Asymmetry
  hemispheric
    in epilepsy, 165
  ventricular
    in epilepsy, 165
Ataxia
  after myelotomy, 26
  after thalamotomy, 137
  after tractotomy, 25
  after trigeminal tractotomy, 189
Athetosis, 10
  thalamotomy for, 10
Atlantooccipital space, 185
Atlas. *see* Stereotactic atlas
Automatism
  sexual
    in seizure, 167
Axolotl embryo
  transplantation of eye primordium in, 39

B

Backlund instrument, 37
Bacterial endocarditis
  after ventriculostomy, 35
Basal ganglia
  stereotactic interventions upon, 18
  stimulation for pain, 27
Beam knife, 211
Behavior disorders
  amygdalotomy for, 31
  in children
    hemispherectomy for, 31
    radiosurgery for, 216
Bennett frame, 19
β-endorphin, 153, 225
  CSF levels of
    in stimulation-produced analgesia, 27
Bioheat transfer equation, 228
Biopsy, 73, 251–252
  arc settings for, 78
  CT-guided, 36, 37, 64, 79f, 100
  data processing in, 78
  digital subtraction venous angiography (DSVA) in, 74
  entry point selection, 77–78
  instrumentation, 78–82
  magnetic resonance imaging (MRI) in, 74, 100
  methodology, 74
  multiple tract, 120
  open
    indications, 101
  operating room perspective, 75f
  patient position in scanner, 78f
  patient preparation for, 80f
  phantom target in, 78
  point access, 75–77

positron emission tomographical scanning (PET) in, 74
stereotactic, 105, 221
  case evaluation in, 99
  case selection in, 99
  in epilepsy surgery, 32
  failed diagnosis in, 99
  image-directed, 74–101
  inflammatory response in, 99
  necrosis in, 99
  target selection in, 99–101
stereotactic robot for, 225
target scan in, 77
target selection in, 79f
target slice, 80f
technique, 82–93
tract, 100
xylocaine with epinephrine in, 76f
Biopsy devices, 82f
Bleeding
  after radiosurgery, 205
  intracranial
    CT-stereotactic surgery for, 11
Blindness
  after proton beam hypophysectomy, 45
Brachium conjunctivum, 135
Brachytherapy, 211, 251
  catheter array in, 243
  catheter array in
    multiple, 101–102
  critical dose per cycle, 41
  CT-guided, 64
  dose distribution in, 104–105
  dose rate, 40, 115, 241
  with hyperthermia, 122
  implantation technique, 242–244
  interstitial, 40–42, 241–246
    advantages of, 241–242
    computer assisted, 119
    surgical technique in, 104, 105–115
  intracystic, 42–43
  NIH protocol for, 42
  parallel trajectory in, 42
  patient selection for, 242
  radionuclide selection in, 104
  short-term results of, 42
  survival times following, 42
  target, 241
  treatment planning in
    computer assisted, 242
    computer simulation of, 243f
Bradykinesia, 133
  after thalamotomy, 144f, 146
  in Parkinson's disease, 134
  thalamotomy for, 18
Bragg curve, 12
Bragg peak, 45, 124–125, 212
Brain
  -particle irradiation of, 125
  biopsy of, 74–101
  biopsy of
    stereotactic robot for, 225
  tolerance to radiation, 102
Brain atlas, 55, 59, 219, 220. see also Stereotactic atlas

Brain tumors. see also Neoplasia
  biopsy of, 62
  brachytherapy for, 40
  deep
    radiosurgery for, 215–216
  interstitial radiation of, 7
  radiation therapy for, 40
  stereotactically implanted radionuclides in, 41
  treatment of, 5
Brainstem
  lesions in
    for pain, 26
Brainstem atlas, 192
Breast cancer
  pain of
    hypophysectomy for, 28, 29, 30
Bronchopneumonia
  after stereotactic operations, 19
Brown-Roberts-Wells (BRW) apparatus, 3, 36, 42, 61, 64, 65f, 65–66, 74–81, 172, 242, 243
  base ring assembly, 75–77
  base ring components, 75f
  base ring positioning, 76f
  CT-guided, 59, 66, 125
  in CT-stereotactic surgery, 11
  data processing in, 118f
  localizer system in, 77f
  methodology, 127–128
  MRI-guided, 69, 172, 173
  used in colloid cyst aspiration, 36–37
Burr hole-mounted systems, 3, 3f

C

C-fibers, 190
C-fibers
  in pain, 149
Calibration
  system
    digital, 234
Californium-252 (^{252}Cf), 103
Campotomy, 7, 18
Cancer. see also Neoplasia
  prostatic
    pain of
      hypophysectomy for, 28
Cancer pain, 224
  ablative procedures for, 8
  glossopharyngeal nerve lesioning for, 26
  hypophysectomy for, 28–30
  mesencephalotomy for, 24
  metastatic
    hypophysectomy for, 30
  thalamic targets for, 27
  thalamotomy for, 23
  transsphenoidal cryohypophysectomy for, 29
  transsphenoidal RF coagulation of pituitary for, 29
  vagus nerve lesioning for, 26
Cannula
  introduction of, into target, 85f
  passage through catheter track, 107f
Capsulotomy
  in epilepsia partialis continua
    focal motor seizures of, 31
  with Gamma Unit, 44

Carcinoma. *see also* Cancer; Neoplasia
  choroid plexus, 96
  embryonal, 97
  lung
    oat-cell, 96
  metastatic, 95–96
  yolk sac, 97
Cardiac complications
  after stereotactic operations, 19
Carotid amytal examination
  in epilepsy, 164
Catheter
  afterloading with seeds, 112f
  antibiotic application to, 114f
  array, 111f
  drainage, 91f
  insertion
    stereotactic guidance for, 243
  introduction of, 111f
    into calvarium, 107f
  placement of, 110f
    CT-guided, 228
  Silastic, 106f, 228
  for therapy, 91f
Catheter array
  antibiotic application to, 112f
  multiple
    in brachytherapy, 105
  parallel
    in brachytherapy, 105
Catheter-cuff complex, 109f
Catheter marker
  application, 108f
Caudal perithird ventricular gray (PVG)
  stimulation for pain, 27
Causalgia
  cingulotomy for, 32
Cell
  endocrine, 252
  glioma
    radiosensitivity of, 105
  hypoxic
    effects of hyperthermia on, 121
  neuroblastoma
    transplantation of, 39
  neuronal, 252
Cell cycle
  phases of
    sensitivity to radiation, 40
Cell division
  interference, 211
Central cord lesion (CCL), 189–190
  analgesia from, 189f
Centromedian (CM) nucleus
  as target in pain surgery, 222–223
Cerebral landmarks, 2, 5. *see also* Stereotactic atlas
Cerebral palsy (CP)
  thalamotomy for, 20, 134
Cerebral topograph, 55
Cerebral tumors. *see* Brain tumors
Cerebroscopy, 84
Cerebrospinal
  fluid, 248
Cerebrospinal fluid (CSF), 182
Cerebrospinal fluid leak
  after aneurysm surgery, 34
  after brachytherapy, 42
  after hyperthermia, 230, 231
  after hypophysectomy, 29
  prevention of, 30
Cervical cord
  torsion of, 186f
Cervical cordotomy, 25
Chemode, 252
Chemotherapy, 239
  cytotoxic
    for glioma, 227
  interstitial, 124
  potentiation
    by heat, 227
    by hyperthermia, 121
Chessboard
  for robot, 222, 225
Choreoathetosis, 6
Choriocarcinoma, 97
Cingulotomy, 10
  for angina, 32
  for anorexia nervosa, 32
  for anxiety, 32
  for causalgia, 32
  for drug addiction, 32
  for dysesthetic pain, 32
  for obsessive-compulsive neurosis, 32
  for pain, 32
  for paraplegia pain, 32
  pneumographically guided
    for pain, 32
  for psychiatric illness, 32
  for psychic suffering, 32
  in psychosurgery, 32–33
  therapeutic effects, 32, 33
Circular accelerator, 211, 213
Cisternography
  target localization
    in radiosurgery, 44
CNS transplantation, 39–40
Cobalt, 241
  source, 213
Cobalt-60 (^{60}Co), 40, 44
Cognitive deficits
  in epilepsy, 164
  reversal of
    with fetal septal grafts, 39
Cold spot
  in radiobrachytherapy, 102
Collimator, 196, 204
Collimator helmet, 200f, 201
Commissure, anterior
  as target in epilepsy, 31
Compton effect, 212
Computations
  volumetric
    stereotactic, 117
Computed tomography. *see* CT
Computer-aided design/
  computer-aided manufacture (CAD/CAM), 249
Computerized tomography. *see* CT
Computers
  in operating room, 9
Confina Nuerologica, 8, 9
Confusion
  after seizure, 167

Contralateral hypalgesia
  after trigeminal tractotomy, 26
Convection
  thermal, 228
Cordotomy, 190
  anterolateral, 150
  cervical, 150
  contraindications for, 188
  for pain, 151
  percutaneous, 185, 188
  stereotactic, 188
Corpus callosum, 169
Corticosteroids
  after hyperthermia, 230
Corticotomy
  laser, 67
Cranial nerve(s), 185
  palsy of
    after tractotomy, 15
Cranial nerve(s), V, VI, VII
  palsy of
    after tractotomy, 25
Craniopharyngioma, 42, 43, 97–98, 207f
  cyst puncture for, 43
  cystic, 7, 98
  radiosurgery for, 124, 126, 205–206, 214
  single-photon beam therapy for, 215
  ^{90}Yt for, 43
Craniopharyngiomas
  Gamma Unit for, 44
Craniotomy, 46, 133–134
  computer-assisted, 236
  following CT-guided diagnosis, 36
  stereotactic techniques for, 249
Creutzfeldt-Jakob disease
  transmission of, 19
Cryoprobe, 5
CT, 92f, 204, 220, 233, 234f, 247, 251
  single extension of
    in epilepsy, 175f
  contrast enhanced, 249
  coordinates, 10
  data
    transposition of, 62
  in epilepsy treatment, 162
  guidance
    in foreign body surgery, 36
  ^{125}I source in, 244f
  images
    axial, 39
    coronal (reformatted), 38–39
  intraoperative, 68
  localization, 199f, 201
    manual, 199
  in pain surgery, 157
  in radiosurgery, 195
  scan
    functional targets, 38
    scout-view image, 10
  slice, 235f
    reconstruction of, 139f
    relationship to stereotactic apparatus, 10, 11
  in stereotactic biopsy, 100
  target localization
    in radiosurgery, 44
  translational image, 10

CT-cisternography
  target localization
    in radiosurgery, 44
CT-guided endoscopy
  in hydrocephalus, 35
CT-guided functional stereotactic surgery, 38–39
CT-guided stereotactic surgery, 3, 9–12, 61–69, 137, 138–140, 139f
  for electrode implantation
    in deep brain stimulation, 38
    in depth EEG, 38
  frames for, 36
  history of, 10–12
  instruments for, 63
  N-shaped localizer system in, 11
  for pain, 157
  for thalamotomy lesions, 38–39
Cuff-catheter complex
  Hemoclip application to, 113f
Cuff-catheter-source complex
  fixing at scalp, 113f
Culture
  in tissue diagnosis, 93
Curitherapy, 211
Cushing's disease
  radiosurgery for, 206
Cyclotron, 201, 211
Cylinder-arc stand, 182f
Cyst. see also Craniopharyngioma
  colloid, 98
    aspiration of, 249
      CT-guided, 36–37
    differential diagnosis, 98
    stereotactic aspiration of, 36
  dermoid, 98
  epidermoid, 98
Cyst aspiration
  CT-guided, 36
Cyst puncture
  in biopsy, 87–91
Cysticercosis, 98
Cytology
  aspiration, 91
Cytotoxicity
  of chemotherapeutic agents, 227
  thermal
    in acidotic cells, 227
    in hypoxic cells, 227
    in nutritionally deprived cells, 227
    in S-phase, 227

D

Data management
  digitalized, 100
Data processing
  programmable calculator in, 81f
Deafness
  contralateral
    after mesencephalotomy, 24
Death
  after brachytherapy, 41, 43
  after electrode implantation, 156
  after hypothalamotomy, 33
  after intracerebral hematoma aspiration, 37
  after laser resection, 238–239

Death—*continued*
    after mesencephalotomy, 24, 152
    after trigeminal surgery, 183
Deep brain stimulation (DBS)
    complications, 28
    CT-guided, 38–39
    of PAG-PVG, 27
    for pain, 8
    side effects, 27
    stereotactic robot for, 225
    stimulus parameters, 27
Delta-nociceptor, 149
Dentatotomy
    for cerebral palsy, 20–21
    for dystonia, 21
Depression
    psychosurgery for, 10
Depth EEG
    results in epilepsy, 163*f*
    before seizure surgery, 30
Depth electrode implantation
    electrode array in, 171*f*, 172*f*
    for epilepsy, 172–173
Depth electrode localization
    in epilepsy, 163*f*
Depth electrode recording
    in epilepsy, 161–162, 162–165
Depth electrode study
    in epilepsy, 164–165
    global, 167
    justification for, 164–165
    three-dimensional, 167
    timing of, 164–165
    whole brain, 167
Deuteron, 212
Diabetes
    hypophysectomy for, 45
Diabetes insipidus (DI)
    after hypophysectomy, 29, 30
    after transsphenoidal RF coagulation of pituitary, 29
Diagnosis
    histological, 251
Digital subtraction angiography (DSA), 169, 201
Digital subtraction venous angiography (DSVA)
    in stereotactic biopsy, 100
Diplopia
    after mesencephalotomy, 24, 152
    after proton beam hypophysectomy, 45
    after PVG stimulation, 154
Dizziness
    after PVG stimulation, 154
DNA
    recombinant techniques
        with grafted source, 39
    synthesis stage (S-phase)
        effects of hyperthermia on, 121
Dopa. *see* L-dopa
Dopamine
    from grafted source, 39
    levels in rat nigrostriatal pathway, 39
    striatal, 135
Dorsal column
    stimulation of
        for pain, 8

Dorsal horn
    synapse of
        in pain, 149
Dorsomedial nucleus
    as pain target, 23
Dorsum sella
    in ventriculostomy, 35
Dose profile
    of ionizing radiation, 195
Dosimetry
    computer-assisted, 40
    of light, 124
    stereotactic, 196
Dressing
    application, 114*f*
Drill
    twist
        in biopsy, 84*f*
Drug addiction
    cingulotomy for, 32
Drugs
    psychoactive
        and psychosurgery, 32
Dyes
    in phototherapy, 123
Dysarthria
    after thalamotomy, 19
Dysesthesia
    after mesencephalotomy, 24, 152
    sensory
        after thalamotomy, 137
Dysesthetic-deafferentation pain syndrome
    PAG-thalamic stimulation for, 28
Dysesthetic facial pain syndromes
    trigeminal tractotomy for, 26
Dysesthetic pain
    thalamic deep brain stimulation for, 28
Dysfluency
    in epilepsy, 165
Dysmetria
    after myelotomy, 26
Dysphagia
    after thalamotomy, 19
    after tractotomy, 25
Dysphonia
    after thalamotomy, 137
Dystonia
    after thalamotomy, 18
    dentatotomy for, 21
    pulvinotomy for, 21
    stereotactic surgery for, 21
Dystonia musculorum
    thalamotomy for, 10, 21
Dystonia musculorum deformans
    thalamotomy for, 134
Dystonia musculorum deformans (DMD), 21

E
Ectopic pinealoma, 97
Edema
    after hyperthermia, 231
    brainstem
        after laser resection, 239
    cerebral
        after brachytherapy, 245

Electrical activity
  recording of, 142f
Electrical discharge
  in schizophrenia, 162
Electrical stimulation
  for glossopharyngeal neuralgia, 182
  for pain, 153–158
  in thalamotomy, 137–138
  for trigeminal neuralgia, 182
Electrocoagulation
  for glossopharyngeal neuralgia, 182
  for trigeminal neuralgia, 182
Electrode carrier, 2
Electrode implantation
  CT-guided, 39
Electrode position
  in spinothalamic tractotomy, 186
Electroencephalography (EEG), 231
  array
    of seizure onset, 174f
  in epilepsy, 161, 164, 168
  before stereotactic surgery, 30
Ellis Formula, 1225
Embolization
  distal
    after aneurysm surgery, 34
Emotional suffering
  with pain
    ablative lesions for, 152
Empyema
  subdural
    after electrode implantation, 156
Encephalography
  for target localization, 199
Encephalometer, 55
Encephalopathy
  after thalamotomy, 19
End effector
  probe guide as
    on stereotactic robot, 221
Endocurietherapy, 225
Endogenous opioids, 150, 153
Endorphins. see also β-Endorphin
  in stimulation-produced analgesia, 27
Endoscopy
  CT-guided, 35
  fiberoptic, 34
  in hydrocephalus, 34–36
  system, 90f
  technique, 84–91
Energy
  deposition of, 228
Ependymoma, 95
Epilepsia partialis continua
  capsulotomy for, 31
Epilepsy, 30–32, 250
  CT-stereotactic surgery in, 11
  diagnosis
    stereotactic, 162–165
  electrical potential recording
    dipole effect in, 161
  electrophysiological study of, 176f
  extratemporal focus in, 164
  ictal
    spiking in, 162

management
  stereotactic methods of, 161–176
onset
  unitemporal lobe, 164
psychomotor, 167
  temporal lobectomy for, 31
radiosurgery for, 201, 216
recording sites
  stereotactic localization of, 173f
stereotactic surgery for
  patient evaluation in, 164–165
  stereotactic technique in, 168–177
temporal lobe, 164
treatment history, 161–164
treatment of, 7, 10
workup, 164
Epileptogenic zone, 30–31, 165, 168, 169
Equatorial line, 185
Equinovarus foot deformity
  after thalamotomy, 18
Ergotropic triangle
  in hypothalamotomy, 33
Essential tremors, 20
Etopalin
  used in lesion production, 5
Extralemniscal myelotomy, 26
Extrapyramidal system
  lesions in, 133
Eye movement disorder
  after deep brain stimulation, 28
  after electrode implantation, 157
Eye primordium
  transplantation of
    in axolotl embryo, 39

F

Faces
  perception of
    in epilepsy, 165
Facial numbness
  after radiosurgery, 44
Facial pain
  atypical
    mesencephalotomy for, 23
  dysesthetic
    trigeminal tractotomy for, 26
Facial weakness
  after radiosurgery, 44, 203
  after tractotomy, 15
Failed-back syndrome
  PAG-thalamic stimulation for, 28
  pain of, 22
Fever
  after hypophysectomy, 46
  central
    after hypothalamotomy, 33
Fistula
  arteriovenous
    radiosurgery for, 124
  carotid-cavernous
    after trigeminal surgery, 183
Fistulas
  carotid-cavernous
    radiosurgery for, 126

Fluoroscopy
  in foreign body surgery, 36
  in hypophysectomy, 28
  short-distance, 59
  in trigeminal neuralgia, 182
Focal phenomena
  in epilepsy, 165–167
  prestereotactic
    in epilepsy, 166f
Focal-point stereotactic apparatus (Todd-Wells), 58f
Focal seizures, 161
  surgery for, 31
Foramen of Monro, 84
Foramen ovale, 179
Forceps
  bronchoscopy, 83f
  flexible
    introduction of, into target, 85f
Forceps complex
  cannula, 84f
Foreign body
  removal of, 7
  stereotactic surgery for, 36
    CT guidance in, 36
Forel's field
  as target in epilepsy, 162
Forel's field H, 7, 18
Formalin, 93
Fornicotomy
  for epilepsy, 31
  for psychomotor seizures, 31
Fornix
  as target in epilepsy, 31
Frozen section
  in specimen processing, 93
Functional deficits
  in epilepsy, 165
  treatment of
    Gamma Unit in, 198
Functional stereotactic surgery
  CT-guided, 61–62
  targets, 38–39

G

Gait disturbances
  after thalamotomy, 144f, 146
  in Parkinson's disease, 134
Galvanometer, 234
γ-aminobutyric acid mediated (GABA-mediated) pathway, 135
γ emitter
  biological effect of, 103
γ knife, 211, 250
γ-Med unit
  radiotherapy with, 41
γ ray, 212
  in radiosurgery, 44
γ Unit, 44, 69, 195, 196, 197f, 198, 198f, 201, 204, 207, 208, 211, 214, 216
  heavy particle beam therapy with, 215
Gammacapsulotomy
  for psychiatric disease, 201
Gammathalamotomy, 196f, 211

Ganglionectomy
  for pain, 151
Gate hypothesis
  of pain, 150
Germinoma, 96–97
  differential diagnosis, 97
Glial-fibrillary acidic protein (GFAP), 98
Glioblastoma, 41, 42, 227
  brachytherapy for, 245
Glioblastoma multiforme, 94
  response to treatment, 115
  treatment of, with Gamma-Med, 41
  treatment of, with interstitial implants, 41
Glioma
  deep
    radiosurgery for, 216
  of hemispheres, 41
  hypothalamic, 41
  low-grade
    radiosurgery for, 216
  malignant
    hyperthermia for, 230
    radiosurgery for, 216
    treatment, 115
  midbrain, 41
  parietal
    radiosurgery for, 216
  pineal
    radiosurgery for, 216
  radiosurgery for, 214–216
  radiotherapy for, 102
  stereotactic robot for, 225
  thalamic, 41
    radiosurgery for, 216
Glioma cell
  radiosensitivity of, 105
Gliosarcoma, 96
Gliosis
  reactive, 94
Globus pallidus, 19, 134
  epileptic discharge in, 31
  lesions in, 6
Glossopharyngeal nerve
  lesioning
    for cancer pain, 26
Glossopharyngeal neuralgia, 179–184
  target, 181f
Glycerol treatment
  for trigeminal neuralgia, 182
Gold-198 (^{198}Au), 40, 242
Goldfish
  optic nerve regeneration in, 39
Gouda-Gibson instrument, 60
Grafting
  of mammalian tissue, 39
Grafting-cross
  of avian species, 39
Guiot instrument
  Turner-Shaw modification of, 59
Gyrantum, 68
Gyrus
  in epilepsy, 161

H

Hardware malfunction
  after electrode implantation, 157

Hartenberg-Denavit parameters, 222, 225
Hassler terminology
    of stereotactic thalamic surgery, 135
Hearing loss
    after radiosurgery, 203
Heat. see also Hyperthermia
    antineoplastic effects of, 120–121
    potentiating effects of, 121
    therapeutic index for, 121
Heat delivery systems, 121–122
    local
        ferromagnetic seeds in, 122
        microwave antennas in, 122
        radiofrequency needle electrodes in, 122
    regional
        magnetic induction in, 122
        microwave in, 122
        radiofrequency in, 122
        ultrasound in, 122
    whole body, 121–122
Heat shock, 121
Heifetz instrument, 46
Helium
    ion, 250
Helium nuclei, 212
Hematoma
    after brachytherapy, 42
    after thalamotomy, 19
    aspiration of
        CT-guided, 38
        suboccipital transcerebellar route, 38
        transfrontal route, 38
    aspirator, 38
    brainstem
        aspiration of, 38
        intraaxial, 38
    CT-stereotactic surgery for, 11
    intracerebral
        after brachytherapy, 43
        stereotactic evacuation of, 37
    pontomedullary
        aspiration of, 38
    pontomesencephalic
        aspiration of, 38
    recurrent
        after intracerebral aspiration, 37
Hematoporphyrin (Hp), 123
Hematoxylin and eosin (H&E) technique, 93
Hemianopsia
    homonymous
        after laser resection, 238
Hemiballismus, 135
    after thalamotomy, 18
    thalamotomy for, 10
Hemiparesis
    after mesencephalotomy, 24
    after thalamotomy, 18–19
    after tractotomy, 15, 25
Hemiplegia, infantile
    hemispherectomy for, 31
Hemoclip
    application to catheter cuff, 113f
Hemorrhage
    after brachytherapy, 41
    after electrode implantation, 172
    after hypophysectomy, 46

    after proton beam therapy, 45
    intracranial
        after brachytherapy, 245
        after electrode implantation, 156
    subarachnoid
        after brachytherapy, 43
        aneurysmal, 33
Heschel's gyrus, 168
Hippocampus
    in epilepsy, 31, 161, 164
    rat
        lesions in
            cognitive defects after, 39
    as target in epilepsy, 31, 168
Histological diagnosis
    CT-guided, 36
Histological preparation
    review of, 89f
Hitchcock apparatus, 25, 26
Horseradish peroxidase (HRP), 150
Horsley-Clarke apparatus, 1, 2, 2f, 55, 56f, 219
Horsley-Clarke atlas, 4
Huntington's chorea, 6
Hydrocephalus, 34–36
    endoscopy in, 34–36
    noncommunicating, 35
    relief of, 7
    shunts in
        glial scarring of, 34–35
    target, 35
6-Hydroxydopamine (6-OHDA)
    injection into rat substantia nigra, 39
    lesions of nigrostriatal pathway, 39
Hydroxyurea
    as radiosensitizer, 245
Hyperactivity
    hypothalamotomy for, 33
Hyperkinetic phenomena
    after thalamotomy, 18
Hyperthermia, 120–123, 227–231. see also Heat
    biological
        effects of, 121
    with brachytherapy, 122
    effects of
        on hypoxic cells, 121
    externally applied, 227
    history, 120
    interstitial, 228
    interstitial microwave, 115
    magnetic-loop induction system for, 122
    microwave
        for brain tumors, 5
    potentiation of chemotherapy by, 121
    with radiotherapy
        patient selection, 117
    selectivity of, 121
    techniques, 227–230
Hypesthesia
    facial
        after radiosurgery, 203
Hypophysectomy, 28–30
    absolute alcohol injection in, 29
    for acromegaly, 45
    complications of, 29
    for diabetes, 45
    with stereotactic proton beam, 45

Hypophysectomy—*continued*
 transcranial, 29
 transfrontal
  fluoroscopic control in, 29
  impedance monitoring in, 29
  RF heating in, 29
  stalk section effect from, 29
  stimulation techniques in, 29
 transsphenoidal, 29
  metastasis remission rate from, 29
  yttrium-90 (^{90}Yt) implanted during, 29
Hypophysis
 as target in radiosurgery, 45
Hypopituitarism
 after hypothalamotomy, 33
 after transsphenoidal RF coagulation of pituitary, 29
Hypothalamotomy
 for aggressive behavior, 33
 complications of, 33
 ergotropic triangle in, 33
 for hyperactivity, 33
 moral objections to, 33
 for sexual criminality, 33
 therapeutic effects of, 33
 for violent behavior, 33
Hypothalamus, 190
Hypotonia
 after dentatotomy, 21
 after tractotomy, 25
Hypoxic cells
 radiation dose rate
  to kill, 41
 in radiobrachytherapy, 102

I

Ictus, 164
Image-directed stereotactic surgery, 73f, 73–128
Image-guided systems, 61–69
Imaging
 in epilepsy, 164
Immune response, 121
Immunohistochemistry
 for diagnosis, 98–99
Immunoperoxidase study
 in tissue diagnosis, 93
Immunotherapy, 123
 adoptive measures of, 123
Impedance recording, 182
Implantable drug delivery systems
 for pain, 26
Implantable neurostimulation systems
 for pain, 26
Incontinence
 after hypothalamotomy, 33
Inderal
 for tremor, 134
Induction
 magnetic, 227
Inductive heating, 5
Infarction, lateral medullary
 mesencephalotomy for, 152
Infection
 after brachytherapy, 245
 after electrode implantation, 156

 focal, 247
 shunt
  after ventriculostomy, 35
 subcutaneous
  after electrode implantation, 157
 subgaleal
  after electrode implantation, 156, 157
 ventricular
  after laser resection, 239
Infection, deep
 after deep brain stimulation, 28
Inflammation
 focal, 248
Information recall
 in epilepsy, 165
Intention tremor, 20
 after thalamotomy, 137
Intercommissural line, 58
 in hypothalamotomy, 33
 relation to functional targets, 38
Interleukin-2 (IL-2), 123
Internal acoustic canal (IAC), 204
Internal capsule (IC)
 posterior limb
  stimulation of, for pain, 27
Interstitial microwave antenna arrays (IMAA), 228
Interventriculostomy
 for cerebral aqueduct reconstruction
  Teflon prosthesis in, 35
 to treat hydrocephalus, 35
Intracerebral hematoma aspiration
 indications for, 37
Intracerebral neoplasm
 diagnosis of, 93–99
Intracranial mass lesions
 biopsy of, 11
Intracranial pressure (ICP), 230
Intraoperative recording
 in pain surgery, 157
Intraventricular surgery
 for hydrocephalus, 34–36
Inverse kinematic problem, 222, 225
Inverse square law
 of radiation dose, 40, 241
Iodine-125 (^{125}I), 40–42, 103, 104, 228, 242, 243, 245, 251
Ionization
 direct, 212
Ipsilateral ataxia
 after trigeminal tractotomy, 26
Iridium-192 (^{192}Ir), 40–42, 103–106, 115, 122, 225, 228, 231, 242, 251
Iron powder
 to induce thrombosis, 33
Irradiation
 interstitial, 211, 228, 251
 for lesion production, 5–6
 photon, 251
Isodose
 in radiosurgery, 214
Isodose contour, 242
Isodose curves, 42
 for collimator, 213f
Isodose invelope, 120
Isotherm
 distribution of, 228

Isotope
  for brain tumors, 40
  choice in brachytherapy, 242
  gamma energies of, 40
  half-life of, 40
  implantation
    interstitial
      traditional, 36
Isotopes
  tissue penetration characteristics of, 40

J

Journal of Neurosurgery, 8
Journal of Stereotactic and Functional Neurosurgery, 8
Joystick, 234

K

Kandel frame, 34
Karnofsky scale, 117
Kaufman-Gildenberg device, 62
Keratin, 98
Kirschner device, 55
Kluver-Bucy-like effects
  after amygdalotomy, 31
Kluver-Bucy syndrome
  after temporal lobectomy, 31

L

L-dopa, 18, 133
  injection of, into basal ganglia, 9
  in Parkinson's disease management, 9, 145
L-dopa/carbidopa, 133
L-tryptophan
  for pain, 28
Language disturbance
  after thalamotomy, 19
Language mapping
  in epilepsy surgery, 165
Laser
  CO_2
    stereotactically directed, 233
  energy
    light generated by, 124
Laser surgery, 67
  stereotactic apparatus for, 235f
  for tumors, 233–239
Lateral polaris (LPO), 135
Lee, Arnold, 5
Leksell apparatus, 2, 6, 10, 57f, 60, 61, 157, 169, 182, 195, 196f
  CT-guided, 60, 62–63, 63f
  MRI-guided, 60, 64, 69
  tomographically-guided, 60
  used in colloid cyst aspiration, 36–37
  x-ray-guided, 60
Lesion
  ablative
    for pain, 150–143
  atrophic
    in epilepsy, 165
  brainstem
    radiosurgery for, 46
  in epilepsy surgery, 165

intracranial
  Gamma Unit for, 44
  laser resection of, 233
  treatment of, 61
language area
  radiosurgery for, 46
mass
  CT-guided treatment of, 36–39
metastatic
  treatment with combination hyperthermia and radiotherapy, 117
production
  in thalamotomy, 141–143
production
  by alcohol injection, 5
  history of, 5–6
  mechanical methods of, 5–6
radiosurgery for, 44
subcortical, 249
Leukotomy, 32
Libido loss
  after amygdalotomy, 31
Light, 212
  blue, 124
  penetration of, 124
  in phototherapy, 123
  red, 124
Limbic system
  stimulation for pain, 27
LINAC
  linear accelerator, 46
Linear accelerator, 125, 200f, 211, 213
Linear accelerator (LINAC)
  for stereotactic radiosurgery, 46
Linear accelerator ring, 128f
Lobectomy
  for epilepsy, 31
Lobotomy
  prefrontal, 32, 58
Localization
  stereotactic, 199–201
Lymphokine-activated killer (LAK) cells, 123
Lymphoma, 96
  malignant, 95
  primary cerebral
    treatment with combination hyperthermia and radiotherapy, 117

M

Magnetic resonance imaging (MRI), 100, 169, 204, 233, 247, 248, 251
  guided stereotactic surgery
    advantages, 69
    disadvantages, 69
  in epilepsy treatment, 162
  in functional stereotactic surgery, 39
  localization with, 199f, 201
  in pain surgery, 157
  in radiosurgery, 214
  in stereotactic surgery, 69–70
  of thalamus, 39
Mammal
  tissue grafting of, 39
Mammilary bodies
  in hypothalamotomy, 33

Manual dexterity
 in epilepsy, 165
Mayfield adapter, 80
Mechanical analogue, 59
Medial pulvinar nucleus
 as target in pain surgery, 22–23
Medulla
 adrenal
  autologous transplantation of, 252
 in pain, 149
 stimulation for pain, 27
Melanin, 95
Memorial Hospital stereotactic apparatus, 220*f*
Memory deficit
 after temporal lobectomy, 31
Memory loss
 after thalamotomy, 137
Meningioma, 97
Meningitis
 after brachytherapy, 42
 after hypophysectomy, 29, 30
 bacterial
  after hyperthermia, 231
Mental deterioration
 in Parkinson's disease, 134
Mental retardation
 amygdalotomy in, 31
Mental symptoms
 after thalamotomy, 144*f*
Mesencephalic tractotomy, 25
Mesencephalotomy, 188
 for cancer pain, 24
 with cingulotomy
  for cancer pain, 24
 complications of, 24
 effects of, 24
 for facial pain
  atypical, 23
 indications for, 152
 for pain, 7
 paraqueductal
  for post brainstem stroke facial pain, 24
 for phantom pain, 23
 for post-stroke thalamic pain, 23
 side effects of, 24
 for spinal cord injury pain, 23
 for tabetic crisis pain, 23
 for zoster ophthalmicus pain, 23
Metastases
 bone
  pain of, 22
 hypophysectomy for, 28–30
Methanol
 in smear preparation, 93
Methodology
 stereotactic, 59
Metrazol, 162
Microadenomas
 endocrinologically active
  microsurgery for, 45
Microelectrode
 recording
  for target localization, 138
 in thalamotomy, 140–141

Microscopy
 electron
  in tissue diagnosis, 93
Microsurgery, 202
 laser, 233
 in tissue grafting, 39
 transsphenoidal
  for microadenomas, 45
Microwave antenna
 placement of, 228
Micturition
 spinal pathways of, 187
Midbrain
 in pain, 149
 targets
  in pain surgery, 23–25
Mitotic death
 with interstitial radiation, 102
Mitotic delay
 after radiation, 41
 with interstitial radiation, 102
Monitoring
 intraoperative, 233
Monoanalgesia
 after tractotomy, 25
Mood disorder
 cingulotomy for, 32
Motion disorders. *see* Movement disorders
Motor cortex
 epileptic discharge in, 31
 extirpation of, 133
Motor deficits
 after thalamotomy, 19
 after tractotomy, 25
Motor neglect
 after thalamotomy, 22
Motor signs
 tonic
  in seizure, 167
Motor stimulation
 unintended
  after electrode implantation, 157
Movement disorders
 extraocular
  after mesencephalotomy, 24
 involuntary, 17–22
 targets for, 25
 thalamotomy for, 133–147
  results, 146
  treatment procedures, 146*f*
Multiple sclerosis
 intention tremor of
  thalamotomy for
   side effects, 20
 thalamotomy for, 134
Mundinger apparatus, 2, 3
Mussen apparatus, 55
Myelotomy, 190
 cervical, 189–190
 commissural, 190
 extralemniscal
  for pain, 26
 lumbosacral, 190
 for pain, 151
 procedure, 190

N

Narabayashi apparatus, 2
Narcotic infusion
　for pain, 151
Necrosis
　induced
　　in radiobrachytherapy, 102
Neocortex
　in epilepsy, 164
Neoplasia, 247, 248
　astrocytic, 93–95
　cerebral
　　malignant, 103
　　radiotherapy for, 115
　choroid plexus, 96
　CNS
　　treatment with hyperthermia, 120
　effects of hyperthermia on, 120
　glial, 93–95
　　nonastrocytic, 95
　intraaxial, 67
　　stereotactic biopsy of, 133
　intracranial, 73–128, 239
　metastatic, 95–96
　　differential diagnosis of, 96
　pineal, 96–97
　primary
　　glial, 239
　resection of, 249–250
Nerve ending
　free
　　in pain, 149
Neural
　pathway, 252
　transplantation, 39
Neuralgia
　postherpetic
　　mesencephalotomy for, 152
　　trigeminal tractotomy for, 189
Neurinoma
　radiosurgery for, 214
Neuroblastoma cells
　as graft source, 39
Neuroimaging, 198
Neurological
　side effects
　　after thalamotomy, 23
Neurological deficits
　after hyperthermia, 230, 231
　after proton beam therapy, 45
　after radiosurgery, 45
　after thalamotomy, 19
　after VPL lesioning, 152
Neurological examination
　in epilepsy, 164
Neuronal loop
　in Parkinson's disease, 135
Neurons
　dopaminergic
　　in rat, 39
　gonadotrophin-releasing
　　transplantation of, in rats, 39
　vasopressin
　　transplantation of, in rats, 39

Neuropathology
　surgical, 91
Neurophysiological investigations, 135
Neuropsychological deficits
　in epilepsy, 164
Neurosurgery, 8
Neurosurgery
　functional, 250
　　radiosurgery for, 214
　stereotactic
　　future developments in, 247–252
　　team, 106f
Neurotoxin
　injection of
　　into rat substantia nigra, 39
Neurotransmitter, 252
　from grafted source, 39
Neutrons
　fast
　　killing effect of, 103
Nigrostriatal lesions
　in rat, 39
NIH protocol
　for brachytherapy, 42
NMR spectrometer, 70
Nonspeech sounds
　identification of
　　in epilepsy, 165
Nuclear subgroups
　ventrolateral, 141f
Nucleotomy, 188–189
Nucleus raphe magnus
　in medulla, 27
Nystagmus
　retraction of
　　after mesencephalotomy, 152

O

Obsessive-compulsive disorder
　cingulotomy for, 32
　psychosurgery for, 10
　radiosurgery for, 195, 201
Ocular deviation
　tonic
　　after mesencephalotomy, 152
Oculomotor deficits
　after hypophysectomy, 29
Oculomotor palsies
　after hypophysectomy, 30
Oligodendroglioma, 236
　diagnosis, 95
　prognosis, 95
Oophorectomy
　for pain relief, 29
Operating room
　perspective during biopsy, 75f
　setup, 88f
Opiates
　for pain, 150
Optic nerve
　goldfish
　　regeneration after crush injury, 39
Optical
　encoder, 234

Orchiectomy
 for pain relief, 229
Orofacial neoplasms
 cranial nerve pain in, 26
Oscillopsia
 after PVG stimulation, 154
Oxidation
 photoinitiated, 123

P

^{32}P (NaPO$_4$), 42
Pain, 126. *see also* Cancer pain
 ablative lesions for, 151–153
 afferent system of, 150
 after electrode implantation, 157
 after limb amputation, 22
 after spinal cord injury, 22
 after stroke, 22
 brain stimulation for
  advantages of, 153
 cingulotomy for, 32
 in cranial nerve sensory territories, 26
 deafferentation
  central, 22
  deep brain stimulation for, 27
  electrical stimulation for, 153
  thalamic targets for, 26–27
  trigeminal tractotomy for, 189
 denervation
  mesencephalotomy for, 25
  thalamotomy for, 25
 destructive operations for, 22–27
 dysesthetic, 22, 25
  cingulotomy for, 32
  deep brain stimulation for, 27
  targets for, 24, 153
 electrical stimulation for, 149
 emotional accompaniments of, 149–150
 facial
  nucleotomy for, 189
  trigeminal tractotomy for, 189
 in failed-back syndrome, 22
 implantable drug delivery systems for, 26
 implantable neurostimulation systems for, 8, 26
 neural basis for, 149
 nociceptive, 22
 oophorectomy for, 29
 orchiectomy for, 229
 perception
  pathways in, 150
 persistent
  after tractotomy, 150
 pneumographically-guided cingulotomy for, 32
 pontine spinothalamic tractotomy for, 25
 radiosurgery for, 124, 201, 216
 recurrent
  after tractotomy, 25
 sensory qualities of, 150
 somatic, 22
 stereotactic ablative treatment for, 150–153
 stereotactic surgery for, 7–8, 58, 250
 suppression
  central control mechanism for, 150
 targets, 22–30
  cervical cord, 185
  dorsomedial nucleus (DM), 23
  PAG/PVG, 27
  PAG/PVG-IC, 28
  PAG/PVG-thalamic/IC, 28
  PAG/PVG-thalamus, 28
  somatosensory relay nuclei (VPL, VPM), 23
  spinal cord, 26
  thalamotomy for, 133
  tractotomy for, 26
 traditional understanding of, 149
Pain therapy
 stereotactic robot for, 225
Pair production, 212
Pallidoansotomy
 stereotactic, 134
Pallidothalamic connections
 epileptic discharge in, 31
Pallidothalamic tract
 destruction of
  for rigidity, 134
  for tremor, 134
Pallidotomy, 6
 ansotomy with, 18, 134
Pallidum
 as target in epilepsy, 162
Panhypopituitarism
 after hypophysectomy, 229
Pantopaque
 as target in brain abscess aspiration, 37
 used in ventriculostomy, 35
Pantopaque cisternography, 26
Parafascicularis (PF) nucleus
 as target in pain surgery, 22–23
Parahippocampal gyrus
 as target in epilepsy, 168
Paraplegia pain
 cingulotomy for, 32
Paresis
 after capsulotomy, 31
 after trigeminal tractotomy, 189
 third nerve
  after brachytherapy, 43
  after ventriculostomy, 35
Paresthesia
 after myelotomy, 26
Parietal cortex
 in pain, 150
Parinaud's syndrome
 after mesencephalotomy, 24, 25
 after ventriculostomy, 35
Parkinsonism. *see* Parkinson's disease
Parkinson's disease, 6–7, 250. *see also* Tremor
 radiosurgery for, 124, 126, 201
 surgical therapy for
  results, 143–147
 targets, 18
  globus pallidus, 18
 thalamotomy for, 19, 133–147
 tissue transplantation in, 39, 252
 treatment of, 9–10, 17–19
 tremor in, 9
Particle
 alpha, 211
 charged, 250

Pelorus frame, 68
Penumbra
  in radiosurgery, 212, 213
Performance intelligence quotient (PIQ)
  in epilepsy, 165
Periaqueductal gray (PAG), 190
  stimulation of
    for pain, 7, 150, 153
  as target in mesencephalotomy, 24
Periventricular gray (PVG)
  stimulation of
    for pain, 150, 153
Periventricular gray stimulation
  electrodes in, 155f
Phantom, 3
  measurements
    in hyperthermia, 228
Phantom base
  targets, 110f
Phantom data
  translation of, 127f
Phantom limb pain
  mesencephalotomy for, 152
Phantom pain
  mesencephalotomy for, 23
Phantom system, 59, 64, 106
Phantom target device, 57, 58f
Phantom unit, 106
Phloxine-eosin technique, 93
Phosphorus-32 (^{32}P), 40, 42, 43
Photodynamic effect, 123
Photoelectric effect, 212
Photon, 212
  high-energy, 211
Photoradiation, 239
Phototherapy, 123–124
  biophysical aspects, 120
Pia/electrode adhesion, 186
Pinealoma
  radiosurgery for, 214
Pineoblastoma, 97
Pineocytoma, 97
Pituitary gland destruction
  by alcohol injection, 29
  by cryosurgery, 29
  by radioactive isotope implantation, 28
  by radiofrequency (RF) thermal coagulation, 28
  for breast cancer pain, 29
  for prostate cancer pain, 29
Pituitary insufficiency
  after proton beam hypophysectomy, 45
  after radiosurgery, 207
Pituitary tumors. see also Adenoma, pituitary
  lesion production for, 7
Pneumoencephalography, 220
Pneumography
  in hydrocephalus, 34
  in interventriculostomy, 35
  target localization
    in radiosurgery, 44
Pneumonia
  after stereotactic operations, 19
Pneumotomography, 61
Polar coordinate system, 55, 57f, 58–60, 64–66

Pons
  electrode traversing, 192
  lesions of
    for pain, 185–192
  in pain, 149
Pontine spinothalamic tractotomy
  for pain, 25
Pontine tractotomy, 25
Porphyrin, 123
Positron emission tomography (PET), 169, 201, 245, 247, 248, 250
  in epilepsy treatment, 162
  in stereotactic biopsy, 100
Posterior column homonculus, 187
Postural gait disorder, 190
Procarbazine, 245
Prolactinoma
  single-photon beam therapy for, 215
Proton, 250
Proton beam therapy, 195
  for AVMs, 45–46
  Bragg peak, 215
Psychiatric disorders
  radiosurgery for, 124, 201
Psychic suffering
  cingulotomy for, 32
Psychomotor seizures
  amygdalotomy in, 31
  stereotactic fornicotomy for, 31
Psychosurgery, 10, 32–33, 216
Ptosis
  after tractotomy, 25
Pulmonary embolism
  after laser resection, 239
Pulmonary complications
  after brachytherapy, 43
Pulmonary embolism
  after stereotactic operations, 19
Pulvinotomy
  for cerebral palsy, 20–21
  for dystonia, 21
  medial
    for pain, 23
Putamen
  epileptic discharge in, 31
  as target in epilepsy, 162

Q

Quintothalamic tract
  as target in mesencephalotomy, 24

R

Radiation
  annihilation, 213
  dosimetry, 251
  ionizing
    enhancement by heat, 121
    for glioma, 227
Radiation necrosis, 40, 41
  after brachytherapy, 245
  after isotope implantation, 42
  after radiosurgery, 45, 205
  of sellar floor
    after hypophysectomy, 30

Radiation necrosis—*continued*
  symptomatic
    after combination hyperthermia and radiotherapy, 115
Radiation surgery, 124
Radiation therapy, 239
  for cerebral tumors, 40
  dosimetry, 40
  external beam, 40, 42
Radiation toxicity
  after brachytherapy, 115
  after teletherapy, 115
Radioactive implantation
  stereotactic robot for, 225
Radiobiology, 40
Radiobrachytherapy, 102–120
  cell cycle-sensitive phases in, 102
  dose per cell cycle, 102
  dose rates in, 102–104
  history, 102
  hypoxic cells in, 102
  sublethal damage repair in, 102
  volume irradiated in, 102
Radiofrequency heating
  see radiosurgery
Radiogangliothomy, 216
Radiographic guidance, 57
Radiography, 179–180, 236
  for glossopharyngeal neuralgia, 179–184
  in hypophysectomy, 28
  for trigeminal neuralgia, 179
Radioisotopes
  boundary dose, 231
  implantation of, 7
    into brain tumors, 40
  interstitial implantation of, 62
Radionecrosis. *see* Radiation necrosis
Radionuclide seed
  graphic depictions, 119*f*
Radionuclides, 102, 251
  activity of, 104
  distribution of, 104
  energy of, 104
  half-life of, 105
  implanted in brain tumor, 41
  interstitial implantation of, 102
  number of, 104
  selection of, 103–104
Radiosurgery, 5, 64, 250–251
  for AVMs, 206*f*
  characteristics, 211
  clinical studies, 126
  dose in
    diminishing of, 213
    distribution of, 212
  dose profile in, 196*f*
  dose rate, 202
  functional, 216
  functional applications of, 201
  indications for, 198
  instrumentation, 44
  linear accelerator technique, 124–125
  multiple arc technique, 125
  nonfunctional applications of, 201–207
  operative procedure, 201
  for pain, 201
  rationale for, 125
  single-beam photon, 211–216
  stereotactic, 43–46, 120, 195–198
    history of, 195–198
    therapeutic effects, 44–45
Radiotherapy
  dose homogeneity, 115
  external beam, 115
  with Gamma-Med unit, 41
  for gliomas
    survival rate in, 41
  high dose, 115
  interstitial
    patient evaluation, 115
  linear accelerator for, 120
  permanent implants in, 41
  personnel protection in, 115
  toxicity of, 115
Radium-226 (^{226}Ra), 40
Rebleeding
  after radiosurgery, 45
Reichert apparatus, 2, 3
  in CT-stereotactic surgery, 11
Reimplantation techniques
  in tissue grafting, 39
Resectoscope, 67
Respiration
  spinal pathways, 187
Reticular formation
  brainstem
    in pain, 149
  mesencephalic
    in pain, 152
Reticular system
  mesencephalic
    as target in epilepsy, 162
Retrocollis
  thalamotomy for, 134
Rhinorrhea
  after hypophysectomy, 30
Rhizotomy
  for pain, 151
Rhodes-Glenn apparatus, 66
Riechert-Mundinger apparatus, 26, 35, 58–59, 59*f*, 60, 61, 64
Riechert-Mundinger CT-guided apparatus, 42
Rigidity
  of Parkinson's disease
    thalamotomy for, 134
Robot
  absolute accuracy in, 224
  calibration of, 224
    with chessboard, 224*f*
  chessboard for, 222, 224*f*
  computer keyboard, 221
  error
    compensation for, 225
  flexible arm movement of, 223
  homogenous transformation T in, 221–222
  relative accuracy of, 221, 224
  repeatability in, 224
  stereotactic procedure with, 222–226, 223*f*
  for stereotactic surgery, 221–226
  surgical field, 222

Unimation Puma 200, 221–226
  watermelon experiment with, 222
Rosomoff cordotomy guide, 26
Rostral mesencephalic reticulotomy (RMR), 24–25

S

S100 protein, 98
Sarcoma
  α-immunoblastic, 96
  meningeal, 96
  metastatic, 96
Schaltenbrand-Bailey atlas, 4, 136
Schaltenbrand-Wahren atlas, 140
Schizophrenia
  electrical discharge in, 162
Seizure disorders
  non-temporal lobe
    surgery for, 31
Seizure onset
  EEG array of, 174f
Seizures, 250. *see also* Epilepsy
  after cingulotomy, 32
  after colloid cyst aspiration, 37
  after hypophysectomy, 46
  clinical
    in epilepsy, 164
  epileptic
    frontobasal-cingulate type, 167
    opercular type, 167
    posterior neocortical temporal type, 167
    temporal pole type
    temporobasal-limbic type, 167
  focal
    diagnosis, 161
  focus of, 167
  grand mal, 162
  onset of, 167
  pathway of, 162
  petit mal, 162
  treatment targets for, 162
Seizures, in children
  hemispherectomy for, 31
Sella turcica
  as target in hypophysectomy, 28, 29, 45
Semielectrode recording
  for target localization, 138
Semiology, 167
Sensation loss
  after VPL lesioning, 151–152
Sensory deficits
  after thalamotomy, 18
Sensory loss
  after tractotomy, 25
  nondermatomal
    after myelotomy, 26
Serotonergic inhibitory pathway, 27
Sexual criminality
  hypothalamotomy for, 33
Silastic cuff
  sutured to scalp, 108f
Silicone
  used to prevent CSF leakage
    after hypophysectomy, 30

Skull base neoplasms
  cranial nerve pain in, 26
Smear
  in specimen processing, 93
Somatosensory potential, 143f
Somatosensory relay nuclei (VPL, VPM)
  as targets in pain surgery, 23
Spasmodic torticollis
  thalamotomy for, 21
Specimen
  open-brain biopsy, 93
  stereotactic biopsy, 93
  tissue, 86f, 87f
Specimen inspection
  by pathologist, 88f
Speech
  melodic quality of
    in epilepsy, 165
Speech disturbances
  after thalamotomy, 144f, 146
  in Parkinson's disease, 134
Spiegel-Wycis apparatus, 1, 2f, 5, 57, 219
Spiegel-Wycis atlas, 4, 136
Spiegel-Wycis stereoencephalotome, 58, 59f, 60
Spinal cord
  lesions of
    for pain, 185–192
  stimulation of
    for pain, 8, 150
Spinal cord injury pain
  mesencephalotomy for, 23
Spinal surgery
  stereotactic, 185–192
Spinomedullary junction
  stereotactic surgery at, 26
Spinothalamic coordinates, ff
Spinothalamic fibers, 187
Spinothalamic homonculus, 187, 188f
Spinothalamic tract
  brainstem coordinates, 191f
  in pain, 149
  as target in mesencephalotomy, 24
  as target in pain, 185–186
  as target in pain surgery, 151
Spinothalamic tractotomy
  stereotactic, 186–188
  target, 187
Stereoelectroencephalography (SEEG), 161
Stereoencephaloscope, 34
Stereoencephalotome, 58
Stereoencephalotomy, 1, 32
Stereognosis
  in epilepsy, 165
Stereoguide, 214
Stereophotogrammetry, 199
Stereotactic angiography, 33, 61, 62
Stereotactic apparatus, 1–2, 219, 247
  arc-quadrant
    for laser resection, 235f
  arc-radius, 55
  Bradford, 60
  Cooper, 60
  CT-compatible, 36, 138, 234f
  CT-guided, 220
  focal point, 55

Stereotactic apparatus—*continued*
  history of, 1–3
  Hitchcock, 25
  Kandel, 60
  phantom target, 55
  polar coordinate, 55
  types of, 1–3, 3*f*
  Walker, 60
Stereotactic aspiration
  of intraaxial brainstem hematoma, 38
  of intracerebral hematoma, 37
Stereotactic atlas, 1–5, 4*f*, 33, 58, 60, 135–137, 154, 162
  computer resident, 138, 139*f*
  Schaltenbrand-Wahren, 140
  standardized, 247
Stereotactic biopsy
  angiography guided, 36
  CT-guided, 36
  traditional, 36
  ventriculography guided, 36
Stereotactic cyst aspiration, 43
Stereotactic data base, 100
Stereotactic depth electrode placement
  before seizure surgery, 30
Stereotactic fornicotomy
  for psychomotor seizures, 31
Stereotactic hematoma aspirator, 37
Stereotactic instrumentation, 33
  cylindrical system, 59
Stereotactic instruments
  CT-directed
    Brown-Roberts-Wells (BRW) apparatus, 74–81
  plane-of-target, 68
  radiosurgical, 44
  target point
    depth setting, 60
Stereotactic radiosurgery, 43–46, 198*f*, 211
  CT-guided, 36
  standards for, 195
  traditional, 36
Stereotactic surgery
  anatomical applications, 17, 33–36
  brachytherapy, 40–43
  for cerebral palsy, 20–21
  CT-guided, 36–39
  destructive
    at cervical cord, 25, 26–27
    at medulla, 25, 26
    at pons, 25–26
  for dystonia, 21
  for epilepsy, 10*f*, 30–32
  for foreign bodies, 36
  functional
    CT-guided, 38–39
    MRI-guided, 64
  functional applications, 17–33
  history of, 1–12, 7
  for hydrocephalus, 34–36
  hyperthermia in, 227–231
  image-directed, 73*f*, 73–128
  indications
    targets, 58
  indications for, 6–10
  instrumentation, 55

  meetings about, 8–9
  modifications, 117–120
  MRI-guided, 69–70
  new directions in, 117–120
  for non-parkinsonian tremor, 20
  for non-temporal lobe seizure disorders, 31
  open, 68
  for pain, 22–30, 185–192
  for Parkinson's disease, 17–19
    results, 143*f*, 143–147
  pituitary ablation, 28–29
  present status of, 9–10
  professional organizations for, 8–9
  for psychiatric illness, 32–33
  publications about, 8–9
  radiosurgery, 43–46
  robotic methods, 219–226
  for spasmodic torticollis, 21–22
  targets, 6–8
    for pain, 22–30
  techniques, 1
  thalamic
    Hassler terminology for, 135
  traditional, 17–36
  trajectory, 219
  vascular applications, 33–34
Stereotactic systems
  history, 57–61
Stereotactic targets
  in psychosurgery, 32, 33
Stereotactic trigeminal tractotomy, 26
Stereotactic work station, 117–120, 118*f*
Stereotaxis. *see* Stereotactic surgery
Steroid drugs, 123
Stimulation-produced analgesia, 8, 150
Stroke
  brainstem, 22
  CNS transplantation in, 40
  ischemic
    after trigeminal surgery, 183
  pain after, 22
  thalamic, 22
Stump causalgia (phantom pain)
  thalamotomy for, 23
Stupor
  after hypothalamotomy, 33
Sublethal damage
  molecular, 227
Sublethal damage (SLD)
  repair between dose fractions, 40
Subnucleus ventrointermedius
  as target for tremor, 7
Substantia nigra, 135
  as target in epilepsy, 162
  transplants, 39
Substantia nigra, rat
  dopaminergic neurons in
    selective destruction of, 39
Suicide
  after cingulotomy, 32
Sulcus
  in epilepsy, 161
Surgical microscope, 202
Synchrocyclotron, 195
Syringomyelia, 190

T

Tabetic crisis pain
  mesencephalotomy for, 23
Tachycardia
  after hypothalamotomy, 33
  after PVG stimulation, 154
Talairach apparatus, 2, 61, 168, 169
Talairach atlas, 4, 136, 170
Tantalum-182 (^{182}Ta), 40
Target localization, 219–220
  CT-guided
    in functional stereotactic surgery, 38–39
  in epilepsy
    subcortical recordings for, 162
Target selection
  for pain, 153–156
Targeting
  stereotactic, 117
Targets
  data coordination for, 199
  in epilepsy, 168
  in hypophysectomy, 28, 29, 30
  neurophysiological localization of, 137
  in psychosurgery, 32, 33
  in radiosurgery, 44, 45, 46
  stereotactic localization of, 199–201
  subcortical, 249
  in thalamotomy, 18. see also specific targets; Thalamotomy, targets
  thalamus as, 220
  visible by x-rays, 28
Tasker atlas, 4
Technetium-99 (^{99}Tc), 43
Telecobalt therapy, 211
Teleradiographs
  anteroposterior (AP), 58
  lateral, 58, 233
  stereotactic, 236 f
Teleradiography, 239
Teleroentgenograms, 59
Teletherapy, 40, 115
Temperature
  distribution of, 228
    effects of blood flow on, 229 f
    effects of frequency on, 229 f
    during hyperthermia treatment, 231
  mapping of, 228
  measurement of, 228
Temporal lobe cortex
  as target in epilepsy, 31, 164, 168
Temporal lobectomy, 31
Tension athetosis
  thalamotomy for, 134
Teratoma, 97
Thalamic fasciculus, 18
Thalamic fasciculus (Forel's field H)
  as target in thalamotomy, 22
Thalamic nuclei VPL
  as target in pain surgery, 151
Thalamic nuclei VPM
  as target in pain surgery, 151
Thalamic nucleus
  dorsomedial
    in pain response, 150
  in pain, 149
Thalamic pain
  post-stroke
    mesencephalotomy for, 23
Thalamic recording
  stereotactic, 143 f
Thalamic syndrome, 151
  after thalamotomy, 18
  deep brain stimulation for, 27
  mesencephalotomy for, 152
  pain of, 7–8
    IC stimulation for, 28
  thalamotomy for, 23
Thalamocortical activating system
  in epilepsy, 31
Thalamotomy, 6, 250
  for athetosis, 10
  basal
    to treat cancer pain, 7
  centromedian
    for epilepsy, 31
  CM
    for spasmodic torticollis, 22
  CT-guided, 38, 39
  data acquisition in, 138
  dorsomedial
    for emotional overlay, 23
  first, 57–58
  for pain, 32
  in psychosurgery, 32
  for dystonia musculorum, 10
  electrical stimulation in, 137–138
  Gamma Unit in, 44
  for hemiballismus, 10
  infectious complications of, 19
  intralaminar
    for cancer pain, 7
    for epilepsy, 31
  for pain, 23, 201
  side effects, 18–19
  for somatic pain, 224
  for spasmodic torticollis, 21
  stereotactic, 133–147
  targets, 18, 135
    centromedian (CM) nucleus, 22–23
    intralaminar nuclear complex, 22–23
    medial pulvinar nucleus, 22–23
    parafascicularis (PF) nucleus, 22–23
  therapeutic effects, 18
  for tremor, 10
  unilateral
    for spasmodic torticollis, 22
  ventralis lateral (VL), 133–147
  VIM
    for spasmodic torticollis, 22
VIm (ventrointermedius), 18
VL (ventralis lateral), 18, 20
  for cerebral palsy, 20
  for dystonia, 21
  indications for, 134
  procedure, 138
  for spasmodic torticollis, 22
VL/VIM complex, 20
  for cerebral palsy, 20
VOa (ventralis anterior), 18

Thalamotomy—*continued*
  VOI
    for spasmodic torticollis, 22
  VOp (ventralis posterior), 18
Thalamus, 22
  electrical stimulation of
    for pain, 153–157
  parafascicularis complex of
    in pain, 152
  somatosensory system
    stimulation of, for pain, 27
  stereotactic interventions upon, 18
  as target in epilepsy, 162
  as target in pain, 27
  targets in
    for tremor, 134
  ventral, 144f
Therapy
  fixed-field, 213, 214
  heavy particle beam
    Bragg peak, 215
  intralesional, 73
  proton beam
    Bragg peak, 215
  rotation, 213
Thermal tolerance, 121
Thermocoagulation
  stereotactic instrument for, 134
  for trigeminal neuralgia, 182
Thermometry
  multiple sensor, 228
Thrombosis
  intraluminal
    current used to promote, 34
  vessel, 211
Tissue
  adrenal medullary
    transplantation in human, 39–40
  attenuation of, 228
  brain
    biochemical protectors of, 120
  electrical properties of, 228
  evaluation, 91–93
  half-value layer (HVL), 104
  perfusion rates of, 228
  staining, 89f
  sublethal damage in, 214
  temperature elevation in, 227
  transplantation of, 252
    adrenal medullary, 39
    in mouse, 39
    from peripheral nervous system, 39
    in rat, 39
    sympathetic ganglia, 39
  withdrawal, 86
Todd-Wells apparatus, 2, 38, 58f, 60, 66, 138, 168–170, 170f, 185
  in CT-stereotactic surgery, 11
  ventriculogram with, 155f
Topectomy, 32
Torticollis
  thalamotomy for, 134
Toxoplasmosis
  differential diagnosis, 96

Tracer
  techniques
    in pain, 150
Tractotomy
  for pain, 26, 151
  pontine, 188, 190–192
    procedure, 192
    targets, 25, 192
  spinothalamic, 25, 150, 185–186
  subcaudate
    for drug addiction, 32–33
    for pain, 32–33
    in psychosurgery, 32
  trigeminal, 26, 188–189
Transformation
  spatial
    with CT scan, 249
    with MRI scan, 249
Transmission tomography, 247
Transplantation
  of cell lines
    to CNS, 40
  of eye primordium
    in axolotl embryo, 39
  of fetal brain tissue
    in mouse, 39
    in rat, 39
Transsphenoidal cryohypophysectomy
  for prostate carcinoma pain, 29
Tremor
  essential
    thalamotomy for, 134
  familial
    thalamotomy for, 134
  intention
    of multiple sclerosis
      thalamotomy for, 134
  non-parkinsonian, 10
    thalamotomy for, 133–147
    treatment, 20
    target, 20
  parkinsonian, 250
    thalamotomy for, 133–147
  resting
    after thalamotomy, 137
Trigeminal anesthesia
  trigeminal tractotomy for, 26
Trigeminal nerve, 149
Trigeminal neuralgia, 179–184
  gasserian ganglion coagulation for, 55
  pain after surgery for, 22
  radiosurgery for, 216
  target, 181f
  thalamotomy for, 23
  trigeminal tractotomy for, 189
Trigeminal rhizotomy, 151
Trigeminal surgery
  free-hand, 182–183
  stereotactic apparatus for, 182
Trigeminal tract
  as target for pain, 185–186
Trigeminal tractotomy, 26
Trigeminal tracts
  brainstem coordinates, 191f

Trigeminus stereoguide, 179–184, 180
Tumor
  acoustic, 203f
    radiosurgery for, 202–024, 204f
    stereotactic localization of, 204
    treatment history, 202–204
  benign
    radiosurgery for, 211
  boundary of
    computer reconstruction of, 233
  brain
    brachytherapy for, 241
  breast
    brachytherapy for, 241
  cerebral
    radiation therapy for, 40
  CNS, 102
  contour of, 120
  in corpus callosum, 242
  deep-seated
    laser resection of, 233–239
    radiosurgery for, 214
  glial
    hyperthermia treatment of, 122
    malignant, 251
  gynecological
    brachytherapy for, 241
  head
    brachytherapy for, 241
  histology of, 238f
  intraaxial, 41
  intracranial
    stereotactic surgery for, 146
  laser resection of, 233–236
  locations of, 237f
  malignant
    stereotactic robot for, 225
  metastatic, 41–42, 236
  neck
    brachytherapy for, 241
  neuroectodermal, 95
  pineal
    Gamma Unit for, 44
    radiosurgery for, 44
    stereotactic biopsy of, 36
  pituitary
    radiosurgery for, 206
    single-photon beam therapy for, 215
  posterior fossa
    in hydrocephaly, 35
  primary
    recurrent, 41–42
  progression
    after brachytherapy, 245
  prostate
    brachytherapy for, 241
  radiosensitivity of, 215
  section
    computer-generated display of, 237f
  sellar
    radiosurgery for, 126
  somatic, 102
  therapy
    intralesional, 101–117

Tumor marker
  immunohistochemical, 98f
  lymphoid, 98
Tumor resection
  following CT-guided diagnosis, 36
Turning behavior
  in nigrostriatal pathway
    of rat, 39

U

Ultrasound, 227
  for subcortical lesion production, 5
Unimation Puma 200 Robot, 221–226
Upward gaze limitation
  after PVG stimulation, 154
Urokinase
  installation of
    CT-stereotactic surgery in, 11
  used in intracerebral hematoma aspiration, 37

V

VA thalamic nuclei
  epileptic discharge in, 31
Vagus nerve
  lesioning
    for cancer pain, 26
Van Buren-Borke atlas, 4, 136
Van Buren instrument, 60
Vaporization
  laser
    computer-monitored, 233
Vascular malformations
  stereotactic angiography of, 33
Vasospasm, 33
Ventralis caudalis (VCE and VCI), 135
Ventralis intermedius (VIM), 135
Ventralis internus (VOI)
  as target in thalamotomy, 22
Ventralis lateral/ventralis intermedius (VL-VIM)
  as target
    in non-parkinsonian tremors, 20
Ventralis lateral (VL)
  epileptic discharge in, 31
  somatic organization in, 147
  thalamic nucleus
    lesions in, 6
Ventralis oralis anterior (VOA), 135
Ventralis oralis posterior (VOP), 135
Ventralis postero lateralis/ventralis posteromedialis
    (VPL/VPM)
  implantation of electrodes in
    for pain, 27
Ventralis postero lateralis (VPL)
  in pain, 149, 150, 151
  stimulation of
    electrodes in, 155f
Ventralis posteromedialis (VPM)
  in pain, 149, 150,151
Ventricular drainage
  CT-guided, 36
Ventriculitis
  after electrode implantation, 156, 157
Ventriculography, 58, 59, 62, 135, 138, 154f

Ventriculography—*continued*
  exacerbation of demyelination in MS, 20
  in foreign body surgery, 36
  in hydrocephalus, 35
  intraoperative, 247
  landmarks in, 135
  positive-contrast, 141*f*
    in interventriculostomy, 35
  precipitation of encephalopathy, 19
  stereotactic, 58, 140
  stereotactic stereoscopic, 168
  subcortical structures in, 135
  traditional
    in functional stereotactic surgery, 38
Ventriculoscopy, 84
Ventriculostomy
  catheters for, 91*f*
  endoscopy unit for, 90*f*
  third
    to treat hydrocephalus, 35
Verbal intelligence quotient (VIQ)
  in epilepsy, 165
Vessel clipping
  for arteriovenous malformation (AVM), 34
Vessel occlusion
  after aneurysm surgery, 34
Vincristine, 245
Visual complications
  after hypophysectomy, 30
Visual construction
  in epilepsy, 165
Visual deficits
  after hypophysectomy, 29
Visual field
  deficits in
    after laser resection, 238
Visual perception
  in epilepsy, 165
Von Recklinghausens disease
  radiosurgery for, 204*f*

W

Waltregny-Laitinen apparatus, 182
Wechsler Adult Intelligence Scale, 165

Work station
  stereotactic, 117–120, 118*f*
World Society for Stereotactic and Functional
    Neurosurgery, 8–9
Wound
  breakdown of
    after brachytherapy, 245
Wound irrigation
  in biopsy, 87*f*
Wurzburg suite, 60

X

X-ray computed tomography (CT)
  in radiosurgery, 214
X-rays, 212, 220, 247
  in foreign body surgery, 36
  in radiosurgery, 44
  stereotactic, 233
  for target localization, 199
Xylocaine
  with epinephrine
    in biopsy, 76*f*

Y

Yttrium-90 (^{90}Yt), 40, 42, 43
  in hypophysectomy, 29
    complications of, 30
  implanted in sella, 29
  for nonadenomatous glands, 30

Z

Zernov-Rossolimo device, 56*f*
Zona incerta, 18
Zoster ophthalmicus (HZO) neuralgia, 22
  mesencephalotomy for, 23
  thalamic stimulation for, 27
  thalamotomy for, 23